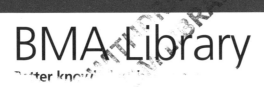

# Biomedical Research
# and Beyond

# Routledge Annals of Bioethics

# Biomedical Research and Beyond

## Expanding the Ethics of Inquiry

### Christopher O. Tollefsen

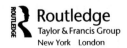

Routledge
Taylor & Francis Group
New York   London

First published in 2008
by Routledge
270 Madison Ave, New York, NY 10016


Simultaneously published in the UK
by Routledge
2 Park Square, Milton Park, Abingdon, Oxon OX14 4RN


*Routledge is an imprint of the Taylor & Francis Group, an informa business*
© 2008 Taylor & Francis

Typeset in Sabon by IBT Global
Printed and bound in the United States of America on acid-free paper by IBT Global

*Library of Congress Cataloging in Publication Data*
Tollefsen, Christopher.
Biomedical research and beyond : expanding the ethics of inquiry / by Christopher O. Tollefsen.
p. ; cm.— (Routledge annals of bioethics ; 5)
Includes bibliographical references and index.
ISBN-13: 978-0-415-96116-5 (hbk : alk. paper)
ISBN-10: 0-415-96116-5 (hbk : alk. paper) 1. Medicine—Research—Moral and ethical aspects. 2. Biology—Research—Moral and ethical aspects. 3. Research—Moral and ethical aspects. 4. Inquiry (Theory of knowledge) I. Title. II. Series.
[DNLM: 1. Biomedical Research—ethics. W 20.5 T651b 2008]

R852.T54 2008
174.2--dc22                                                                 2007036109

ISBN10: 0-415-96116-5 (hbk)
ISBN10: 0-203-93034-7 (ebk)


ISBN13: 978-0-415-96116-5 (hbk)
ISBN13: 987-0-203-93034-2 (ebk)

# Contents

# Acknowledgments

This book has benefited from the good will and assistance of many people. I began thinking about the topic after receiving a grant from the South Carolina Honors College in the summer of 2002 to prepare a class titled "The Ethics of Inquiry." I taught that course in the fall of 2002; I thank the Honors College and its students for much intellectual stimulation.

In the spring of 2004, I taught a graduate course on the work of Alasdair MacIntyre; work from that course has made its way into this book, and I thank the participants in that seminar. In 2004–2005, I was a fellow in the James Madison Program at Princeton University. Much of the writing of this book was done at Princeton; I thank my friends from the program, and especially Robert P. George and Bradford Wilson for an exceptionally stimulating and collegial environment. Parts of this book were read at a seminar of the Madison Program; I thank George Kateb in particular for helpful comments then and afterwards.

Ed Munn, Laurie Tollefsen, and Mark Cherry all read the entire manuscript and provided helpful comments and criticisms. Mark has been extremely helpful in shepherding the book through to its home in the Annals of Bioethics series. I am truly grateful.

Parts of the book have been read at the University of South Carolina, Coastal Carolina University, Princeton University, the University of Catania, and the Metaphysica Conference in Rome, 2003. At all these venues, I have received much help. Thomas d'Andrea, Matteo Negro, and Gabrielle de Anna all made especially helpful comments at a meeting of the International Society of Law and Morality. In addition, many friends and colleagues have read drafts of parts of the book at various times and in various stages, and I have benefited from discussion with members of the Philosophy Department of my own university in particular. I thank all of them for their invaluable assistance.

In 2005, Fr. Juan Velez gave me some advice for finishing the manuscript that proved invaluable. Without his help, it is unclear that there would be a book.

My wife, Laurie, and my children all deserve awards, but will have to settle for my thanks, for their support and patience.

The author would like to thank the following for granting permission to reproduce material in this work:

*Public Affairs Quarterly,* for permission to reprint Tollefsen, C. (2000). "Journalism and the Social Good." *Public Affairs Quarterly* 14: 293–307. © North American Philosophical Publications.

Springer Academic Publishers, for permission to reprint Tollefsen, C. (2002). "Managed Care and the Practice of the Professions." In *The Ethics of Managed Care,* edited by W. B. Bondeson and J. W. Jones. Dordrecht: Kluwer. © Springer.

*International Philosophical Quarterly,* for permission to reprint Tollefsen, C. (2006a). "MacIntyre and the Moralization of Enquiry." *International Philosophical Quarterly* 46: 421–38. © Philosophy Documentation Center.

The American Catholic Philosophical Association, for permission to reprint Tollefsen, C. (2006b). "Persons in Time." *American Catholic Philosophical Quarterly* 80: 107–23. © Philosophy Documentation Center.

# Introduction

Inquiry drives change. It is the means by which human beings move from the world of today into whatever the world of the next century, the next millennium will be. And that world comes about as a result of many factors—social, political, scientific, medical, moral, philosophical—all of which are made possible by the present day's inquiries.

This has always been the case. The transition from the pre-modern to the modern world, a change of political, economic, technological, and religious significance, was mediated by a variety of forms of inquiry: philosophic, scientific, historical. The medieval world was likewise a product of the forces of inquiry, particularly those that emerged from the great universities. And the world we live in today, a world of political autonomy, computer chips, global economies, and communications, exists in consequence of the inquiries of political theorists, computer engineers, a succession of economists, and others. Inquiry—the sustained search for truth—is in each case the agent of change from the old to the new.

This is clearly seen in the present day in the context of biomedical and scientific inquiry. In the world of the next century, medicine and the health sciences will have been radically transformed. Our understanding of disease, and our ability to cure and to prevent it, will have advanced to degrees unimaginable. Our capacity to deal with the accidents of life—the loss of limbs in war, disfigurements in car crashes, inherited disabilities, the diminishments of age—will be similarly transformed. We will be healthier, stronger, longer-lived, and more secure. Inquiry in the biomedical sciences will have made all such changes possible.

The chosen means of inquiry will likewise have great consequences, in particular for our moral culture. For instance, the medical realities of the future may depend on the widespread use of human embryos for research. They may encompass genetic enhancements of human beings, and possibly modifications of human nature. They may have been driven by an ethos of discovery at any cost, and with no restraining hand from traditional morality, politics, or religion. In these ways and others, both the consequences and the conduct of inquiry will change not just what is medically available to us, but who we, as moral beings, are.

The shape of our future thus crucially depends upon the nature and the results of biomedical and scientific inquiry. But similar claims are true in other areas. Consider an area of inquiry seemingly far removed from that of inquiry in the biomedical sciences, that of military investigation. At present, we must decide what sort of a culture of investigation we will tolerate. Will we be a culture that adopts the most forceful and coercive techniques of our enemies, using even torture to discover their plans and prevent their attacks? Or, will we adopt a gentler, more peaceful approach, even if that puts us at more risk? Either choice will determine who we are and what sort of a world future generations will inhabit. But either choice is in part a choice about the conduct of inquiry.

To give another example: Will the world of the future be a world in which all inquiry is driven by a narrow focus on technological or instrumental progress? Or will it be a world in which humanistic inquiry is valued, in which knowledge can be pursued for its own sake, and in which questions about the nature of man, nature, and the divine may be asked and answered in good faith? If humanistic inquiry does exist in our future, will it be genuine inquiry, inquiry in pursuit of truth, or will it be a sham, a mask for the political and moral agendas of those disillusioned with the very notion of truth? Analogous questions can be asked about the natural and biomedical sciences: Will they exist only in service of instrumental rationality, or will we value our understanding of nature for its own sake? Will there be nobility in the life of inquiry?

All such questions have both moral and political dimensions. The state will either help or hinder the course and conduct of inquiry in each of these dimensions, and the political world and culture of the future will be shaped by such decisions, and by the fruits of the inquiries that result from such decisions.

Let us call the domain of philosophy that considers all these questions, and that articulates and argumentatively defends answers to them, the ethics of inquiry. So broadly envisaged, this field of philosophy does not, at present, exist. Rather, the questions, answers, and arguments of the ethics of inquiry are distributed across a range of philosophical subdisciplines. Most dominant among these subdisciplines are the ethics of biomedical research and the ethics of science; also of importance are military ethics, the ethics of the academy, and journalistic ethics. The politics of inquiry, a proper part of the ethics of inquiry, is currently at home in political theory. The question of the value of inquiry, and its role in a well-lived life, is perhaps a part of normative ethics, perhaps a part of metaphysics, or philosophical anthropology. This division of philosophical labor is neither surprising nor intrinsically unfortunate. But there is no systematic area of philosophy that attempts to address all these questions; there is no unified "ethics of inquiry."

This book investigates the possibility of just such an ethics of inquiry. It is centrally concerned with the ethics of biomedical and scientific inquiry; but it is also concerned with military, journalistic, philosophic, and humanistic inquiry insofar as all these have inquiry—its nature and ethics—in common.

This book is, further, an attempt to bring the normative questions of inquiry within the domain of a single systematic moral approach, what I shall call a basic goods approach to ethics and politics. This approach will be described in more detail in Chapter 1, but its unifying focus, that all moral action is action for the sake of human fulfillment and well-being, will allow us to answer not just the narrow normative questions about the conduct of inquiry—in biomedical research and beyond—but the broader questions about inquiry's point and value, for persons and cultures.

Of course an expanded ethics of inquiry must begin somewhere, and there is a natural starting point: the ethics of biomedical research, and the ethics of science. In these areas of practical ethics, philosophers, doctors, medical researchers, and professional scientists have, over the course of the past forty or so years, made considerable progress, and achieved considerable consensus on at least some core matters. There are, for example, few conclusions in ethics, or any other area of philosophy, so widely accepted as that medical researchers must obtain the informed consent of their research subjects.

Still, the issue of informed consent gives us a good indication of the limits intrinsic to the diversity of the discussion. For although there is this impressively widespread agreement as to the importance of consent, many philosophical questions remain unsatisfactorily answered. Is the demand for consent related exclusively to the value of autonomy, as some think, or are its foundations broader and deeper? Must the requirement of informed consent, dominant in the field of clinical research, be expanded to other forms of inquiry on human persons, such as the social sciences, or data collection and analysis? Is the requirement of application only to us, Western subjects, for whom autonomy is a core value, but not to others, such as subjects in developing or primitive countries? Is there any overlap between what is essentially a requirement of a research ethic, and the various other fields, such as military and legal investigation, and journalistic inquiry, that also are inquiries into human persons and their lives? We must ask whether any unity can be brought into these disparate areas of the ethics of inquiry on the matter of informed consent. But the division of labor referred to above has made it difficult to answer questions such as these, distributed as they are across a variety of fields.

While the chapters that follow are centrally concerned with research ethics and the ethics of science, they attempt, in various ways, to move beyond these borders, to see what analogies, contrasts, and discontinuities exist between biomedical research and inquiry, and inquiry in other fields. This is particularly true in the final chapters, in which I address the question of the vocational nature of inquiry. Is it possible to orient one's life around the activity of inquiry, and if so, what sorts of commitments does this require? What, further, are the virtues that an agent who has made such a commitment should have? What is the character of a virtuous inquirer? Answers to such questions should provide guidance not just to those engaged in biomedical and scientific inquiry, but to all who have undertaken a life of inquiry.

# 1 Is There an Ethics of Inquiry?

Some might think the norms of inquiry so obvious that only their constant breach makes their repetition necessary. But inquiry of many forms, scientific, philosophical, biomedical, has often been afforded a status, in theory, and sometimes in practice, that shields it from ethical investigation. This is true not only of inquiry. Consider business. It is obvious to many that businessmen and women should adhere to a set of ethical norms that are authoritative for their profession. Yet some deny this. On one conception of business, held by some businesspeople, the primary aim of business is to make money, and ethics be damned. Considerations regarding the "morality" of money making are merely impositions forced upon business by those outside the profession. Given such conflicts, the business profession must ask itself whether there are genuine and authoritative norms that should govern the making and seeking of money.

A parallel question can be raised about the pursuit of truth: are there genuine and authoritative norms that ought to govern the seeking, sharing, and articulating of truth? Let us start by giving some *prima facie* reasons for thinking that there is an ethics of inquiry, before turning to specific denials that there is such an ethics.

Inquiry is a fundamental part of our lives. Indeed, it seems to be a fundamental part *only* of the lives of human persons: neither animals, nor angels, nor God inquire. It is a peculiarly human activity. It is known by many names: investigation, research, "finding out." It takes place in any number of contexts: medicine, the sciences, history, philosophy, the crime scene, the newspaper, and the fence over which two neighbors gossip. It is an activity that some agents engage in for the whole of their adult lives. Something so fundamental to who and what we are and to the way we live seems a proper subject of ethical consideration.

Moreover, it is an activity that is not simply ubiquitous, but is also commonly thought to be of great importance. Universities and research laboratories exist to foster inquiry, men and women are praised for success, and sometimes scorned for failure in their investigative pursuits, and cultures are judged friendly or hostile to inquiry. In many cases these judgments are simply a consequence of success or failure in the investigation. Jones seeks the cure of a rare disease; we judge the investigation successful and praise him when and if he discovers the cure. Smith pursues research into a question of cell biology. If the question remains unanswered, we might judge his inquiry unsuccessful, or a failure.

But success and failure do not exhaust the possible judgments we might make, nor are they always indicative of what these other judgments would be. Jones might have discovered his cure by testing dangerous possibilities on unsuspecting humans. He might have been reckless with resources. Perhaps the answer to his question was staring him in the face, but because of carelessness or inattention, he neglected it for a considerable period of time. In these cases, we will judge Jones's inquiry negatively, as disrespectful of persons, as inefficient or wasteful, or as lazy and neglectful. We might question whether Jones should have been involved in this rather than some other project, or think that some of Jones's findings have been unduly influenced by the pressures of the pharmaceutical company for which he works. We might question the way, or degree to which, Jones made the results of his inquiry available to other inquirers. We can make a host of ethical judgments about Jones's work that are not correlated to the overall *success* of his project.

Similarly, although Smith's investigation in the end did not succeed, we might be impressed by Smith's diligence and perseverance, his forthrightness about his failures, and his overall integration of his research into the fabric of his life. We may notice that Smith, despite not finding his own work successful, does not for that reason judge it a complete failure, because he might see his work in the larger context of the investigations of an inquiring community for whom he thinks of his work as of benefit. No one else will need to go down these blind alleys, he might think with some satisfaction. Finally, we might judge that Smith was the first to see the significance of the problems he pursued. Our moral judgments will not necessarily correlate to a simple judgment of failure.

Such moral judgments can raise protest. "Leave science to the scientists; don't bring morality, or religion, or politics into it." This sentiment is sometimes expressed by scientists and their defenders, when they seek permission, or even public money, to pursue some new avenue of inquiry. But if inquiry is a human activity, why should it be immune from ethical assessment? If it is in some instances a public activity, with public consequences, why should it not be assessed from a political perspective? Indeed, if inquiry constitutes a link between the human being and the rest of the universe, why should it not be assessed from a religious perspective? If we are unique among all beings in being inquirers, this might raise ethical, political, and religious questions about our responsibilities as inquirers.

Moreover, there is a clear overlap between the ethics of other disciplines, and that of inquiry. No physician is entitled to operate on a patient without first obtaining, if possible, informed consent, nor is she allowed to operate only to serve her own, rather than the patient's ends. Why, then, if

Jones needs to cut open living human beings to perform his experiments, should we be convinced by his demand for liberation from ethics in the pursuit of inquiry?

This is not to deny that inquiry requires some autonomy. This consideration was present in the story of Jones, who, we thought, might have been unduly pressured by the company for which he worked. More questions are available to us concerning the appropriate context for inquiry, and what steps should be taken to ensure that context. But even these questions seem to be questions of ethics, not justification for an escape from ethics.

It seems that inquiry of all sorts is properly subject to ethical appraisal and guided by ethical norms. Yet we do find the opposite sentiment expressed. Steven Maynard-Moody accurately describes views of this sort: "The belief that inquiry is sacrosanct is central to the cultural authority and political autonomy of science. Supporters of scientific autonomy argue that physical, material, and cultural progress are threatened if science is guided by anything but itself" (Maynard-Moody, 1995, p. 7).

It might seem that this attitude is primarily to be found among scientists (and perhaps politicians) seeking practical benefits from research. But even inquirers in the humanities are capable of demanding autonomy from ethical restrictions. The historian Jaroslav Pelikan writes that "scholars in all fields, myself included, have often defined the purpose of research as the single-minded pursuit of truth at any price, and have cited the principle of knowledge its own end in justification" (Pelikan, 1992, p. 43). The view that inquiry possesses an immunity from ethical or political considerations is thus not limited to scientific inquirers.

## THE IMMUNITY CLAIM

There are several possible justifications for this claim to immunity. The first is the view that *success* in scientific research could be jeopardized by the introduction of moral or political constraints. This is true, but not unique to science. Many worthwhile projects could be done more quickly, more cheaply, or more effectively if we did not need to worry about ethical considerations. But this is hardly a justification for ignoring such considerations.

A second source of opposition to ethics in research is the view that science and scientific research are to be judged solely in terms of the practical benefits they promise. If the benefits are great enough, they will outweigh any possible negative effects, and render objections otiose. This consequentialist response depends on the strength of consequentialism as a moral theory. I will critique this sort of theory below.

A third view, expressed in the quotation from Pelikan, is that knowledge is a good in itself, and, in fact, either the only such good, or the highest such good. An Aristotelian, for example, might view the contemplative life as dedicated to the highest possible good; from this somewhat angelic standpoint, other considerations might seem trivial and burdensome. Because of the importance of this Aristotelian standpoint, I will address it too in this chapter.

Two further possibilities both involve theoretical claims about the nature of politics and the state. They are not strictly ethical claims, but they involve claims to immunity from ethical considerations at the political level, and so deserve attention.

The first views the state's relationship to the individuals making it up as being similar to the relationship between an organism and its parts. This view, expressed by both Plato and Aristotle, would justify the state in ignoring person-centered moral requirements in inquiry for the sake of the good of the whole (Plato, 2001; Aristotle, 1984, 1253a18–29). While similar to consequentialism in certain ways, the view should be distinguished as of more limited scope; for consequentialism offers a method by which to judge the actions of all individuals, but the organic-state view offers justification primarily to those acting on behalf of the state (see Aquinas, 1981, II-II, Q. 64, a.2).

Second, one might ground a political immunity to ethical considerations in research by means of some form of political liberalism or libertarianism. On such views, it would be no business of the state to regulate research for ethical reasons except insofar as such research overran the consent of fully competent moral agents. Such an immunity would be considerably more restricted than the immunity of the previous views; harmful research on non-consenting adults would, for example, be impermissible. But the view is still quite permissive. The disputed questions regarding research on stem cells, or aborted fetuses, or cloned embryos would all be outside the realm of political debate, for the most serious ethical issues that they raise do not involve the consent of competent adults.

A variety of claims, then, need to be assessed to judge the demand for immunity for research and inquiry from ethical considerations. But first, we need more rigor in characterizing the notion of "immunity." Often, in political or popular discourse, what is demanded for scientific research is indeed a strict immunity from ethical requirements. Such requirements might be applicable to ordinary folks, but to scientific researchers, they are not.

Strictly speaking, consequentialism offers no such immunity. Rather, consequentialism offers a standpoint for the ethical judging of research from which the considerations of so-called ordinary, or common, morality are inapplicable. According to our everyday ethical practices, it is morally impermissible intentionally to harm an innocent person. Thus, performing hazardous research on him without his consent for the benefit of others is morally impermissible. Consequentialism does not offer immunity from such claims; it straightforwardly denies them. Nonetheless, the appearance is of immunity, of liberation from the demands, or restraints, of ordinary morality.

The Aristotelian position can also be interpreted in this way; as knowledge is the highest good, all actions are to be judged in terms of their efficacy towards the production of knowledge. But it might also be interpreted as offering immunity: not all can pursue knowledge or contemplation; but those who can are exempt from the demands of ordinary morality. Presumably, however, the life of contemplation would be subject to its own moral norms, even if these differed from the norms of the active life.

The organic-state view does offer a kind of immunity. For persons acting in a private capacity, there are straightforward moral norms governing various actions. But those acting in a political capacity may sometimes be exempt from such rules. Thus, one strand of Christian thinking has held that intentional killing may never be performed by a private citizen; but agents of the state have been considered immune from this demand under certain circumstances.[1]

Finally, liberalism and political libertarianism offer an immunity at the political level from ethical considerations, even if, at a moral level, ethical requirements remain in play. Both views argue for a degree of autonomy from the demands of the state, especially when those demands are couched in robust moral language unlikely to be shared by all citizens.[2]

Few of these positions offer a complete immunity from ethical considerations. But all claim that in some contexts of research or inquiry, some ethical claims that many moral agents think of as binding are in fact not binding. For brevity, then, I will continue to speak of these views as making demands for immunity from ethical restrictions. In this chapter, I shall primarily be concerned with the first two positions, consequentialism, and the Aristotelian view about the value of knowledge.[3] In Chapters 8, 9, and 10, I will return to the political question concerning the limits of political interference in inquiry.

## MORALITY AND PRACTICAL REASON

Few theories have been criticized more extensively than consequentialism (Donagan, 1977a, Chapter 6; Grisez, 1970; Williams, 1973; see also the essays in Scheffler, 1988). There are many well-worked-out objections to consequentialism in the philosophical literature of the second half of the twentieth century, but still consequentialism has numerous philosophical proponents. Additionally, it can appear to represent the best reconstruction of much practical deliberation in everyday settings. Agents appeal to the consequences to justify their actions across a variety of contexts.

The Aristotelian claim that contemplation is the highest good, or the only real good, and the claim that those who pursue contemplation or knowledge are immune from ordinary ethical requirements is not as popular as consequentialism.[4] Still, it is worth investigating what is wrong with a view that claims either that there is only one good, or that there is a highest good, and that those pursuing such a good are less subject to ethical demands.

My strategy to address consequentialism and Aristotelianism will be somewhat roundabout. I shall not offer straightforward refutation of either; rather, I shall offer a sketch of the moral theory that I shall utilize throughout the book. I shall then show how the theory is incompatible with both consequentialism and Aristotelianism, and how that theory is more adequate than these alternatives in respect of several important, and widely shared, ethical insights.

I shall call the theory I defend a "basic goods" view.[5] It rests, at its foundations, on two essential distinctions. The first is an understanding of human action as directed by practical, rather than theoretical, reason. The second is an awareness that practical reason's direction is towards certain intrinsic, rather than instrumental, goods. Such goods are ultimately understood as aspects of human flourishing, or fulfillment.

The contrast between practical and theoretical reason concerns the difference between thinking that has as its purpose how the world is, and thinking that has as its purpose how the world is-to-be. Practical reason is directed towards action. Consider the difference this way: One common impetus to directed thinking is the force of a question. A question signifies some lack, some way in which we are unsatisfied. So questions, and the type of thought employed in their resolution, might be distinguished by consideration of the different ways in which questions are satisfactorily answered.

Suppose Jones asks who first circumnavigated the globe. If this question truly reflects a lack he is attempting to fill, then the lack will be filled by an answer: "Magellan." The question asks about a state of affairs, and is answered when the relevant state of affairs is indicated. By contrast, when Jones asks whether he should keep his promise to Smith, his lack will not be satisfied simply by an answer. Were Jones to receive the answer and then do nothing, we would think that in a crucial way the need that led him to ask the question would have been left unsatisfied.

What satisfies Jones's question is action: Jones must not only know the correct response, but act on it. Here we see the difference between theoretical reason and practical reason. Theoretical reason is oriented only towards the answer, whereas practical reason is directive, pointing us towards action as that which will satisfy some lack or need.

What, then, can satisfy this demand that practical reason orient us to action? Practical reason cannot direct by simply indicating the existence of an already obtaining state of affairs; in what way could what already is direct us to what is-to-be? Rather, practical reason must orient us to possibilities, opportunities. And possibilities and opportunities will themselves be understood as calling for action only inasmuch as they are apprehended as in some way or other good, as offering some benefit. All practical reasoning begins, then, with the apprehension of what is good, for only in this way could practical reason end in action.

The second foundational distinction concerned the nature of the goods apprehended by practical reason. The theory here articulated is referred to as a *basic* goods theory, for it holds not just that all practical thinking is oriented to something apprehended as good, but that underlying all practical evaluations are a limited set of basic goods—fundamental reasons for action that underlie all intelligible options. Such goods may be thought of as various aspects of human well-being. Each indicates a way in which human agents can be completed or perfected. They thus offer genuine reasons for action to agents whose lives are always in some way or other characterized by incompleteness, lack of full well-being, and imperfection.

Which goods are basic? I include the following: life and health; knowledge; aesthetic experience; excellence in work and play; marriage and family; friendship; integrity and practical reasonableness; and harmony with the divine. Each of these goods gives a basic reason for action—not a reason, such as "to make money" or "to take that medicine," that is intelligible only by reference to some further good or reason. That such goods are basic, rather than instrumental, may be seen by asking, across a range of cases, why agents act as they do. Rather than give an infinite chain of justificatory reasons, agents are likely to run out of reasons when they reach the basic goods: that something was done for a friend, or to save a life, or to satisfy a desire for knowledge, are often sufficient reasons for an agent's actions.

Human agents, then, are faced with a multiplicity of possible goods, all promising some important aspect or other of human flourishing. This, in turn, presents agents with a deep practical problem. How, in the face of such plurality, is one to order one's pursuit of human goods in a reasonable way?[6] The problem is deepened by the following considerations.

First, the basic goods are goods not just for me, or for you, but for all agents. They offer agent-neutral reasons for action—that your life may be promoted is as much a good as that mine will be, for example. A reasonable response to the goods must acknowledge this fact.[7]

Further, the goods are understood as desirable for pursuit not just now, but over a life. This raises further structural difficulties for an agent attempting reasonably to organize her pursuit of human goods.

What is needed to address these difficulties is some grounding principle of organization, which can be specified so as to make clear which pursuits are reasonable, which unreasonable.

What does it mean to think reasonably about the organization of a multiplicity of goods across lives and agents? What structuring principle could be at work? A comparison with theoretical reason is here instructive. One guiding principle in theoretical consideration of some domain is a principle of completeness: One's theoretical principles should be such that together they are adequate to all the phenomena investigated within the relevant domain. No fact is left unaccounted for.

Taken on its own, this interest of theoretical reason would be of little help for practical reason, for there is an important difference between the two at just this juncture. Theoretical reason really can aspire to completeness in any given domain precisely because it strives to apprehend the facts, the way things are. And there is but one way things are, even if that one way is tremendously complicated. Because theoretical reason is world guided, it can reasonably aspire to the whole of the world. The ideal of a completed science, while probably not a practical possibility, is not conceptually problematic.

This cannot be the case for practical reason. Each of the goods offers possibilities, and indeed limitless possibilities for action. Such possibilities cannot all be instantiated. Inevitably, pursuit of some rules out pursuit of others. But those other possibilities, which were themselves directed at genuine goods, would themselves have been good—they are not ruled out by practical reason as not being good, as false claims are ruled out by theoretical reason as not being true. There simply is no way for practical reason, therefore, to produce a system of directives that is complete in the sense of requiring pursuit of every genuinely good opportunity.

There is an analogue to completeness, though, that seems appropriate to practical reason, and seems to be an ideal of reason underlying even theoretical reason's demand for completeness, namely a demand for a kind of reasonable whole. For theoretical reason, a reasonable whole is complete, because the whole is the world. This is not possible for practical reason, but the ideal of the whole can still play a regulating function for practical reason (Tollefsen, 1997). And as playing this function, it seems that its consequence is the following architectonic demand of practical reason: that in all choosing, agents be directed to an ideal of integral human fulfillment (Grisez, Boyle, and Finnis, 1987, pp. 121–31).

Because completeness is not an option, the ideal of integral human fulfillment is just that—an ideal, not a concrete state of affairs envisaged as a goal. But in striving to make all choices open to this ideal, by striving not to close off options by ignoring the bearing of the goods on other persons, or on other parts of one's own life than the present, or by arbitrarily damaging some goods in favor of others, practical reason respects both its directedness towards human goods, and its regulative ideal of the whole.

It is thus that certain practical principles, which will be of crucial importance in this book, emerge. To reiterate, in a more principled way: In willing and acting, respect the fact that the basic goods are goods for all agents, and not just for some privileged few; hence, do not pursue the goods in a self-preferring or biased way, but fairly. Do not allow individual enthusiasm to deter you from cooperative action for the goods. Pursue the goods by developing a plan of life that allows concentrated and disciplined pursuit of some goods to play a structuring role in the pursuit of other goods. Do not intentionally destroy or damage instances of basic goods for the sake of other goods, basic or instrumental, out of hostility or anger. Pursue the goods with vigor and creativity, not lazily, wastefully, or in a way that accepts mere appearances of the goods (Finnis, 1984, p. 75; Grisez, Finnis, and Boyle, 1987, p. 128). Such practical principles are crucial as premises in moral arguments whose conclusions concern much more specified forms of action. So, for example, because intentionally to kill is intentionally to destroy an instance of a basic good, such killing is morally impermissible, ruled out by practical reason.

While there is more to be said on this matter, enough has been developed to throw some light on the contrast between a basic goods approach, and both consequentialism and Aristotelianism.

## CONSEQUENTIALISM

Consequentialism strives to accomplish with practical reason what is a reasonable goal only for theoretical reason: a completeness that rules out all alternative possibilities as less good. Consequentialism does this by two maneuvers that are foreign to basic goods views. First, it holds that all goods are commensurable with one another; that is, that there exists a common measure or standard by which the goods can be weighed, in their instantiations, next to one another. Second, it posits the goal of action as a state of affairs: that state of affairs in which the most good, or the most good for the greatest number of people, is realized. That state of affairs, and only that state of affairs, corresponds to a demand of practical reason functioning without error (see Tollefsen, 1997).

Basic goods theories deny that the goods are intrinsically commensurable. On their own, and independently of any work of practical reason, no basic good can be said to be better than another. Basic goods cannot be weighed up next to each other. Nor, as the discussion of the *ideal* of integral human fulfillment indicated, does practical reason direct us to a definite state of affairs; there *is* no possible state of affairs in which all the goods are maximally realized.

Basic goods views are superior to consequentialism for two reasons. The first is that basic goods views do, but consequentialist views do not, allow for principled constraints on what may be done in pursuit of the good. Because consequentialism makes only one demand, that the greatest good be pursued, the consequentialist demands that whatever action can bring about that state of affairs should be pursued. In principle, no type of action can be ruled out as intrinsically wrong.

Basic goods approaches do have the resources to rule out, in principle, action types, however, because some forms of action always involve a direction of the will incompatible with the ideal of integral human fulfillment. For example, actions that denigrate some persons as not, intrinsically, deserving of some share of basic goods, or actions, such as intentional killing of the innocent, which always involve intentional damage or destruction to basic human goods, are always incompatible with the ideal. Thus absolute moral prohibitions on slavery and murder are at home in a basic goods ethics.

The fact that basic goods views are capable of generating restrictions should seem like a positive feature of the theory, judged by common intuitions we have about the impermissibility of certain kinds of actions. In the realm of biomedical inquiry, for example, few would think that lethal experimentation on a live and unconsenting adult would be ethically acceptable, even if the possible benefits would be great.

The second difference between consequentialism and basic goods views is itself twofold. In two senses, basic goods views allow for options for action. Consequentialism does not. This might seem surprising, for consequentialism appears liberating in its abandonment of constraints on action. However, recall that consequentialism makes one and only one demand on agents: pursue the greatest overall good.

When this injunction is considered in light of the consequentialist claim that all goods may be commensurated, then options for action disappear in two ways. First, in any given situation of choice, unless there is a tie between options, then one action, out of all possible action possibilities, will be singled out as offering the greatest possible good. This action will be mandatory, for any other action possibility will fail to maximize the good (Kagan, 1989).

By contrast, a basic goods view can hold that because there are a multiplicity of incommensurable goods, each offering beneficial possibilities for action, it is not necessary that for each set of action possibilities there will be one that is best, full stop. Indeed, while some possibilities might be ruled out as not open to integral human fulfillment, there might conceivably be a number of options offering different, incommensurable benefits, all of which might be fully reasonable, each in its own way. This points us back to the lack of a completeness requirement for practical reason: full practical reasonableness underdetermines which options may be chosen, thus preserving, in an ordinary sense, options for agents.

Thus, an agent faced with a choice between pursuing a life of inquiry, or a life of music, might, under many circumstances reasonably choose either; an agent faced with a choice between pursuing medical inquiry or philosophical inquiry might, again, reasonably choose either. By the demands of consequentialism, however, there will be one possible course of action only, in each case, for any given agent, which will maximize the good, and this is the one that must be chosen.

It is not clear, however, that anything else *could* be chosen, and this brings us to the second way in which consequentialism eliminates options. According to consequentialism, the action that is to be chosen is the one that offers the greatest amount of good. Further, it offers the greatest good in the same sense that all other possibilities offered were good, with only this difference, that the choice-worthy option offers more good than any of these other possibilities. But now it becomes impossible to see how an agent could choose anything other than the possibility recommended by consequentialism, for a choice made for some lesser good seems completely irrational. So not only does consequentialism fail to offer morally permissible options for action, it fails to offer any options. In a world in which all goods are commensurable, agents can make no genuine choices (Finnis, Boyle, and Grisez, 1987, pp. 254–60).

Basic goods views, however, respect the phenomenon of choice, and the phenomenon of regret at options not chosen. For options not chosen, whether morally permissible or not, are still options that offered some good, a good incommensurate with, i.e., different in benefit from, the chosen option.

Consequentialism is behind some claims that at least some types of inquiry should be granted an immunity from ordinary moral considerations. Because some forms of inquiry promise such significant benefits to human beings, those pursuing the relevant research should not be hindered by "ethics," for the benefits would outweigh any possible negative consequences of the research. But this notion of future benefits outweighing negative consequences is fundamentally misguided: if the goods basic to human persons are incommensurable, then the good of some agent who might be harmed by research is simply not weighable next to the good of other agents who might be benefited. The proper framework in which to assess such harmful research is not that of the greatest overall good, but of what is reasonable, in the sense of promoting integral human fulfillment. Research whose promised success requires denying some agent the right to live fails precisely by this standard—it fails to treat the damaged agent's good as an aspect of integral human fulfillment.

## THE ARISTOTELIAN VIEW

The basic goods view offers a more reasonable ethical approach than consequentialism, and it should be preferred in addressing an ethics of inquiry. What of the Aristotelian view? Does it similarly suffer by contrast to basic goods views? There are, in fact, two different versions of Aristotelianism that must be addressed; the basic goods view is, I will argue, superior to both.

Let me, then, distinguish the two possible interpretations of the Aristotelian view. The first I shall call the Single Final End view (SFE), the second the Dominant Final End (DFE) view. Each is a position about the relationship between what seem (in some cases only seem) to be genuine goods other than contemplation, or the pursuit of knowledge, and contemplation itself. The generic Aristotelian view claimed only that knowledge is the highest, or the best, or perhaps the only good, and so was neutral between the different interpretations of these claims. But both interpretations have critical difficulties with what Gabriel Richardson Lear calls "mid-level goods," goods such as friendship, virtue, or play that seem important to a well-lived life, but seem jeopardized by Aristotelian monism about the good (Richardson Lear, 2004, Chapter 1).

On the SFE view, what these claims mean is that all other goods are good only to the extent that they instrumentally bring about the possibility or actuality of knowledge. So the pursuit of family, or political life, or leisure, is valuable either as it directly or indirectly brings about the possibility or actuality of the pursuit of knowledge. These pursuits could do this directly by serving causally to bring about knowledge or its possibility; or they could do so indirectly by, for instance, providing the distractions necessary for inquirers to relax, the better to be able to pursue inquiry later.[8]

As a result, these other goods are only apparent goods, of no intrinsic worth themselves. On the DFE view, by contrast, these other goods may be acknowledged to be intrinsically good, and may be pursued for their own sake. However, they must also be pursued for the sake of knowledge or contemplation, which is the highest good. So a life not primarily oriented towards contemplation and the pursuit of knowledge is a lesser life than the life so oriented. A life of family, work, and leisure, for example, if not also directed towards contemplation would either be forbidden, or, at any rate, of morally less value than the life directed at contemplation. The second of these two possibilities appears more likely, as not all seem capable of leading a life of contemplation.[9]

Are either the SFE or the DFE view a plausible starting point for an ethics of inquiry? If so, this would have significant implications. Like consequentialism, for example, the SFE view seems to allow for damage and destruction of persons and goods when necessary to the pursuit of knowledge. But even worse, this view seems significantly to undersell the value that non-inquiring and non-knowledge-related pursuits have for us.

Consider the value of friendship. Few would think that a life without friends was worth living. At the same time, pursuit of friendship for the sake of attaining some other good—knowledge, for instance—seems intrinsically corrupting of friendship. The relationship of friendship seems possible only if pursued because it is thought of as itself good—good to have friends, and this friend, in itself. Instrumentalizing the friendship seems equivalent to instrumentalizing the friend, and thus not really treating him or her as a friend at all. On the SFE view, genuine friendship looks impossible.

Similarly, consider the way the pursuit of knowledge reasonably in many cases is subordinated to other pursuits and activities. A good husband rightly puts aside his lab work to spend time at home, and not simply to be better rested the next day. Ordinary obligations to help others sometimes take precedence over inquiry. If Aunt Millie needs to be taken to the hospital, even though this will cut into one's research time, then abandoning the research is the reasonable thing to do. In this circumstance, human life takes reasonable precedence over knowledge. Similarly, the example of research on an unconsenting subject shows that it is morally wrong to make all other goods second to knowledge. So, like consequentialism, the SFE view does not respect our sense of the range of genuine goods, and the moral demands made by practical reason regarding the pursuit of these goods.

The DFE view seeks to avoid such denigrations of genuine goods, and the radical revision of ordinary morality that such denigrations would entail. Goods other than knowledge, such as family, art, life and health, and friendship, are all to be pursued for their own sake, and not merely instrumentally. This, in turn, should provide some ground for a denial that such goods may be sacrificed for the pursuit of knowledge and contemplation; only instrumental goods seem reasonably sacrificed in this way. But the DFE view seeks to make the case that there is, nonetheless, something special about knowledge, and hence inquiry, that entitles this good to a position at the top of a natural hierarchy of goods, pursued for its own sake only, where other goods are pursued both for their own sake and for the sake of it. St. Thomas gives expression to such a view as follows: "Ultimate and complete happiness, which we look for in a future life, consists entirely in contemplation. Imperfect happiness, such as can be had in this life, consists principally in contemplation, but secondarily in the operation of the practical intellect directing human actions and passions" (Aquinas, 1981, I-II, Q. 3, a. 5).

Why would such a view seem attractive? Two possible answers suggest themselves. One argues from the nature of the knowing agent; the other from the nature of what is known.

Aristotle's function argument in *Nicomachean Ethics* 1.7 seems to be an example of the former sort of argument. Aristotle asks what the function of the human being might be, seeking thereby to discover what will make the human being happy. Aristotle rules out various possibilities—living, as common also to plants, perception as common to animals—and claims that the function of the human being is activity of the reasoning part of the soul, as this is unique to the human being. When understood in light of Aristotle's claims about contemplation in later books of the *Ethics,* it seems that Aristotle is suggesting that because the pursuit of knowledge is something that only man, of the animals, can do, that it is thereby his proper good.

The second argument also has roots in Aristotle (and in Plato, as does also the previous argument). It works by consideration of the possible objects of knowledge. Granted, not all possible objects of knowledge are equal; some are of particularly, and impressively, high status. Knowledge of God, for example, is knowledge of the singularly best thing. Such knowledge raises us up to something far greater than we actually are, and far greater than the things of this world. Thus, in contemplation of the highest things, we are best off, and the best life is the one spent pursuing such knowledge.

There is good sense, on a basic goods view, in saying that the best life demands inquiry into, and contemplation of, the highest things, including God, if such a being exists; for living harmoniously with whatever the ultimate and transcendent source of meaning is, or living harmoniously with one's knowledge of the non-existence of such a being, is itself a basic good, the good of religion. Adequately to participate in such a good, and to achieve the necessary harmony, one must address, and answer, the question of whether there *is* such a being. This, in turn, requires inquiry into the problem.

Moreover, if there is indeed such an ultimate source of value, then one will want, in some way, to organize one's entire life in a meaningful relationship to that being. But such inquiry, and such ordering, is possible without denigrating the various legitimate non-inquiry-related goods, activities and lives. My contention is that the DFE view does denigrate such goods, activities and lives.

To make this clear, it is necessary to understand the distinguishing mark of the DFE view: the claim that knowledge is naturally a greater good than all other goods, even though these other goods may be ends in themselves as well. When I say "naturally a greater good" in this context, I mean that, considered in themselves, apart from any commitments made by an agent, or any other considerations, but looked at only and precisely insofar as knowledge, and the various other goods, are good, then knowledge is recognized as more good, a greater good, a superior good, and so forth.

This claim must be distinguished from three different sorts of claim with which it might be confused. First, this claim is different from other sorts of views that attribute a formal, rather than a substantive, final end to all that human agents do, while also claiming that many of the constituents of that final end are substantive goods-in-themselves. Consider the good of "happiness," which many philosophers have been convinced is the end for the sake of which we pursue all other ends. What sort of an end is happiness? It is not a substantive end—that is, not an end of some definite sort offering a good analogous to knowledge, friendship, life, and so forth, but greater—rather, happiness is constituted by a reasonable pursuit of all these goods. But the DFE view of knowledge is not like this. It does not claim that knowledge is merely a formal good, to be filled out by the pursuit of various other goods. Knowledge is a distinct and substantive good.

Second, it might be the case that some agent or agents may reasonably adopt a commitment to the good of knowledge, and the life of contemplation, such that the agent, after the commitment, treats that good as of dominant importance in his life. Third, it might be the case that all agents ought to give contemplation a kind of priority in their lives, where this priority is demanded by practical reason.

Neither of these latter two views is identical with the DFE, nor do they result in the same sorts of demands on agents as the DFE. They are not identical to the DFE because neither claims that knowledge's and contemplation's dominant part in a good life is demanded by the *goodness* of knowledge as compared with the goodness of other goods. For instance, the first possibility, that some agents might reasonably make a commitment of such a sort that they thereafter treat knowledge as of dominant importance, can emerge from the demand of reason on all agents that they make selective commitments, so that they may pursue with greater depth some goods over the course of a life. This demand presupposes no special goodness to knowledge, and indeed, allows that other goods might reasonably play a similar role in the lives of other agents.

The second view also works from a demand of reason, rather than an initial assessment of some good as "greater." Suppose that there is indeed a God, who has created all things, and hence all objects of knowledge. An agent might reasonably want to direct all that she does towards God in such a way that all her actions possess religious significance. If, indeed, there is a God, then this might be the reasonable thing for *all* agents to do, as demanded by norms of gratitude and piety. An agent might, perhaps, do this by considering all her actions cooperative ventures with God. In doing so, she would be acting "contemplatively," even when engaged in the most "active" of pursuits.

Such a contemplative approach to action would take its start from norms of gratitude or piety, or out of a desire for friendship with God. This shows that the priority given to knowledge (here, of the divine) and contemplation is not a result of a natural assessment of the goodness of such knowledge, in the sense of knowledge defined earlier. Contemplation does not achieve a privileged place on this account in consequence of its greater *goodness* than the other goods, but in consequence of the way in which it can provide a framework of understanding within which one can relate all one's actions to God.

Nor do these views make the same demands on a moral agent as a DFE view. Both, for example, offer a wide variety of possible dominant goods that could alternatively serve as the objects of life-structuring commitments. But, except as one's life is somehow lesser, not as good, it is not clear that the DFE view can allow for pluralism about worthwhile lives, for any life that gives greater priority to some good other than knowledge may be judged from the same standpoint from which knowledge is recognized as a greater good, and seen to be wanting. Despite the fact that it emerges as an attempt to save pluralism of lives from inevitable denigration, the DFE view does not have the resources to do this.

I conclude, then, that a pluralistic theory of basic goods that holds these goods to be intrinsically incommensurable represents our best understanding of the foundations of ethics that takes the notion of "good" to be essential to those foundations: better than all forms of consequentialism, and better than the Single Final End and the Dominant Final End views. That this has consequences for an ethics of inquiry has already been seen: the pluralistic theory can sustain options and restraints, and give good reasons for attributing tremendous importance to the life of inquiry, without privileging that life at the expense of various other worthwhile lives, or at the expense of reasonable moral restraints.

## SOME FURTHER DISTINCTIONS

Having laid out in very rough outlines an ethical theory to serve as the grounding for an ethics of inquiry, and having compared that theory to some other possible ethical approaches, there remain some further clarificatory points to make.

The first point is to distinguish between judgment and inquiry. Judgment is the goal of inquiry. Judgment involves assent to or dissent from some proposition or set of propositions on the grounds of that proposition's truth or falsity, and what I shall call responsible judgment involves assent or dissent on the basis of evidence. In some cases the evidence will be more or less immediate: my evidence for the judgment that it is sunny outside, made when I am looking out the window, is immediate.

Where this immediacy is not present, however, a search must often be made—evidence must be gathered, and by "inquiry" I mean just this: the gathering of evidence with a view towards judgment. Inquiry is directed; I wish to form a judgment on some subject matter, to arrive at the truth in regards to some issue. Random accumulation of facts is not inquiry, and for this reason we might think of inquiry as especially directed by the activity of asking questions.

At the same time, however, the definition allows us to understand inquiry quite broadly. This is important, in terms of the purposes of this book, for it allows us to see biomedical and scientific research as on a continuum with inquiry in other domains. Inquiry as defined here occurs in a wide variety of contexts. Not just medical researchers, and scientists, but also journalists, police investigators, historians, gossips, moral agents, and philosophers all engage in inquiry precisely insofar as they wish to make a judgment on some question, and seek evidence to shape that judgment.

An *ethics* of inquiry is an account of the norms governing, and the virtues shaping, the gathering of evidence with a view to judgment regarding the truth of some proposition. These norms and virtues are themselves of two very general types, and their distinction will determine the structure of this book.

The distinction is between what I will call person-centered norms and virtues, and good-centered norms and virtues. The distinction is somewhat artificial, because persons are protected and harmed via the basic goods. But the distinction is nevertheless helpful.

Inquiry is a human activity; like all activities, it has its particular point, or purpose, which I have specified as judgment with a view to truth. Like many human activities, inquiry involves those agents who engage in it with other human beings in a variety of ways: as subjects of inquiry, as when a scientist performs an experiment on a human person; as beneficiaries of inquiry, as when a medical cure for some disease is made available to someone suffering from that disease; and as persons incidentally affected by inquiry, as when information gained from a subject of inquiry bears in some way or other on a different person, not directly involved in the inquiry.

These two points—that inquiry has its own purpose, and that it is person affecting—track two different types of norms and virtues that have application to inquiry. The first, which we could also call internal norms and virtues, emerge as guiding inquiry precisely because of what inquiry is *for*: the obtaining of the truth. Such norms and virtues are internal because they are structured by the particular nature of the activity itself. They are good centered, or, more specifically, "truth centered" because they emerge from consideration of the good, or point of the activity, which in this case is truth.

The second sort of norm or virtue arises out of the fact that inquiry typically involves persons other than the inquiring agent. Such norms and virtues might also be thought of as external, because they have less to do with the special nature of inquiry than they do with general moral considerations regarding the treatment of persons.

So, to illustrate the distinction, the commitment to truth that is a part of any serious inquiry requires a form of intellectual courage. This virtue is internal to inquiry in the same way that we might think of sympathy as internal to the profession of medicine, considered precisely as a healing profession. On the other hand, researchers and doctors who are careless with the lives of their research subjects or patients have violated a person-centered norm whose application does not depend upon the particular nature of inquiry, or medicine, as such.

This distinction, between a person-centered, or external ethics of inquiry, and a good-centered, or internal ethics of inquiry, informs the structure of the rest of this book. Much of the recent work in biomedical and scientific research ethics has focused on person-centered norms and virtues. We see this in the emphasis on informed consent, for example, or in concerns with privacy or fairness. The first part of this book involves a person-centered, external approach to the ethics of inquiry, beginning, in various ways, with the ethics of medical and scientific research, and working outwards, to determine what overlap in person-centered norms and virtues there might be between these familiar domains of the ethics of inquiry, and other areas of inquiry, such as military or journalistic investigation.

Commitment to the truth as the end of inquiry has not been absent in discussion of research and scientific ethics, but it has been a particular focus of recent philosophy done outside the strictly bioethical and research ethics context.[10] As I will show, the truth-centered ethics of inquiry is best understood as a virtue ethics. The virtues that govern inquiry whose end is the obtaining of truth are, however, virtues that should be widely shared across a variety of inquiring agents; like the external, person-centered ethics of inquiry, application of the internal ethics of inquiry extends beyond the ethics of science and biomedical research.

This distinction, while important, is somewhat flexible. In some cases, it might be difficult or impossible to specify whether a norm is person-centered or truth-centered. Some norms might be grounded in both person-centered and truth-centered considerations. This happens in other domains of ethics. Suppose, for example, that it is intrinsically wrong to execute criminals. If so, this applies equally to all agents for person-centered reasons. But the norm has special application in the case of doctors and other medical personnel, for doctors to engage in lethal practices is a special violation of their professional responsibilities. So the norm against killing is internally related to the goods of medicine as well as being an external person-centered norm. The virtue of honesty and norms about truth telling are also of this dual sort.

To say that a norm or set of norms is a part of the person-centered or good-centered ethics of inquiry is not to make any judgment on the comparative importance of that norm or norms. Arguably, the most important area of the ethics of inquiry right now concerns the person-centered ethics of inquiry, namely, the ethics of human embryonic research. But also, we live in a culture experiencing a crisis of truth, in which researchers manipulate historical research for reasons of advocacy, or invent scientific findings for personal gain.[11] As there can be no genuine inquiry without a commitment to truth, from this point of view the internal ethics of inquiry might be thought the most important.

Rather than make such comparative judgments, I hold only that the ethics of inquiry must be pursued from both person-centered and truth-centered standpoints. In the next chapter, I turn to the initial stages of a discussion of a person-centered, external ethics, by articulating five normative concepts that can be expected to play a major role in ethically sound approaches to inquiry.

# 2 Core Concepts in the Ethics of Inquiry

Events of the twentieth century make clear the importance of a person-centered, or external ethics of inquiry. Moral clarity has emerged in part because of the moral horrors, great and small, of the twentieth century. Thus, the norm demanding that human subjects give informed consent for all research performed on them has become widely accepted; the abuse of this norm by Nazi scientists, the Tuskegee experimenters, and others was too egregious to be ignored by members of the medical and scientific professions.

In other areas, controversy remains. Few issues are as contested, or are of such importance in recent years, as the problem of research involving human embryos. Is it permissible to experiment on embryos left over from in vitro fertilization (IVF)? Is it permissible to create new embryos, whether through IVF, or newer cloning techniques, to investigate the possibly therapeutic value of stem cells, even though such research would result in the destruction of the embryo? The recent report of the President's Council on Bioethics (PCB) reveals that despite an impressive generosity and good will among the panelists, unanimity was not forthcoming (PCB, 2002). At the end of deliberations, several members remained as far away from one another's positions as at the beginning, and some, in personal statements made after publication of the report, seemed not even to understand the rationale of the views of other members with whom they disagreed.[1]

Or consider the increased awareness of issues related to lying. Researchers have lied to gain evidence, in reporting evidence and findings, and in attributing their sources of evidence (see Broad and Wade, 1983). Others have distorted their findings for political purposes. Scientists are not the only guilty parties—newspaper reporters, law enforcement officers, and intelligence operatives have also engaged in ethically questionable behavior.

Consider also animal research. While the number of people adamantly opposed to research involving animals is smaller than that opposed to embryo research, it is equally vocal, and its ranks include numerous philosophers and theoreticians. Thus, this issue has generated considerable, heated discussion in recent years.

What lies beneath these moral requirements, such as the demand for informed consent, or the restrictions on lies and coercion? What norms can help to clarify the remaining areas of controversy? The purpose of this chapter is to articulate several of the concepts and norms most deeply implicated in the person-centered, external ethics of inquiry. Specifically, I shall provide an analysis of the following concepts: autonomy, privacy, bodily integrity, fairness, and personal integrity. These core concepts will give us some purchase on understanding the justifications for norms in inquiry central to biomedical and scientific research, but also for other domains. These justifications and implications will be addressed in subsequent chapters.

The clinical context has, by and large, provided the most fruitful venue for discussion and argument about the necessary conditions for morally legitimate research involving human subjects. As Baruch Brody points out, there is a remarkable consensus in the ethics of research using human subjects, and on the norms that investigators should follow. Brody lists four in particular: that risks be minimized, and that the expected benefit be proportionate to the risks; that subjects be chosen equitably; that their informed consent be obtained; and that their privacy be respected (Brody, 2004). This remarkable convergence has its roots in the continuing authority of the founding documents of the research ethic of the second half of the twentieth century, specifically, the Nuremberg Code, the World Medical Declaration of Helsinki, and the *Belmont Report*.

The *Belmont Report*, however, went further than either of the other two documents in articulating core "principles" underlying this research ethic: the principle of respect for persons, the principle of beneficence, and the principle of justice.[2] Since the publication of the *Belmont Report*, various theorists have attempted to provide the conceptual and normative underpinnings and articulations of these principles.

The *Belmont Report* was essentially concerned with clinical research, as were both the Nuremberg Code and the Declaration of Helsinki, and not with inquiry more generally. My goal is similar to that of the theorists who have attempted to ground the principles of the Belmont Report, but I aim also to broaden the investigation into the ethics of inquiry, including, eventually, the ethics of military, criminal, and journalistic investigation. Moreover, while there is overlap between the concepts and norms that I address, and those discussed by the Belmont Report, there are some differences as well. Finally, my philosophical account of the core concepts of a person-centered ethics of inquiry will be by way of the general goods-based ethic outlined in Chapter 1, rather than, say, principlism or Kantianism.

## AUTONOMY

I turn, first, to autonomy, and its relation to the basic goods theory. Why is the capacity to choose for oneself what one will do and undergo of great normative weight?[3] On the goods-based approach, recall, all genuine human action is directed to basic human goods that offer opportunities for human well-being. But all reasonable human action is directed to integral human fulfillment. Now, by the approach outlined in Chapter 1, the basic goods are good for all, as is human fulfillment. This accounts for the possibility of intelligible, and sometimes obligatory, action on behalf of others. If I see a child drowning in shallow water, and can easily save her, I should recognize that life is a good for her as well as for me, and that life, so understood, is jeopardized by my inaction.

In this case, I am somewhat unusually situated relative to the possibility of another agent's participating in a basic human good, for my action or inaction will make the difference between the child continuing to live or not. But most often, I am best situated to act for my own fulfillment, and the fulfillment of those close to me. Thus my own well-being rightly takes a kind of practical precedence in my deliberations about what to do, for I am best situated to understand and act for the sake of that well-being.

Moreover, some of the goods are such that an agent can only participate in them if the agent has *chosen* to pursue them. While I may save another's life, even if they do not wish me to, I cannot save another's friendship, absent cooperation on his part. Friendship requires a harmony of wills between agents, and this cannot be brought about save by those agents engaging in the relevant acts of will. Nor is another agent's integrity something over which I have control, even though I must act to foster and preserve my own.[4]

Consideration of the first principle of morality, and the need for some basic goods to be pursued with more sustained attention and commitment than others over a life, contributes to this line of thought. In order both adequately to participate in human goods, and to avoid various practical conflicts, all agents must form some sort of life plan. Commitments are morally called for. But, what a reasonable pursuit of certain goods will be will then differ for me in light of commitments I have made. Having made a commitment to marry will entail certain responsibilities, and also certain immunities, not shared by those who have made a commitment to celibacy, or who have made no commitment in these matters yet.

These considerations—that an agent is often best situated with respect to her own good, that some goods can only be participated in by an agent's choosing that participation, and that an agent must make commitments that shape her subsequent obligations—all have as a consequence that autonomy is of considerable importance, for it is the agent herself who is in the best position, and sometimes the necessary position, to deliberate and choose in a way most open to integral human fulfillment.

To see this, consider what a lack of autonomy would result in, or in some historical cases, has resulted in. Take, for example, the first point. Who is in the best position to determine what goods I am suitably situated to pursue? An answer other than "I myself" often leads to serious mistakes, especially if the answer is generalized over many agents. The kind of paternalism inherent in communism, for instance, in many cases put, and continues to place, decisions about what should be done in pursuit of human goods in the hands of those who are not close enough to the situation to really know, even in regard to very banal questions, such as "Should a well be put here?" or "Should the crops be harvested now?"

The problem becomes considerably worse, however, in regard to the second issue. Only the agent can make certain kinds of decisions if the relevant goods are to be participated in. No one can decide who my friends are to be—only I can do that. A full understanding of marriage indicates the same point. While it is possible, through emerging harmony of wills, for arranged marriages to work out well, such marriages are ill devised with respect to the friendship-like good of marital communion. Further, since being practically reasonable seems to be one of these goods that is only participated in by those who themselves strive to be practically reasonable, and being practically reasonable requires a reasonable approach to all the basic goods, even withdrawing control over the pursuit of substantive goods, such as life, or knowledge, seems to block an agent's capacity for participating in the good of practical reasonableness.

This leads to the third point. Agents must make commitments and life plans for at least two reasons. First, none of the goods will be pursued well if they are all pursued equally. So it is reasonable to allot more time and effort to the pursuit of some goods in order that a deeper practical experience of the goods may be had. Second, without making any effort to give structure to their lives, agents will find their lives rife with conflict. Commitments and life plans introduce a necessary order into human life that is consistent, in a way confusion and conflict are not, with the ideal of integral human fulfillment.

Who should make such commitments for an agent? Agents should make them themselves; first, because, again, agents are in the best position to be able to know what a reasonable commitment to make would be. To the external observer, it may seem as if the agent should become a musician. But perhaps the agent feels no love for that, and relishes instead the thought of a steady job that will help him care for his family without the anxieties of a musician's life? The agent is in the best position to consider such factors and bring them to bear on the content of the commitment. Second, that one has made reasonable commitments, and a reasonable life plan, and taken the steps necessary to follow through, is itself a great good for an agent, part of practical reasonableness, and thus something the benefits of which accrue only to those agents who actually deliberate and choose themselves regarding those commitments. Finally, the very notion of a commitment itself introduces a requirement of an act of will—while you can be forced to do something, no one can truly make a commitment for you.

When we come to those obligations that emerge from the specific commitments an agent has made, it once again is clear that the agent herself is in the best position to recognize what those obligations are—after all, she is the one who made the commitment and who knows its full content. Others are often poorly situated to be able to understand the implications of a different agent's commitments, and will therefore poorly understand what she is or is not obligated to do under those commitments.

All of this adds up to an argument for the importance of autonomy. Autonomy, in the relevant sense, just is being able to deliberate and choose on one's own behalf, and agents who are not allowed so to deliberate and choose are deprived of the opportunity to participate well in a variety of important goods. Correspondingly, respect for a person's autonomy requires restraint from making decisions for them when they are capable of making those decisions.

Before continuing, it is worth identifying two claims that this account of autonomy does *not* make. First, there is no claim here that autonomy is the only, or the most important good. Autonomous choices must be oriented towards genuine goods if they are to be humanly fulfilling (see Raz, 1986). Second, there is no claim here that an autonomously made choice is for that reason a valuable choice. That one has chosen to do, or value, such and such is no guarantee that one has made an appropriate choice (see George, 1993). Some autonomous choices are very bad. These qualifications distinguish my account of autonomy from more radical accounts of the value of autonomy (Sartre, 1984; Richards, 1982).

## PRIVACY

Since 1973, when the Supreme Court of the United States justified its ruling in *Roe v. Wade* by reference to the value of privacy, that value has been at the center of one of the most contentious debates of modern life. Judicial discussion of the concept had begun even earlier with the writings of Justice Brandeis at the turn of the century (see Warren and Brandeis, 1984). But there is little unanimity as to what privacy is, and why it is valuable. Some think the right to privacy is a right to be left entirely alone, some think it a right to be free of moralizing legislation, and some think it a right to construct for oneself one's "personal meaning of life."

If there is a right to privacy, however, it will be important for the ethics of inquiry, for to make the activities or actions, or life, or health, or bodily or psychological state of another subject to one's own inquiry typically involves an incursion into that subject's privacy. An understanding of a right to privacy should begin with an attempt to understand the importance of privacy in light of the basic goods approach. My thesis is this: in many cases, the activities, or the conditions for activities, that agents engage in with a view to integral human fulfillment are more successful and sometimes possible only under conditions of privacy, and in some cases are made possible at all only under conditions of privacy. By privacy I mean an exclusive zone of non-observation; non-interference is a consequence of this non-observation. Privacy can thus be violated both by observation or intervention of another agent.

Why might some activities, or their conditions, have their success jeopardized by the observation of another? Consider the following sort of case.

You wish to do something with your friend—to plan a surprise party, perhaps. This requires, in turn, that you and your friend be able to communicate. So conditions conducive to such communication are necessary. Your ability to plan the party with your friend will depend upon the exclusiveness of the communication—if others hear, they might eventually spoil the surprise. Your ability to communicate freely, and to pursue the activities communication is supposed to make possible, therefore depends upon privacy—your ability to communicate with your friend without observation from others.

This reflects a general character of our social life, which Alasdair MacIntyre calls its "game-theoretic character" (MacIntyre, 1980, p. 97). Our ability to carry out our own projects across a wide variety of contexts depends upon our ability to render ourselves unpredictable—too much predictability will stymie our bargaining position, and lead to failure. An agent under constant surveillance and study, such that his every action could be predicted with a high level of success; would be at an immense disadvantage in the social world. Privacy with regard to what he thinks, and what he says, and with respect to many general patterns of behavior he engages in, is highly desirable for him.

Privacy makes possible this advantageous unpredictability. But at another level, privacy makes possible something more than this. Privacy makes possible both an interiority, and a kind of exclusivity necessary for the pursuit of goods that require self-determined self-giving.[5] Not only is my ability to go to the movies with my friend *alone* protected by privacy; so also is my ability to maintain an "inner self" that I can choose to communicate to this, rather than that person, so as to develop and maintain friendship with this person.

Hence the importance of privacy in communication, thought, and patterns of behavior. We can see why the home should have been thought of such importance in the early Brandeisian discussion of privacy, for the home provides a physical context in which planning, thinking, and communicating can all be undertaken in a way preparatory for action. By extension, the home becomes a locus of the value of privacy as the area in which you may be most free to engage in these activities without interference or observation by others.

It should be clear, then, that this defense of privacy understands that concept primarily in the "informational" and "spatial," rather than "decisional" sense (George, 1993, p. 211). Robert George summarizes this "traditional" sense of privacy as follows:

> In the traditional conception of the value of, and the right to, privacy, it fundamentally concerns protected places, and the control of personal information about oneself. Privacy thus conceived is protected by procedural guarantees of freedom from, for example, unreasonable searches and seizures, warrantless searches (except in exceptional circumstances), undue surveillance, wire-tapping, etc. The right to privacy,

as traditionally understood, is not the substantive right to be legally free to perform certain "private" acts, the immorality of those acts notwithstanding. (George, 1993, p. 211)

So privacy, like autonomy, is of great instrumental importance—our likelihood of success is greatly increased if we have a degree of privacy, and know that we can count on having it. With regard to some activities, the connection to privacy is even more stringent. For some activities, privacy is a condition of their full meaningfulness. Foremost among these seems to be sexual activity. Consider a husband and wife who desire to express their marital love through sexual intercourse. It is not just vulgar, nor merely inappropriate, but inconsistent with this end for them to invite friends along to watch. The full giving of self that is characteristic of sexual intimacy is by definition unshareable, and demands privacy as a condition of its success. When guests are invited, and spectators introduced, then neither partner is giving him or herself fully to the other, nor does either partner receive the giving of the other in an exclusive way.

Indeed, our paradigm of debased sex is pornography, sex that is performed entirely for the sake of viewers, and not out of any sense of love or intimacy at all. In the case of sex, then, it is not just the case that privacy renders it more likely that we will be able to achieve our legitimate ends; privacy is a *necessary* condition for that achievement.

One implication of these considerations may be seen in the increasing appreciation of the value of privacy where personal data is concerned. With our increased capacity for collecting and maintaining data about persons, such as medical and genetic data, personal history data, and so on, respect for the privacy of another requires some consideration of the consequences of seeking and publicizing personal data. Failure to respect privacy with respect to genetic data, for example, may lead to unfairness in the workplace, or in the attempt to purchase insurance. Violations of privacy in these areas is instrumentally damaging to an agent's ability to obtain for himself opportunities for well-being, or instrumentalities necessary for flourishing.

On the other hand, with regard to many activities, and various forms of information, the right to privacy is limited in various ways. While I will address some of these limits in more detail in the next chapter, it is worth pointing out some of them here. First, the right may be limited by where I am—it is not reasonable to expect a high degree of privacy in a conversation undertaken in a public place. There, one's right to it is limited. Privacy may be limited by what I am doing. Certain activities, because they impinge upon the public good, or are undertaken by those in some public capacity, are subject to legitimate scrutiny. If I am engaged in activities that might be quite damaging to the public good, as opposed to merely my own good, then my right to privacy is limited. Information also can lose its protected status if it is of crucial importance to the public good—as when I am infected with a highly contagious and dangerous disease.

It is possible, in many cases, for me to limit my own right to privacy through consent. I may invite others into my home, and indeed, allow them to scrutinize it in ways that they could not do without my consent; I can invite people to participate in my plans, and also to observe me making them. I will return to this in the discussion of informed consent: in those cases in which my right to privacy is not for some *other* reason limited (public space, public activity, or public information), those who wish to observe or interfere in activities that would otherwise be entitled to privacy must obtain my consent. So if someone wishes to inquire into how often I clean my kitchen, I must first consent to various interventions and observations with a view to making that knowledge possible.

## BODILY INTEGRITY

We not only have a sphere of privacy, within which we may remain uninterrupted in our thoughts and plans, we have an actual physical sphere of immunity from the actions of others, a sphere more or less identical with the space occupied by our bodies. The basic claim underlying the importance of bodily integrity, and so also a right claim to bodily integrity, is that human persons are essentially animals. Not *just* animals, since we are also rational, but animals nonetheless. I will argue for this claim in Chapter 5. But its basic import in the context of this chapter is clear. If you and I are essentially animals, then any injury sustained by our animal body is an injury to our self, and incursions into our bodily "space" are violations of our bodily integrity.

Not all bodily contact constitutes an injury. Moreover, much bodily contact that is not consented to is morally acceptable, appropriate, or even sometimes obligatory. Strangers brush against one another on the subway, or one taps the other on the shoulder to inform him that he has dropped his wallet. The mere fact of bodily contact is insufficient to require informed consent. On the other hand, "mere" bodily contact is not utterly insignificant. If there is plenty of room on the subway, yet you insist upon standing very close to me, I may find this threatening or stifling. If so, then you have wrongfully invaded my bodily space. It is not necessary that injury result from contact or proximity for such actions to be considered wrong.

In general, bodily contact seems acceptable when it is incidental and shows reasonable concern, or when it is directed to the good of the one touched, or to some mutual good (Grisez, 1993, pp. 549–61). If I brush you in passing by, without intending to, and I have shown ordinary signs of giving to people the room they deserve, then there is no wrong in what I do. Again, the tap on the shoulder to inform someone that he has dropped his wallet falls into the second category. Finally, in certain contexts in which mutual pursuit of a good or good is presumed, such as between colleagues working together, ordinary bodily contacts are also acceptable. On the other hand, any kind of intentional injury, damage, or destruction of another's body is injury to that person. Since it is impermissible directly to harm a basic good, and bodily life is a basic good to human beings, it is thus impermissible to intend bodily harm to another. Moreover, it is likewise impermissible to accept as a side effect unfair amounts, or unfairly distributed bodily harms.

## FAIRNESS

Fairness, the point behind the norm "Do unto others as you would have them do unto you," is central to the notion of justice. Human agents are often inclined to take something, do something, or behave in some way towards someone else *simply* because of the bearing their action would have upon themselves. *I* want to have the book that is on reserve, so I remove the note indicating that it is saved for someone else; *I* want to have a nice yard, so I water it despite the drought-related restrictions; *I* do not like my student's appearance, so I treat him poorly in class, and fail to read his papers with an unbiased eye.

In each of these cases, emotional attachment to goods insofar as they have a bearing on me leads me to ignore the bearing that those goods have on others. In the case of the reserved book, the other has a prior claim, but this is not always necessary: my student does not have a prior claim to something over me, he simply has a claim as a human being to be properly treated whether I wish to so treat him or not. What has gone missing in my practical reason or in my will in each case is that each human good is a good equally for all human beings; none specifically have my name on them. Moreover, as beings perfected by the basic goods, each human being is a being of intrinsic worth; their value is not measured by their value or disvalue to me. Thus each is deserving of equal respect in my actions.

This principle of equal respect is not just a negative principle, urging me not to act in certain ways towards others. Rather, since the goods are goods for all, and promotion of the goods in an ideal community is the point of reasonable action, I respect the equal worth of others by promoting their good, not simply by refusing to violate it. But when bias, emotion, or desire interferes, then I am tempted to set aside the just claims of others and behave selfishly and unfairly.

Many philosophers, concerned with justice, have proposed aids to the imagination for the purpose of understanding with more specificity what fairness demands. John Rawls's notion of a veil of ignorance, behind which we do not know what party we are in some situation, is a fair approximation of the sort of de-privileging of oneself that must be accomplished if one is to be fair to others, provided that the goods one is considering in assessing what to do are the thick basic goods, not a set of thin or instrumental goods (Rawls, 1999; see also O. Tollefsen, 1987; Finnis, 1984, pp. 48–50). A more homely mechanism is the demand that one think what it would be like to be in another's position. One might accept that others should bear some burdens in a project from which one will benefit—often this *is* fair. But would one be willing to accept those same burdens if one were in the situation of the other, or would one object? By such considerations we can begin to assess the role that desire and bias play in our decisions.

Fairness is a crucial part of a person-centered ethics of inquiry. Fairness will also be critical in the discussion of the truth-centered ethics of inquiry, for inquiry, I shall argue, is a cooperative activity. Fairness is at the foundation of any cooperative endeavor, and thus, at the foundation of any genuine community. Because the pursuit of truth demands cooperation, it also demands fairness among the cooperating agents.

## PERSONAL INTEGRITY

The final foundational concept is personal integrity, for which there is both a narrow, and a broad, sense. In the narrow sense, personal integrity is dependent upon one's own choices for its existence and erosion. Unlike bodily integrity, which can be directly damaged by others, personal integrity in this narrow sense is deeply under the control of agents. In a broader sense of integrity, however, the integrity of the person can be threatened, manipulated, or assaulted in ways that go beyond threats to and assaults on the body. Other agents can work to break down not only the physical, but the mental, spiritual, and moral integrity of an agent in various ways. Integrity in this sense will be the focus of the later discussion, in Chapter 7, of torture. The purpose of this section is to explore the nature and value of the narrower sense of personal integrity, and to see how it can be put at risk

Human beings are complex; were we angels, or pure substances, we would not be faced with as many ways of coming apart as we are. We are rational, volitional, and passionate; each of these aspects of the human being may come into conflict with the others. Thus, Smith judges that it is best to give blood, but, fearing pain, does not choose to give; there is a lack of harmony between judgment, on one hand, and choice, action, and emotion on the other. But even if Smith does indeed choose, and act, she may continue to feel a strong aversion. This conflict is a form of disharmony between reason and choice on the one hand, and emotion on the other.

Moreover, Smith's various emotions may be in internal conflict; she may not have considered well various aspects of her life, resulting in conflicts between judgments and commitments. By contrast, if Smith has made wise structuring choices, is of good character, and has educated her passions adequately, she will be a person of integrity: in internal harmony across the various aspects of her person.

Some think integrity is possible for agents of bad character—surely a Nazi, or Don Giovanni, may be of high integrity, with judgment, will, and emotion all operating as one (McFall, 1987). In one sense this is true—very corrupt characters are unified in their corruption. But in another sense it is false. The reasonable life is a life spent in structured pursuit of some genuine human goods, and openness to all. Immorality involves in all cases some form of hostility or closedness with respect to basic goods. Those who attack human life, or art, or the good of friendship, have for that reason, avenues towards the fullness of human flourishing closed to them; rejecting genuine goods limits their opportunity for human flourishing.

In consequence, any integrity that is purchased through immorality is bought at the price of a radical limiting of the scope of opportunity for human well-being. This obtains unity in the wrong way for integrity. Consider the integrity of a work of art. An excellent painting has its integrity through a unity in multiplicity—multiple parts are structured into a pleasing whole. A single speck of paint has a kind of unity, but of a diminished sort; we would not say it has artistic integrity.

One aspect of human well-being is found in society—in friendships, marriages, and sociable and cooperative relations with others. This diverse good is itself a form of harmony, so again, human well-being is damaged if this form of harmony is rejected, denied, or damaged. But, further, social goods, such as marriage, can provide a vocational focus for agents, around which their life centers. This vocational focus is central to the shape that integrity will have for such agents. This requires explanation.

A good life, as I have argued, is fully reasonable not just at a time, but through time. A good life must take on a certain structured shape. The contours of this shape are provided by those commitments an agent makes to pursue and foster some goods, and projects, rather than others—to get married rather than remain single, to marry this person rather than that. Or, to become a philosopher rather than a doctor, to pursue this branch of philosophy rather than that. Such commitments are more or less architectonic, playing a structuring role in the agent's life, raising new demands, but also limiting other considerations that would have been important given other commitments.

It follows that vocational commitments, which I shall discuss further in Chapter 11, are central to an agent's integrity, for the agent recognizes what is morally appropriate for her in light of these vocational commitments. But many of these commitments, such as marriage, are social in nature. So the forms of harmony one pursues socially are often centrally defining of what integrity would be for an agent.

This intersection of the individual and society can also create challenges to personal integrity. These challenges exist because of the general lack of moral rectitude found in human beings and societies, conjoined with the fact that *societas* is a basic human good, for the immoral and irresponsible purposes and instrumentalities shared by many create pressure on individuals who wish to maintain harmony with the social world around them. A husband urges his wife to lie on taxes about part-time work; a business encourages its employees to engage in minor acts of fraud for the company well-being. In such cases, it is tempting to pursue a fraudulent form of sociability—the mere appearance, rather than the reality—by acquiescing to the demands made on one by society. In this way, society can threaten an agent's integrity.

The final form of harmony is harmony with the transcendent source of all meaning, God. This form of harmony is crucial because of its tendency to play a vocationally defining role in an agent's life. This role is normatively demanded of all Christians, for example, whose lives are supposed to be shaped throughout all their concerns and pursuits in relation to this fundamental option—a commitment to put God first in all they do. Violations of this commitment result in radical disruption of integrity. So the martyr, in refusing to deny God, not only continues to give to God what is due, but also, in that very act, maintains her integrity in relation to her most central and important commitment.

I will argue in Chapter 12 that such forms of harmony are important to the truth-centered ethics of inquiry, for inquiry has both vocational and social aspects. It is additionally of crucial importance in a discussion of the wrongfulness of lying, which will be addressed in Chapter 4, and in its extended sense, in the account of the nature and wrongfulness of torture given in Chapter 7.

These five core concepts, autonomy, privacy, bodily integrity, fairness, and personal integrity, play various roles in the variety of theoretical attempts to unify the ethics of clinical research, and the ethics of science; they are also critical, as we shall see, to the professional ethics of law enforcement and journalism. I have argued that each of these concepts can find a home in a basic goods ethics, as crucial, in some way or other, for human flourishing and fulfillment. I now turn to the project of showing how each of these core concepts plays a role in generating widely, and sometimes not so widely, accepted norms governing permissible inquiry.

# 3   Questions of Consent

There is, at present, no unified "ethics of inquiry." Rather, the various questions of such an ethics have been distributed across a variety of sub-fields in philosophy. But to the extent that there is something like the ethics of inquiry, it is to be found in the ethics of medical research. This field is notable not just because it has transformed the professional ethics of medicine and medical research in the past fifty years, but also for the unanimity that has been generated within the field. In particular, ethicists in this area, whether they come from philosophy, theology, law or the medical profession itself, have agreed, almost without exception, that the requirement of informed consent constitutes the core of the ethics of medical research. For this reason I begin the discussion of the external ethics of inquiry in this chapter with an account of the importance of informed consent.

The requirement of informed consent is relatively easily stated. Before engaging in an intervention upon another human being, an agent must inform the patient concerning what he wishes to do, the patient must understand what the agent wishes to do, and the patient must voluntarily consent to the agent's performing the intervention (Donagan, 1977b; Faden and Beauchamp, 1986).

This requirement is of widest application in a medical context, where patients must consent to surgical and other therapeutic interventions. It is crucial also in the context of research, much, but not all of which, is medical, involving human subjects. But the requirement has its roots in concerns whose implications extend even beyond these limited contexts. Central to its justification is the value of autonomy, and it is on this that most discussions of informed consent have focused.[1] My discussion follows that trend, although I argue that privacy and bodily integrity are also crucial to understanding the requirement. And I shall give a broader picture of the normative implications of autonomy, privacy, and bodily integrity by looking at the need for informed consent in non-medical research contexts, such as social science research, and by considering analogues to the consent requirement in non-scientific investigations such as those carried out by law enforcement agents and journalists.

The centrality of autonomy can be seen by looking at informed consent in a context that is not primarily about inquiry, the context of decisions regarding medical treatment. Joseph Boyle and Germain Grisez have discussed the notion of informed consent in light of considerations of autonomy and vocation (Grisez, 1993, pp. 519–45; Boyle, 2002). Suppose that an agent's doctor recommends some treatment as offering certain benefits—an increase in amount of time lived, for example. There will also be various disadvantages; perhaps the agent will have to receive frequent, invasive, and costly treatments. To a physician looking dispassionately at the matter, it might seem obvious that she should accept the treatment.

Boyle and Grisez point out, however, that there is no natural commensurating standpoint, from which the advantages naturally outweigh the disadvantages. The standpoint from which they are to be judged, reasonably, is that of the agent, with her life plan and commitments, her personal vocation. From that perspective, aspects of the case take on new notes of salience: She may have obligations that she must fulfill, so that remaining alive seems quite important. Or, she may be concerned not to leave her dependents in debt, and be averse to the invasiveness of the technique. It is the agent who is in the best position to determine what sorts of treatment are unreasonable given her commitments and previous choices. It is not for the doctor to decide; informed consent thus emerges as a requirement before the intervention may be performed.

A similar line of reasoning can be applied to the issue of research. Agents asked to participate in research are always asked to do two things. First, they are asked to participate in the pursuit of knowledge. Insofar as the research is also potentially of therapeutic benefit to the patient, they are offered the possibility of certain health benefits as well. But in both therapeutic and non-therapeutic research on human subjects, knowledge is always a primary end of the intervention. Because knowledge is a basic good, agents requested to participate in such research, therapeutic or not, can understand the importance of the research, and find that importance to be a motivating factor, even when its benefits will not straightforwardly apply to them.

But agents are always also asked to make certain sacrifices, or accept certain risks by participating in such research. The sacrifices may be as minimal as the sacrifice of time that comes from participation. But the risks may be in some cases significant, particularly when the research is tied to experimental medical procedures that might or might not harm the agent. So the case is structurally similar to the earlier medical intervention case; it is the agent who is best situated to make a determination of what is a reasonable risk to accept, and what benefits are reasonably pursued given the sacrifice and risk for her. Thus, informed consent for research performed using human subjects is a reasonable demand of the ethics of medical research, just as it is in the broader context of therapeutic medicine.

Informed consent is thus grounded in the need to respect subject autonomy. But it is also important to recognize both privacy and bodily integrity as core concerns underlying the necessity of informed consent. Much of what one consents to involves what would otherwise be a violation of one or the other of these values. Because one autonomously gives up certain rights over one's privacy or body, it becomes permissible for a researcher to undertake otherwise invasive investigations; but this indicates the point in question. It is because of the significance of these values, and of threats to them, that it is necessary to seek a subject's consent where these values are implicated. While research may affect other important values, research involving human subjects almost inevitably affects either privacy or bodily integrity because it involves an investigation into something about the subject: her thoughts, her desires, her physical ailments, her patterns of behavior, her bodily nature, and so on. So privacy and bodily integrity are specially implicated in research involving humans.

This analysis suggests various further questions. For example, the ethical problem regarding consent to research seems to have shifted. The explanation of the importance of autonomy rested on the claim that it is the agent who is best situated to make a reasonable choice about what risks are appropriate in exchange for possible benefits. The questions of research ethics seem thereby to have been moved, in part, to the sphere of the subjects of research.[2] Are there any norms by which the potential *subjects* of research should govern themselves?

Further, our paradigms of research requiring informed consent are those in which there is either risk or sacrifice demanded of the subjects. But not all research involves sacrifice or risk. Suppose that I am counting the number of people who cross a certain intersection during rush hour. I surely do not need their consent. Suppose, however, that I wish to monitor how often you enter and exit your house on a daily basis. I require no participation from you, and there seems to be no sacrifice and no risk. Unlike the street-crossing case, though, this looks rather suspicious. Can concerns for privacy here generate a requirement of consent?

A third sort of issue raised by the analysis concerns the question of possible exceptions. In the area of medicine and medical treatment, there are some cases in which the need for informed consent is overridden. In a life-or-death situation, when there is no time or ability to obtain consent, consent to medical treatment can often be assumed, in the absence of evidence to the contrary. In the case of those who cannot consent, a proxy's consent is sometimes considered adequate.

Such cases raise analogous questions about research. Are there cases in which researchers may continue with their work despite a lack of informed consent from their subjects? Is consent necessary in all forms of research, including social science research? Is it necessary in the developing world, for example, in drug trials aimed at finding cures for AIDS, or can the high stakes, or the alienness of a culture, justify trials where consent seems not fully possible? In the next several sections, I address such questions.

## CONSENTING TO RESEARCH

The ethics of clinical and scientific research is largely focused upon the researchers themselves. But the strong emphasis on informed consent raises a natural question, one that has been inadequately addressed: On what grounds should a subject decide to participate or decline to participate in such research? Are there norms to aid these subjects in their decisions? In this section I sketch an answer to these questions.

Consider first the case of those who are asked to participate in medical research; such research might, without their consent, be inimical to their right to privacy, or to their bodily integrity. It might bring with it the risk of injury or illness, or involve other inconveniences. What principles can guide those who are asked to participate when deciding whether or not to give their consent to medical research?

Among the major sources of guidance for a moral agent on such questions should be her previous commitments and obligations. Suppose the subject is considering participating in research which is highly risky. It seems irresponsible for the subject to agree if she has dependents counting on her, or other serious obligations to fulfill. Jesse Lazear was a microbiologist who allowed mosquitoes fresh from yellow fever infected bodies to bite him, to discover whether mosquitoes were the transmitter of the disease. Lazear, who died at the age of thirty-four leaving behind a wife and two children, is often presented as a hero for his participation. However, it seems at least questionable whether such behavior was responsible, given his previous obligations.

On the other hand, subjects already ill, and with little chance of recovery, might responsibly agree to participate in very hazardous trials. Or, as Grisez suggests, subjects with no other responsibilities might, as a work of mercy, agree to participate in some risky experiments (Grisez, 1993, p. 534). The principles guiding the decision flow from the same rationale that demands that the potential subject be the one to make the decision in the first place. But all this presupposes an important condition: the experimentation itself must promise great benefits to others. To risk one's life, even with no prior obligations, for little possible benefit to self or others is unreasonable.

Consideration of the subject's responsibilities here leads to a reconsideration of one of the basic principles of clinical research ethics apart from informed consent: that proposed experiments must offer a reasonable balance of risk to benefit. Both the Declaration of Helsinki and the *Belmont Report* are somewhat ambivalent about the distribution of risks and benefits. The Declaration, for example, states in regard to non-therapeutic biomedical research that the interest of science and society should "never take precedence over considerations related to the well-being of the subject" (Barnbaum and Byron, 2000, pp. 30–32).

But the *Belmont Report* holds that " . . . the risks and benefits affecting the immediate research subject will normally carry special weight. On the other hand, interests other than those of the subject may on some occasions be sufficient by themselves to justify the risks involved in the research, so long as those subjects' rights have been protected" (Barnbaum and Byron, 2000, p. 40).

I suggest that risks may reasonably be accepted by some agents in some circumstances even though the promised benefits will not accrue to the patient herself; subjects may permissibly consent on occasion to what will only be in the interest of science or society and not, or not foreseeably, in their own when this is consistent with, or even demanded by, their status in life, their previous commitments, and their personal vocation.

These considerations apply in other research contexts. Consider those asked to participate in sociological or anthropological investigations, by answering questions, or allowing observation of their lives. What sorts of concerns should be kept in mind by these potential subjects? Such research typically differs from medical research in that the promised benefits are less significant from a practical point of view. While anthropological knowledge might be of some long-range benefit, it is, more frequently than medical knowledge, knowledge that is being pursued for its own sake. When anthropologists enter the communities of the West African village, or the Amazon rain forests, those agents who are asked to cooperate with them in their research will not be able, typically, to justify their actions as works of mercy.

Still, if the risks are not too great, as often they are not, members of such communities may reasonably consent simply to foster the growth of knowledge. Even in the absence of external benefits, anthropological knowledge is a good, and contributes to human flourishing.

But subjects of such research, and the researchers themselves, should be sensitive to the way in which the information they disclose has a bearing on others. Much of the information that a subject could provide to a researcher will imply facts about others; it may thus, in some circumstances, constitute a violation of the privacy of other members of the tribe, village, or community (Wilkinson, 2004). Moreover, some types of observation, or too much observation, might be destructive for the subject of the types of goods privacy fosters. While much might be learned from twenty-four-hour videotaping, for example, of consenting subjects, this sort of continual scrutiny is likely to have deleterious effects on their domestic life. Spousal relations, even apart from sex, and other familial relations all require a degree of privacy. So subjects often should not consent to research that will be inappropriately invasive into their lives or the lives of others, nor should researchers pursue such knowledge. Further, those invited to be kept under close and continued observation should not do so if the primary purpose of the observation is the satisfaction of a prurient curiosity. This, however, applies less to genuine research than to the sort of "reality" TV show that seeks to gratify "inquiring minds" (on the vice of curiosity, see Chapter 12).

These considerations should be brought to bear by potential subjects of research who are considering whether or not to participate. There is no algorithm to provide to such subjects by which they could determine what to do, for each such decision requires attention to the particulars of the subjects' commitments and circumstances. They are morally serious choices nonetheless.

## PRIVACY AND CONSENT

Some inquiries involve neither risk nor sacrifice. Can we distinguish between morally acceptable and unacceptable forms here? Consider three cases. In the first, sociologists monitor a busy street crossing to study the habits of those crossing the street: How many look both ways before crossing? How many wait for the walk signal? How many cross only at the approved location? In the second, the same researchers study your house: How many times a day do you exit and return? How many people a day enter and exit your house? At what times is traffic in and out of your house heaviest? In the third case, a researcher, or her agent, pretends to be in need of medical assistance on a busy street. How many people will stop and offer to help? How many will not even look at the person in need?

Can such research legitimately continue without the informed consent of those under observation? Neither autonomy nor bodily integrity seems jeopardized. But privacy is critically at stake. This seems to be the case in many situations in which it is claimed that consent is not necessary because of the lack of risk involved; something about the agent is under scrutiny in these cases, and this inevitably raises the issue of privacy.

This is obvious where your house is under observation. You are entitled to a sphere within which you may plan, think, discuss, and collaborate in these activities with others, and in which you may carry out the acts that are mandated by your planning, thinking, and collaborating, because otherwise your reasonable hope for success in these activities is jeopardized. This space reasonably, and, apart from your body, paradigmatically, includes your home; thus, it is an unreasonable infringement on your right to privacy for a researcher to put you or your home under the sort of scrutiny described above. (Whether law enforcement officials can put your home under such scrutiny will be addressed later.)

As discussed in Chapter 2, however, your right to privacy is limited to a certain extent in public places. A busy street corner is one such place. Of course, not just anything may be legitimately observed or monitored in public—eavesdropping in public is still an invasion of privacy. But your public bodily movements seem to be a legitimate part of the public space, and may be monitored or observed, without your consent, as part of the pursuit of knowledge. Thus, many non-invasive and non-participatory observations may be performed in public areas for research purposes. This probably extends to the taking of photographs or videotapes.

Suppose, next, that Jones is the researcher, and Smith one of the passersby. Jones's interest in Smith is legitimate, and not invasive of Jones's privacy, if it is an interest in Smith precisely insofar as she is a passerby, and, presumably, one of many, and it is Jones's purpose to make a study of certain behavioral features of passersby. Jones's research takes account of Smith only insofar as Smith's public behavior puts her in a certain category with publicly identifiable criteria for membership, and those criteria are determined on the basis of some inquiry-related interest.

Suppose, however, that Jones's interest is only in, and precisely in Smith— it is Smith that Jones is studying, albeit only when Smith is in a public place. This does not seem acceptable—Smith is a person, entitled to her sphere of privacy, which cannot be entered without her consent; to make a study of a person seems definitely to enter that sphere. For Jones to follow Smith around taking pictures of her, or videotaping her, would be overstepping important boundaries.

This distinction is, I believe, part of what is behind concerns with allowing videotaping or photographing of persons in public places for research— a concern that the researcher's interest, or the interest of those viewing the tape or picture, will not stay bound to Smith under a public description. If Smith is beautiful, she will worry that pictures taken of her will arouse salacious interest; if she is handicapped, she will worry that they will arouse unwanted sympathies or revulsions. What is important is the guarantee that the interest be taken in Smith only under an impersonal and public description.

This is best understood as an aspect of the professional ethics of researchers involved in this form of inquiry; at all times, they must maintain their interest in the doings of the subjects of their research only as members of a publicly identified class (persons crossing this street at noon) and not as individuals (that good-looking woman), or members of some irrelevant class (good-looking women crossing the street). Moreover, they must ensure that any photos or videos be used only by legitimate researchers, and not sell or give them to others whose interest might be illegitimate.

This indicates the direction to take in discussing privacy and personal data, especially medical data. By collecting patient records, and using various types of data analysis, researchers can learn a considerable amount about epidemiological trends, or institutional procedures in the medical profession, or success rates in screening or treatment procedures for certain diseases, and so on (Cassell and Young, 2002). Some such knowledge is extremely important and socially beneficial, but its accumulation is accompanied by fears that gathering it involves an invasion of privacy. Moreover, there is considerable worry that the information gathered will be used in ways harmful to the patients themselves. Yet there is no need for patient involvement or awareness for investigators to acquire the knowledge; the subjects of the research are not being acted upon, although information about them is being obtained.

One kind of abuse in this area can be easily addressed, namely, the providing, or sale, of patient records for use, not by researchers, but by insurance companies and employers. This is a violation of privacy, and is morally impermissible. But the question of use of medical records for legitimate research purposes is less clear.

The previous discussion of public and private monitoring provides the key: insofar as the data gathered is wanted or needed with respect to the person or persons whose data it is, it is an invasion of privacy to gather it without obtaining consent. If the information is desired because it is information about Smith, or about Jones, then it is impermissible to get it without permission by Smith or Jones. But when there is an important need for the knowledge, and the knowledge can be gained, articulated, and disseminated without the cooperation of, or reference to, the individuals in question, then I believe the information can be considered part of the public realm, and can be gathered without consent. Procedural precautions are necessary to enforce such distinctions, but these seem in principle to be possible. However, if some of the most obvious procedural safeguards, such as anonymisation, would jeopardize the quality of scientific knowledge itself, then the demand for informed consent would stand.

What of the third case mentioned above? In that case, again, subjects are observed in public settings, but they are observed to see how they will respond to certain staged events. Muggings, for example, or physical collapses, are staged, to measure the degree of altruistic response when a stranger is seen to be in trouble (Piliavin and Piliavin, 1972).

Even apart from the issue of lying, such studies are problematic. One might think that the problem is again with privacy—the subjects' right to privacy extends to protect their reactions, thoughts and decisions, and forbids attempts to elicit these reactions without consent. This captures part of the problem, but the reference to the attempt to "elicit" a reaction indicates a more significant issue. For, unlike the busy street intersection case above, experimenters in the cases under discussion are not just observing public behavior in a public place, but are creating experimental conditions that are designed to induce reactions from those involved. The subjects are thus (covertly) induced to become participants in the study on the terms dictated by the researcher. Such studies are not, then, non-invasive as the intersection-observation case was; they constitute threats to autonomy of potential subjects in the same way that medical experimentation does. Subjects should therefore be given the choice of whether or not to participate in such studies, and informed consent should be first obtained.

In such experiments, obtaining informed consent will effectively render the experiment impossible; if you know you are being tested to determine your altruism quotient, you will probably behave altruistically, rather than meanly. But sometimes the cost of ethical behavior is a scientific slowdown.

## INFORMED CONSENT AND ALIEN CULTURES

The third set of problems involves difficulties related to special classes of research subjects. Children, for example, are incapable of giving consent; provided their parents or guardians are reasonably thought to be acting in their children's best interest, then proxy consents may be given. More radically, some wonder whether the same standards of informed consent should be applied to research subjects in developing or primitive cultures. The denial of the need for informed consent here can turn on either the nature of the research, or the nature of the subject, or a combination.

Consider first anthropological or sociological research and observation (I shall consider medical research in developing countries afterwards). Some would deny the need for informed consent here. When the Western anthropologist arrives in the native village, where few if any have ever seen Westerners, and none have the concept of informed consent at their disposal, why is it necessary for the researcher to obtain consent, and is it even possible?

The alternative approach is one that has been adopted on occasion by researchers in the social sciences; the researchers give some other reason for their presence, saying, for example, only that they wish to stay and live with the natives. It may later come as a shock to some when they discover that their "friend" was really working on a dissertation, but most will never know about it; what they don't know won't hurt them.

Let me begin with the question of capacity. Are those studied by cultural anthropologists or sociologists capable of giving informed consent to those who wish to study them and their ways? In some cases, including some in which consent was not sought, the answer is clearly affirmative. In a case in the Virginia tidewater region, sociologist Carolyn Ellis spent many years, as an undergraduate, graduate student, and assistant professor, visiting, befriending, and talking to members of a closed fishing community, the Guineamen, without informing them of her research purposes (Ellis, 1986; Allen, 1997).[3] It would be laughable to suggest that they were incapable of providing informed consent (or denying it); had any been diagnosed with cancer during that time, they would have been expected to give informed consent to any suggested procedures. More plausibly, they were not asked for permission because it was doubtful that they would give it. But this is hardly a good reason for failing to seek informed consent.

Cultural anthropologists sojourning in remote regions of the world, and among less developed or sophisticated peoples might argue that their cases are different. Primitive tribesmen have no concept of informed consent. Leaving aside the question of whether this might mean that anthropologists should therefore not engage in such research at all, there is reason to question the claim. It is true that primitive cultures cannot be expected to have a word or phrase that translates directly into our phrase "informed consent." But the question is whether they have the conceptual resources for understanding the notion in roughly the way that we do. I believe the answer to this must typically be affirmative.

To begin with, most, and probably all primitive peoples do indeed recognize the difference between actions consented to or agreed to, and actions not consented to or agreed to. Any society in which members are occasionally coerced, whether wrongly or rightly, into doing something, can make sense of the concept of consent.

That concept need not be limited in its application merely to cases of coercion; trickery is a frequent theme of the oral tradition of some primitive peoples—heroes and villains both trick others into doing what they want, in circumstances in which the dupe would not have agreed to do it (Hynes and Doty, 1997). From such resources can be developed the idea that agreeing to something requires understanding it, or knowing about it—in other words, the concept of informed consent can emerge. From this vantage point, the primitive people can no doubt see that even if the dupe said "yes," he did not agree in full awareness—did not give, in other words, informed consent.

Moreover, it requires a relatively small amount of sympathy on the part of members of the culture to recognize that the dupe often would object to being duped. So a sense of the value of informed consent can easily be part of, or emerge from, a primitive people's ordinary understandings and sensibilities.

This does not mean that that culture has anything like our culture's robust sense and appreciation of the *value* of informed consent. Some cultures might delight in trickery and think there is nothing wrong with hoodwinking others, or encouraging them to make decisions and participate in activities without really knowing what they are doing. Informed consent will not be valued by such a culture as it is by ours.

However, the repudiation of slavery might also be a value not shared by some other culture. This would not justify us in taking such people as slaves. On the contrary, we might have, with respect to such a culture, an obligation to educate them into the value of persons, and the evil of slavery. But even if we did not have such an obligation, we would hardly have moral permission to enslave such peoples, essentially taking advantage of their moral difference from us.

The basic goods view, and the understanding of human flourishing which that view posits as foundational for ethical thought, gives good grounds for thinking that the very same values that underwrite *our* conception of informed consent are of intrinsic importance for all peoples of *all* cultures, whether they recognize such values or not. It is true of primitive peoples, just as it is true of us, that autonomy is necessary for the pursuit of some goods, and significantly improves the chances of participating in others. Members of primitive peoples still have friends and personal projects, even when their lives are very tightly bound up with that of the tribe. Were we to find a primitive tribe in which one ruler made every single decision for all the tribe's members, we would not simply shrug this off as a cultural difference; we would consider it significant burden for the members.

Similarly, both privacy and bodily integrity are important goods for all persons, regardless of their cultural circumstances. Indeed, these values seem universally recognized, even though the scope of the recognition is often limited, and the demands of these values often violated. It would be surprising to discover even one culture in which marital relations were carried on entirely in public, or in which assault was not considered a grave crime. Since these goods, especially privacy, are implicated in almost all research on human subjects, they remain important considerations in this context too.

We thereby arrive at the following conclusion: social sciences research on alien peoples, cultures, and groups requires their informed consent. This might involve a considerable degree of explanation, as the researcher would need to make the potential subjects aware both of what he wished to do and of his need for their agreement to it. In some circumstances, it might also be necessary to explain why it was thought that the agreement was necessary, in order that the subjects might be better able to deliberate about whether or not to participate.

Occasionally, researchers will not obtain the consent they seek, either because it is denied, or because they are, in the end, unable to make themselves clear to the desired subjects. In such cases, unfortunately, the research may not be done, just as it could not be done in the West. Such a conclusion is unlikely to please members of the social sciences. Christopher Shea, summarizing much sentiment on the matter, writes that "human subject rules may be . . . less appropriate in sociology and anthropology, where research often involves hanging out and getting to know people. If a sociologist whips out a consent form . . . people might run—or laugh" (Shea, 2000, p. 31). It is true that the willingness of people to let others get to know them *can* be compromised by the discovery that the primary purpose of the acquaintance is knowledge, not friendship. But this is a justification for informed consent in these contexts, not a reason against it.

The discussion of informed consent among primitive cultures so far has concerned only research in the social sciences, research that neither offered much benefit beyond the (still quite important) good of knowledge for its own sake, nor threatened much in terms of risk. But in the area of medical research involving underprivileged subjects of developing countries, neither condition obtains in many cases.

The most pressing current example of this is research in Africa on experimental AIDS drugs and potential AIDS vaccines. The possible social benefits of such research are great; Africa has a high AIDS rate, with over a quarter of the population of some countries infected. Medical research into AIDS is required to rein in this disaster. On the other hand, the potential benefits to participants are typically much more tenuous, and there are considerable risks. Yet many worry that those who participate in AIDS drug trials in Africa have not given their fully informed consent.

One of the most famous examples of controversial AIDS research concerns experiments in Thailand and Africa designed to test whether a smaller dose of AZT than used in the West would be effective in slowing the transmission of AIDS from mother to newborn. In those experiments, mothers were given either the reduced doses of AZT or a placebo. In this, and in other AIDS-related experiments in Africa, there are often significant doubts about whether the research subjects were given information that they could understand and in such a manner and time frame that they could understand it. Among other difficulties, cultural considerations often lead to a situation in which it is assumed that the "doctor" is primarily attempting to help the patient; the assumption is then that any pill given is for the benefit of the patient. Evidence suggests that many of those who participate in such trials believe that they are being given medicine that will help them get better; they seem not to be fully aware that they are participating in a medical experiment, nor do they seem to be aware that some of them will receive only placebos (French, 1997; Moodley, 2002; Resnick, 2006).

The requirement of informed consent has roots in values such as autonomy, privacy, and bodily integrity that are of universal importance. But could the requirement of informed consent here be bypassed because of the emergency nature of the situation? I believe not. Such a position would run too close to consequentialism, and would justify far more than is desired. Moreover, I will argue in Chapter 4 that there are resources on which researchers may draw in encouraging potential research subjects to consent to risks for the sake of social benefits. It might thus turn out that the most ethical course will in fact result in research conditions close to those desired by Western scientists.

I conclude that informed consent is a legitimate requirement of all scientific research on human subjects, regardless of what part of the world, or what branch of the sciences it involves. The only exceptions involve cases in which the research essentially involves no more than monitoring persons in public places, with no attention to those persons as individuals, or gathering and analyzing data on groups, again, with no attention given to those persons as individuals. Informed consent thus rightly has its place among the foundations of the ethics of inquiry.

## THE ETHICS OF INVESTIGATION

The previous discussion focused on the role and justification of informed consent in the context of scientific research, whether in the social sciences or medical research. But these are not the only areas of inquiry in which concerns for autonomy, privacy, and bodily integrity can be raised. All three values may be jeopardized in the course of inquiry carried out by law enforcement officials, spies, or journalists. Does inquiry that threatens these values require, in these areas, something at least analogous to informed consent? If so, under what conditions and why?

There are, in fact, analogues to the requirement of informed consent in some of these fields—the Miranda rights, for example, seem to make something like informed consent a necessary condition for obtaining certain kinds of information from a suspect in a crime;[4] and journalists are, in a wide variety of cases expected to inform those whom they are questioning of the nature of their work.[5] On the other hand, police surveillance and the surveillance and investigation of possible terrorists by federal investigators have recently come under criticism for being carried out in an overly permissive environment. Journalists have often concealed their identities as journalists in ways similar to social scientists.[6] Finally, the use of force in the obtaining of information from suspected terrorists raises questions about threats to bodily integrity.

In this section, I will provide justification for some broad principles that are widely, though not universally, accepted regarding the ethics of investigation. One important goal is to uncover the reason for the apparently greater degree of flexibility that law enforcement agents have in their investigations than do scientific investigators. The former, it is widely acknowledged, can investigate in some circumstances covertly, can use a degree of force in uncovering information, and can investigate aspects of someone's private life, to a degree that is typically unacceptable for other investigators. At the same time, there are also limits to this flexibility, and I shall identify some of the reasons for these limits. In the next section, I shall argue that the reasons that underlie this greater flexibility do not bear on the issue of journalism at all; in consequence, the ethics of journalistic inquiry, as regards the autonomy, privacy, and bodily integrity of those from and about whom journalists attempt to obtain information, should be seen as very continuous with the ethics of medical and scientific research.

Before laying the groundwork for the discussion of police and intelligence investigation, a quick distinction is in order. In these sorts of investigations, there are often two parties other than the investigators whose interests are at stake—those in whom the investigators have a direct interest, such as the suspected criminal, and those from whom the investigator attempts to obtain information about the primary subject—friends, neighbors, business associates, and so forth. This is unlike the various forms of research discussed so far. In AIDS drug trials, although the subject of the research is of interest because of what she can "tell us" about other persons, she is nonetheless the primary subject of the research, rather than a witness or a source of testimony. But the difference between a subject of an investigation and a witness in an investigation is important. Police may not treat a criminal suspect's neighbor in the same way it is sometimes permissible to treat the suspect. It might sometimes be acceptable to spy on the criminal suspect, but it will not be acceptable to tap the neighbors' phones to obtain their testimony about him. Similarly, when a journalist asks a neighbor for information about her primary subject, the neighbor will need to consider the subject's privacy as a value to be respected, even if she herself does not mind answering the journalist's questions.

Let us call the area of ethics concerned especially with the inquiries of law enforcement agents, spies, and journalists the "ethics of investigation." Two foundational notions for understanding the ethics of investigation are the related notions of authority and responsibility for the common good. These two notions explain many of the ways in which police or intelligence investigators are freed from the restrictions of scientific researchers. The fact that journalists, while they undertake a responsibility to the common good, do not have the same sort of authority as do law enforcement authorities explains why the ethics of journalism should be considered closer in substance to the ethics of science than to the ethics of criminal investigation.

Every community has a set of needs precisely as a community, a common good that must be promoted and protected for the community and its members to flourish. But the decisions necessary to foster this common good require the existence of authority. Without such authority, there is a danger that decisions will not be made, and that resolution between competing conceptions of what should be done for the sake of the common good will not be resolved. Yet this authority too must be fair and impersonal, rather than arbitrary and tyrannical; hence the desirability of a *political* authority, an authority itself governed by law, a rule of law and not men.

Again, what is needed is political authority—some person or persons who, because they have been entrusted under the law with certain kinds of care for the community, also have authority to make and carry out decisions regarding that care (Aquinas, 1981, II-II, Q. 60, a.6; Finnis, 1998, pp. 245–52).

Such authorities are entrusted with various responsibilities, responsibilities that are correlative to the necessities of the community, and that cannot be provided for without that authority. The making and promulgating of new laws, collection of taxes, and mustering of defensive forces against attacks are all necessary for the survival of a community, but none can adequately or fairly be carried out without political authority. It follows from this that those with the requisite authority are enabled to do certain things that no one could legitimately do in a private capacity or in the absence of such authority.

This justification of political authority also brings with it certain restrictions on how it can be utilized; since fairness is part of the rationale for the creation of political authority, such authority cannot be utilized randomly, or to prosecute grudges or personal agendas. Thus authority makes laws while at the same time it must be subject to them. Moreover, there should be political safeguards to protect citizens against the lawless application of political power.

Among those purposes for which political power exists is the defense of the citizenry, not simply from external attack, but also from dangers that exist within the bounds of the state. In between law and punishment there must be the discovery and apprehension of those who break the law; this is an essential feature of the common good of any state. And thus the state becomes inextricably involved in the process of inquiry—police investigation is necessary to discover when the law has been broken, or if it is going to be broken, and, when it has been broken, who is responsible.

This chapter has detailed some of the restrictions that exist in regards to inquiry into the activities of people—restrictions having their justification in autonomy, privacy, and bodily integrity. But in some cases, certain of these restrictions may be lifted: when (a) such lifting is necessary for the public good, (b) these restrictions can be fairly lifted, and (c) the restrictions are not expressive of moral absolutes.

This last restriction has not yet been mentioned. If it is permissible for public authority to use a certain amount of force, or to take away certain rights, then the use of force must not itself be intrinsically illegitimate, nor the rights absolute or inalienable rights. No one can be sentenced to slavery, for example, for this would be to have an absolute right taken away. But autonomy rights and privacy rights are instrumental, and can rightly be considered contingent upon an agent's not misusing those rights for the sake of evil; and force and restraint may be applied without intending to harm; so force and restraint may sometimes be used by those with political authority. The crucial point is this: with regard to some of the restrictions on inquiry that have been advanced, the restrictions exist for agents precisely considered as private citizens; while with regard to others, the restrictions exist for agents considered as human beings.

It follows that for those with the appropriate authority, who are charged with protecting certain aspects of the common good, some invasions of autonomy and privacy, and some use of force, might be permitted in furthering their inquiries. At the same time, some restrictions remain, and certain procedural limitations must be observed on any lifted restrictions. So, on the one hand, in investigating a serious crime police may engage in inquiry without the suspect's permission, even when the inquiry goes to the heart of a protected area, such as the suspect's house; but, on the other, hand, in a well-regulated society, such inquiry cannot be carried out with regard to just anyone, in any circumstances, but requires a determination that there are good reasons for the search, and, under most circumstances, a judicial warrant granting the power to search. The Fourth Amendment of the United States Constitution specifies precisely this: "The right of the people to be secure in their persons, houses, papers, and effects, against unreasonable searches and seizures, shall not be violated, and no Warrants shall issue, but upon probable cause, supported by Oath or affirmation, and particularly describing the place to be searched, and the persons or things to be seized." Nevertheless, a search of a home or car that would be illegitimate if carried out by a private citizen can under some circumstances legitimately be carried out by an officer of the law.

Such procedural requirements cut to the heart of recent debate over provisions in the Patriot Act for warrantless searches and surveillance (including telephone and email communications), and the seizure of records. With regard to private records, for example, the Patriot Act gives broader powers to the government than it previously possessed. Dahlia Lithwick and Julia Turner summarize:

> Previously the government needed *at least* a warrant and probable cause to access private records. The Fourth Amendment, Title III of the Omnibus Crime Control and Safe Streets Act of 1968, and case law provided that if the state wished to search you, it needed to show probable cause that a crime had been committed and to obtain a warrant from a neutral judge. Under FISA—the 1978 act authorizing warrantless surveillance so long as the primary purpose was to obtain foreign intelligence information—that was somewhat eroded, but there remained judicial oversight. And under FISA, records could be sought only "for purposes of conducting foreign intelligence" and the target "linked to foreign espionage" and an "agent of a foreign power." Now the FBI needs only to certify to a FISA judge—(no need for evidence or probable cause) that the search protects against terrorism. The judge has no authority to reject this application. (Lithwick and Turner, 2003)

Similar provisions exist in the bill extending permissions for warrantless searches of homes and, in some cases, radical diminishment of the procedural requirements for certifying probable cause. By the guidelines outlined above, such provisions seem illegitimate: the very necessities, in terms of fairness, that generate the need for a public authority seem jeopardized in these cases.

On the other hand, some measures that are objected to on privacy grounds might be legitimate. Consider the dispute over encryption technology. Amitai Etzioni has argued that it is necessary for the government to have access to the code keys of deeply encrypted communications when those communications are implicated in terrorist or other criminal activities (Etzioni, 2000). At the same time, he points out, in response to objections, that this does not mean that the government should have arbitrary or complete access to the keys of all encoded messages. Rather, the ability to obtain the key and decrypt communications should be subject to the same sets of considerations that govern other legitimate investigative incursions into privacy, such as wiretaps and house searches, specifically, a warrant given in response to evidence.

Just as there may be legitimate limits to privacy rights against those in authority, so, within certain limits, may some of the restrictions regarding bodily integrity be lifted for those with certain kinds of public authority— police officers may forcibly restrain and apprehend suspects, even when they are not actively committing a crime. Such use of force might have as a side effect various harms to criminal suspects. When such harms are not intended, but are mere side effects of otherwise permissible uses of force, police officers may morally cause them. Those with information material to the case may be legally compelled to provide testimony, and incarcerated if they do not acquiesce.

Several points must be reiterated, however. First, these permissions are possible only because some agents have authority for pursuing the common good. Second, such authority is in part necessary in order that the common good be *fairly* promoted, and so the lifting of restrictions must be procedurally constrained. And third, there are limits to the extent to which these restrictions can be lifted, limits dictated by moral absolutes that cannot be violated by any agent.

## JOURNALISTIC INQUIRY

Journalists have often been tempted to think that inquiry-related restrictions in their field are more like restrictions on the police than like restrictions on scientists. Journalists have, on occasion, engaged in activities that would, if committed by anyone else, be considered an invasion of some other agent's privacy, obtaining, by subterfuge or stealth, access to non-public records, maintaining surveillance on a person's home and activities, and developing relations to sources who could provide "off the record" information—sometimes illegally (Bezanson, 2003; Lewis, 2003).

The justification offered for such activities is that journalists, like police officers, are engaged in an important work for the common good. Journalists play an important watchdog function for society; they point to the stories that would not have emerged but for their activities—the Watergate cover-up, abuses in various industries, the criminal records of political candidates, and so on. As Anita Allen puts it,

> A free press . . . fulfills societal obligations implied by the public's right to know. Journalists have assumed the professional responsibility of channeling news and information to the general public, which has grown reliant on their newspapers, radio stations, television stations, and computer services to provide information. Journalists seeking justification for privacy intrusions can turn to the right to know as a defense against almost any condemnation for invasion of privacy. (Allen, 2003, p. 75)

These points should be acknowledged, and the importance of journalism to the social good recognized; I will give a further account of the nature of this good in Chapter 10. However, there is a clear difference between journalists and police officers: the former have no more public authority than do scientists, who are also engaged in important work for the common good. One consequence of this is the frequent perception of unfairness in the ways journalists pursue the truth—they are not subject to the procedural safeguards that the police are, and thus their invasions of privacy often seem illegitimate. Journalists ultimately remain private citizens, and the ways in which they can infringe upon the privacy of others are normatively limited in much the same ways. Journalists should have no more rights to surreptitious recording of conversations than ordinary citizens, nor should they be able to search a man's home or possessions. Such "intrusions" are, in fact, considerably less protected by law than are "revelations," which are protected by the First Amendment. As Rodney Smolla writes, "The First Amendment provides no license to trespass, engage in fraud, or breach contracts" (Smolla, 2003, p. 91).

Moreover, it seems that something analogous to the notion of informed consent should apply to journalists' dealings with sources—sources should always be informed that the information is being sought by a journalist and given the opportunity to refrain from giving information. Nor should potential sources consider themselves immune from ethical considerations. In particular, the privacy of others remains an important value to be respected by those offering information to journalistic investigators.

Considerations similar to those relevant to the police govern what sorts of information journalists may seek, and what sorts of persons they may seek information about. Distinctions must be drawn between those objects of journalistic inquiry who are to be considered public figures, and those who are not, and those aspects of people's lives, whether those people are public figures or not, that should remain private and those that need not. These questions are a matter of journalistic ethics; even if journalists do not have more rights than other private citizens, it is still the case that their job involves in many cases the investigation of persons that few others would investigate. This involves a necessary incursion into the lives of others, when journalists report an untimely death, or a criminal prosecution, and so on. These are matters of public import, and it is good that there be a class of people whose profession it is to investigate. But the ethics of such investigations should make use of the distinctions above.

For example, some facts about the life of an agent are intrinsically public—facts about their birth and death, or about criminal convictions. Some facts bear on public matters, and are of public importance. They may rightly be reported by journalists, provided they are obtained in morally permissible ways. Other facts about some people's lives become matters of public importance because of some public role played by the agent in question. So, while it is no matter of public importance what the results of my latest physical were, it is reasonably thought of public importance to know what the results of the president's latest physical are.[7] But even public figures are entitled to private lives; not every fact is rightly pursuable and publishable, even if obtainable by legitimate means. This is an obvious implication of the earlier discussion of privacy: privacy is of great instrumental value in leading a flourishing life, and public officials do not sacrifice their claim to lead such a life on taking office. Since privacy is especially important in domestic and family matters, these areas should be specially respected by journalists.

This section has certainly not provided a definitive solution to all of the practical difficulties facing members of the police or journalism professions; some additional issues related to privacy and journalism will be addressed in Chapter 10. However, I hope to have shown that the core concepts for research ethics of autonomy, privacy, and bodily integrity, understood in light of the basic goods, also play a role in investigative ethics. The next chapter will return us to the discussion of research ethics in the biomedical setting, moving beyond the discussion of informed consent with its grounding in autonomy, privacy, and bodily integrity, in order to see what role fairness plays in scientific, and especially biomedical research. I will then address the issue of truth telling and lying in research and investigation. I shall argue that the fifth of the core concepts, personal integrity, generates an argument against all forms of lying in inquiry.

# 4  Fairness and Truth-Telling

I return in this chapter to scientific research performed on human subjects, in particular clinical research in biomedicine and related fields. My initial focus will be on the importance of fairness. I then turn to the issues of lying and deception. After providing a number of accounts of the wrongfulness of lying, all of which permit *some* lies, I argue that the real ground for the moral wrongness of lying is to be found in the value of personal integrity. This value grounds an *absolute* prohibition on lying. Such an absolute prohibition has significant consequences for the ethics of inquiry, in clinical research, but also in social science research, and police, military, and journalistic investigations.

## FAIRNESS

Given the role of informed consent in most research with human subjects, is there need, or even room, for any further ethical considerations? If an adequately informed agent is willing to participate in an experiment, why should that not suffice to justify continuation of the research? The answer is that what an agent may or may not consent to is a function of the options with which he is presented. But under some circumstances options may be presented that are unfair, and thus to which the agent has intrinsic reason to object, even if, under the circumstances, it makes sense for the agent to consent to one of the options.

Suppose that Smith is given the option of going behind enemy lines to take out an artillery gun at great personal risk, or refusing and suffering the consequences. Suppose further that the choice has been unfairly offered to Smith: he is given the high-risk choice, rather than Jones, who would have been more likely to succeed, because Jones is well-liked and is a relation to a high-ranking officer, who wishes to protect Jones from harm. Smith has reason to protest his options as unfair. Yet he also has good reason to consent to the mission, insofar as the good of his unit requires that the mission be performed. The unpalatable option can be reasonably chosen, even though it was not fairly offered.

The example demonstrates that it is necessary not just to respect the informed decisions of potential research subjects, but also to present them with options that are themselves reasonable. Many ethical guidelines for researchers, especially medical researchers, are of this nature: they do not wait on the subject's refusal to mark out some options as unacceptable, but rather front-load ethical concerns in an attempt to ensure that potential subjects are presented with reasonable options, or even that potential subjects are not singled out on the basis of unjust considerations (see the *Belmont Report,* p. 41 in Byron and Barnbaum).

Several overlapping guidelines are of interest here, which can all be given an explanation in terms of the core concept of fairness. One set of guidelines concerns the assessment of potential experiments in terms of both the benefit-to-risk ratio the distribution of benefits and risks. A second and related set concerns the selection of subjects. Another involves methodological constraints that overlap the areas of good ethics, and good science such as randomization, blindness, and equipoise. And a final set considers the obligation to care for the subjects of research. These norms are usually treated under a diverse group of headings. In the *Belmont Report,* for example, "Assessment of Risks and Benefits" is presented as a demand of the principle of beneficence, whereas subject selection is treated as a question of justice. Randomization, blindness, and equipoise are typically thought of as demands of good science; and the obligation to care for subjects flows from the nature of the doctor-patient relationship. I believe that there is a unifying explanation for all these "front-loaded" norms: they are all grounded in considerations of fairness that emerge from the dual nature of the community established between researcher and research subject.

Some writers have argued that tensions arise in research ethics from two conflicting demands. On the one hand, doctors and patients have a particular sort of relationship characterized by a focused concern on the part of the doctor for the well-being of the patient. This concern is supposed to be overriding of a wide variety of other considerations, such as financial reward; it is thus a concern that does occasionally conflict with other interests of doctors (Pellegrino and Thomasma, 1988).

The second concern is of the researcher qua researcher, whose goal is a systematic truth ("generalizable knowledge") about the subject matter at hand. From this perspective, patient-subjects are a means to the end of socially important knowledge. Tension arises from seeing the agent qua doctor as engaged in a kind of cooperative relationship with the patient, while the agent qua researcher is engaged in utilitarian relationship with the subject. Moral concerns are natural to the agent from the first point of view, but not the second (Hellman and Hellman, 1991; Miller and Brody, 2003).

But this misdescribes the relationship that exists between researcher and subject, whether or not they are also in a doctor-patient relationship. For researchers and their human subjects, unlike researchers and their animal or sub-animal subjects, are themselves in a kind of community, namely, a community of inquiry. The division of labor is certainly extreme, but researcher and subject are engaged in a cooperative pursuit of scientific knowledge and thus constitute a community, together with the variety of other researchers and research subjects working on the same or related problems.[1]

If the researcher is also medically responsible for the subject as a patient, then the community is twofold: it is a community of inquiry and a doctor-patient community. But recognizing the relationship as a *community* of inquiry means that we should not divorce the scientific relationship from all relationships of fair care, *even* when the relationship is not also a medical relationship. This is a consequence of the relationship between fairness and the nature of any community.

In Chapter 2, I argued that fairness is both a positive relationship of benefit and constitutive of a community. Likewise, consider the following description by John Rawls of political community:

> Citizens are reasonable when, viewing one another as free and equal in a system of social co-operation over generations, they are prepared to offer one another fair terms of social co-operation (defined by principles and ideals) and they agree to act on those terms, even at the cost of their own interests in particular situations, provided that others accept those terms. For these terms to be fair terms, citizens offering them must reasonably think that those citizens to whom such terms are offered might also reasonably accept them. (Rawls, 1996, p. xliv)

The existence of a community, as opposed to a relationship of dominance, or mere coordination, depends upon the willingness of participants mutually to offer and accept fair terms; it is this willingness, in fact, that signals the openness to community. Likewise, damage to those fair terms would inevitably result in treating some better than others, the dominance of some by others, and the like.

What Rawls says here in regard to political community seems true of any cooperative engagement of agents, any attempt to establish a relationship of community. But this shows also that fairness is not a matter of merely avoiding certain kinds of behavior. A community is structured by pursuit of some common good, and if the terms of the pursuit of that good are fair, then they will require work by each on behalf of others in service of that common good. A mutual pact to stay out of each other's way is insufficient to form a community, but an engagement to work together will be unfair if each does not offer fairly of himself on behalf of others. Someone who works only for himself, even if he does not obstruct others, or take from them, has hardly offered fair terms of cooperation.

The medical relationship has in part been seen in light of such considerations, despite the obvious imbalance of power and capacity between doctor and patient. Doctors often think of themselves as being not in a primarily contractual relationship—although they are also in this—but as being in a covenantal relationship with their patient (May, 2000). The doctor makes an offer of time, resources, and care to the patient. Of course, some compensation is required for the well-being of the doctor. But doctors who are in medicine exclusively for the money are thought to be corrupt. Doctors and patients share a common good—the patient's physical health, and, it is to be hoped, offer each other fair terms of cooperation in pursuit of that good.

Breach of these fair terms could occur, however, in such a way that the patient would still consent to some procedure. If a doctor refuses to provide aid except at an extortionate rate, the patient will no doubt consent to the best of grim options. Concern for fairness, and for the establishment of a just and cooperative community among persons equal in dignity, thus generates up-front norms about initial grounds of the community.

We should similarly see the invitation offered by researchers to potential research subjects to participate in research as an invitation to enter into a kind of community, here, a community of inquiry. This community might overlap with an already established medical relationship, and also with membership in a political community. But the researcher qua researcher should not view herself, any more than should the doctor, as an agent making use of a research subject in service of a unilaterally pursued good. Rather, she should think of herself as offering fair terms of cooperation in a common project—the pursuit of important scientific knowledge.

Such fair terms are not offered by those who offer to run risky experiments on others for trivialities, or for dimly conceived, or unlikely benefits. However, it need not be the case that the benefits sought are exclusively, dominantly, or even expectedly, for the research subject. Potential research subjects may see themselves as offering a contribution to pursuit of a cure for a disease that will inevitably kill them. This willingness becomes more intelligible when we view the relationship as a community of inquiry established on fair terms of cooperation, for some of those fair terms might include the promise to provide aid, when possible, to other members of what we could call the ground community of the subject.

Many of the various restrictions currently accepted as guiding research on human subjects can be seen in these terms. They comprise a kind of package of terms that together may be fairly accepted. But variations on the standard package may also be fairly offered and accepted in certain cases.

Consider those methodological considerations that overlap the boundaries of ethics and science: the demand for randomized and blind trials, and for equipoise. From the point of view both of the researcher and of the subject, these may typically be seen as fair terms of cooperation in a scientific venture. By creating a context in which sound research may be done, researchers and research subjects are assured within reason that their time is not being wasted; subjects are assured that they are given a fair shot within a trial of benefit, and a fair shot at avoiding harm, while researchers are assured of a superior methodological approach. Of course, the information that the research will be randomized and blind, or that the subject may be given a placebo, must be made available to the subject prior to consent. But this seems like a reasonable option, rather than an unreasonable option that it is reasonable to choose.

Elizabeth Wager and her collaborators express similar considerations in their discussion of the terms that should be offered to prospective subjects:

> Explaining the concepts of randomization . . . is not easy . . . Randomization may sound less threatening if you explain that it ensures the hoped for benefits and unknown risks are spread fairly between groups of patients. You might also explain how randomization reduces bias. For example, in an unrandomized study comparing a new drug with an established treatment, patients who had not responded to available treatments might be more likely to choose the new drug, causing this group to include more cases of treatment resistant disease. Most patients can appreciate the need for double blind procedures if you explain that results could be affected by either patients' or the doctors' expectations. (Wager et al., 2000, p. 109)

Such considerations might still seem to favor the researcher rather more than the research subject, although, as mentioned, it is in the interests of the subject that good science be performed, lest the endeavor be a waste of time. After all, the researcher is more or less guaranteed to get what she wishes: knowledge of some sort or other. But other considerations common in Western science attempt to balance this concern.

For example, the radical separation of burdens from benefits that characterized the Tuskegee experiments is now recognized to be morally unacceptable, as is the choice of research subjects who might easily feel coerced into participating, as with prisoners. Moreover, compensating consideration has been given to the well-being of the research subject when he or she is ill or dying. The invitation to participate in medical research typically brings with it a commitment to provide care to the subject in a variety of ways—medical care, for example, in respect to other ailments, and palliative care. As well, researchers are expected to step in if it is clear that there is a superior course of treatment to the one being taken, or if the treatment is causing harm. The research subject, in other words, is guaranteed care in the course of the experimentation, even at some risk to the outcome of the experiment itself.[2]

If these commitments are indeed part of the fair terms of cooperation offered by the medical or other researcher to her subject, then the degree of tension that *does* exist when the medical researcher is also the patient's doctor could perhaps be mitigated somewhat; for now in both relationships the doctor-researcher should think of herself as engaged in a community, and committed to fairness and to care for another. On the other hand, the research subject also need not be in an antagonistically self-centered relationship to the researcher, but may make a commitment to the common good of scientific knowledge, understanding that some sacrifices could reasonably be accepted to this end.

This model is normative, not descriptive of what historically has been the case. Large numbers of researchers have been insufficiently concerned to provide adequate information, adequate time for a decision, or adequate sympathy for their subjects' conditions, nor have subjects seen themselves as voluntarily entering into a community of inquiry. Sandra L. Titus and Moira A. Keane, commenting on their study of researcher attitudes and actions in obtaining consent write, "The researchers did not appear to extend an invitation to participate to their potential subjects, as if researchers thought that the subjects would already know that the researcher was extending an invitation. Yet, to the subjects, the professional was likely to appear commanding and demanding of participation" (Titus and Keane, 2000, p. 123). It seems overly charitable to suggest that researchers thought that subjects must "already know" that they were extending an invitation. Rather, the notion of extending an invitation on fair terms to cooperate as free and equal subjects, albeit with a radical division of labor, in a community of inquiry seems to have insufficiently taken root in the minds and hearts of researchers.

If this is the case in the West, the problem is greatly exacerbated in the developing world. In Chapter 3, I discussed the AZT trials performed in Thailand and Africa, from the standpoint of the need for informed consent. Evidence exists, in these and other trials in Africa and Asia, that many subjects have not given what would count as informed consent in a meaningful sense. But there are other difficulties as well.

In the AZT trials, subjects were divided into two groups, one receiving a dosage of AZT lower than that typically used in the United States, the other receiving a placebo. Such a trial could not have been performed in the United States where it was already known that the full dose of AZT works in preventing vertical transmission of the HIV virus, whereas its absence does nothing. But in Africa, the standard of care for HIV mothers did not include provision of AZT. So researchers were able to argue that they were meeting the local standard of care, and not leaving anyone worse off than they would otherwise have been. Against this, some have argued that the relevant standard of care is not relative to the area in which the experiment is performed, but is, rather, absolute: the best care provided anywhere (Wolf and Lurie, 1997; Angell, 1997).

In another study, discussed in the *New England Journal of Medicine*, "several hundred people with HIV infection were observed but not treated," to determine "whether sexually transmitted diseases such as syphilis and gonorrhea increase the risk of HIV infection" (Angell, 2000, p. 967). This involved giving antibiotics to some participants to reduce the prevalence of non-HIV sexually transmitted diseases (STDs), and asking participants questions about their sexual history. As Marcia Angell, who has been critical of Western scientists' treatment of research subjects in the developing world, writes, "Such studies could not have been performed in the United States, where it would be expected that patients with HIV and other sexually transmitted diseases would be treated. In addition, in most states it would be expected that caregivers would see that sero-negative partners were informed of their special risk" (Angell, 2000, p. 968).

Angell argues that the discrepancy between approaches comes from two different perspectives the researcher can take on her subjects. She can see them as individuals, for whom she has a professional responsibility, or she can see them in the context of the population to which they belong. Seen in the former light, researchers will "assume broad responsibility for the welfare of the subjects they enroll in their studies—a responsibility analogous to that of clinicians" (Angell, 2000, p. 968). Seen in the latter light, subjects will be considered to be no worse off than they otherwise would have been; thus, certain standards necessary to ethical research in the United States, such as the requirement to care for the subjects of one's research, will seem unnecessary.

But this second approach, on which research subjects are seen merely as members of a "population," is deeply at odds with the notion of an invitation to participate in a community of inquiry, and is, ultimately, unfair. To see this, we might compare the situation of HIV-infected mothers, or other HIV patients seeking experimental treatment, or high-risk subjects seeking an experimental vaccine, to our hypothetical soldier earlier, who was offered the choice to go behind enemy lines or not, or our suffering patient who was offered a cure by her doctor on extortionate terms. In each case, the subject has reason to consent, given the circumstances in which he or she finds him or herself. The problem is that the circumstances themselves, which are part of the offer made by the commanding officer or doctor, are themselves unfair.

In order to make an assessment, we need to look at the overall situation, and ask whether, as terms offered for a *cooperative* endeavor, they are fair or not. In the second study criticized by Angell, involving monitoring of HIV patients with and without other STDs, researchers cannot be thought to have offered fair terms of cooperation for a community. In particular, keeping members of a community in ignorance about their conditions is deeply unfair; as is the consequent putting at risk of all those with whom the subjects might subsequently have sexual intercourse. It is important to see that this research was not relevantly similar to the forms of impersonal and public research described in the previous chapter, namely, population research based on public data or public observation. Researchers were actively involved with their subjects, and thereby implicitly undertook obligations to those subjects, obligations that seem not to have been met in this case.

Does the preceding analysis support Angell's criticism of the AZT trials in Asia and Africa? To answer this question, let us first ask more broadly: must the "standard of care" practiced in the West be the automatic starting point for all research done in developing countries? No; there will be circumstances in which it genuinely would be difficult for researchers to provide that care. But it must be the case that in such circumstances, the researchers make clear the reasons for this to potential research subjects and give them good reasons why it would still be reasonable for them to enter the experiments. One such reason would be that the experiments promised significant benefits that would then be made widely available among the subject's own people, their "ground community."

One must leave open the possibility that subjects in developing countries will, in their circumstances, freely accept an invitation to join certain studies that others in the developed world would not consent to, and that the initial conditions of the offer might still be fair. Several thinkers, in discussing various aspects of South African traditional worldviews, for example, have drawn attention to the concept of *ubuntu*, a concept with parallels in other parts of AIDS-suffering Africa (Tutu, 2000; Moodley, 2002).

The concept of *ubuntu* is strongly communitarian, indicating that persons are and become persons through other persons. The life and personality of each member of a traditional tribe is thus bound up with the lives of other tribal members, resulting in a strong sense of communal responsibility. This may be seen in a small way in the tendency of members of many African societies to refer to one another by familial names—brother, sister, mother, father—even when there is no blood relation.

Given the importance of this traditional notion, and the significance of the AIDS threat in Africa, there is reason to think that potential subjects could accept as initially fair the terms of some studies in which it is genuinely impossible to offer a higher standard of care, even though that higher standard is currently met elsewhere. Nonetheless, the burden will be on researchers to show that such a standard genuinely cannot be met here, and that a real commitment exists to the future well-being of those in the developing world. "Fairness" in such a context, the fairness of "fair terms of cooperation," will be understood somewhat differently by the relevant subjects in developing and AIDS-plagued countries, for the benefits offered in the cooperation will be more communally distributed than in the West. But this difference in understanding is legitimate; it involves no exploitation if researchers enter into a community of inquiry with research subjects holding this conception, provided they do so in good faith, intending to honor the promised conditions even after the subjects themselves have died.

What this analysis leaves out, however, when it comes to the particular AZT trials in question, is the role to be played by the infants in the trial. In the case in question, mothers were not just deciding for themselves, but for their children. The risks accepted by mothers did not, therefore, extend merely to themselves, but to their infants, some of whom would not be protected from AIDS. Of course, what mother would not see this as a providing a chance at medicine for her child, and accept? The question is, again, was it fair for researchers to offer mothers *that* choice?

In this particular case, I am not convinced that the offer was fair. I have argued that subjects may accept risks for themselves for the sake of benefits for others in their community, and that under some circumstances, research-ers may legitimately, that is, fairly, ask for subject participation in such stud-ies. In hopes of a cure for the next generation, the present generation may reasonably consent to risks without much hope of personal benefit. But mothers could not accept risks to their children for the sake of benefits to future generations. Such a choice violates the responsibilities of parents to their children. Mothers who accepted the risk to their children of receiving nothing did so only in hopes that those children would in fact be the ones to get the real medicine (assuming full knowledge of what was going on). The situation was, therefore, not one of a fair community of research, but a state of at least implicit competition; any given mother who fully understood the situation would need to hope that her child would receive the benefits at the expense of some other child. The researchers who offered, therefore, to establish a community of inquiry on such terms were certainly not offering fair terms of cooperation. Those experiments, despite their social benefits were unethical.

## LYING

I turn now to the morality of lying in inquiry. The use of lies and deception in medical research was once more prominent than it is now; the emphasis on informed consent has had a significant impact of the extent to which deception is thought permissible. There is evidence to suggest that lies and deception in the social sciences are still somewhat common; in Chapter 3, I gave some examples of deceptive social scientific research. To the extent that informed consent takes hold as a deep principle of social scientific research, a similar progression can be expected.[3] But lies in investigative forms of inquiry such as police work and journalism seem quite common.

## FOUR APPROACHES TO LYING

Four paradigms govern most philosophic consideration of lying and truth telling. They are, from least restrictive to most restrictive, the consequential-ist approach, the autonomy approach, the communication approach, and the integrity approach. The first two approaches are prominent in the justi-fication of lies in non-scientific inquiry, but, I shall argue, it is the integrity approach that should give us the last word on the matter (Finnis, 1998, pp. 154–63; Boyle, 1999).

The consequentialist approach is familiar: it states that the criterion for determining whether an agent should tell the truth or lie is whether either will contribute to the greatest good. Thus, when by telling a lie, a police officer can find out whether a suspect has committed the crime or not, and the discovery will promote the greatest good, the officer should lie. Similarly, journalists will be permitted to lie in pursuit of information of public importance, particularly if the information will be unobtainable in any other way.

The negative consequences of lies must also be weighed in the balance. These are chiefly judged by consequentialists to be ruptures in the fabric of society—if trust is eroded through lies, society will be less stable, less able to rely on contracts, and so on. Henry Sidgwick sums up the general consequentialist approach: "But if the lawfulness of benevolent deception in any case be admitted, I do not see how we can decide when and how far it is admissible, except by considerations of expediency; that is, by weighing the gain of any particular deception against the imperilment of mutual confidence involved in all violations of truth" (Sidgwick, 1907, p. 316).

We need here to make a distinction. The ethics of truth telling concerns at least the following two different sorts of consideration, viz., the question of whether and when lying is permissible; and the question of whether and what truth to disclose. The two sorts of concerns are not identical: if it is morally impermissible to lie, this will not in every case mean that one is required to volunteer the truth. One may remain silent, or indicate one's refusal to give certain information. So, while the consequentialist justification for lying may fail, it may still be the case in some circumstances that one does not have a positive duty to tell the truth, and this might be related to the negative consequences of volunteering the information.

I have already argued that consequentialism is deeply flawed as a moral theory. Among other things, it denies the existence of rights, including the rights of those to whom we lie. So consequentialist justifications of lying generally fail. However, although the ethics outlined in the earlier parts of this book is non-consequentialist, this does not mean that a consideration of the consequences should never have any bearing on our decisions. So, absent other considerations, it might sometimes be permissible to lie for fear of the consequences, and sometimes permissible to refrain from offering the truth for similar reasons. The final word on these matters must wait: identifying the other three paradigms for the understanding of the ethics of truth telling can help us to see what sorts of considerations consequentialism overlooks in this area.

The second paradigm revolves around the notion of respect for persons, and in particular, respect for their autonomy. If my doctor lies to me, he reduces my autonomy, for I am no longer in a position where I can decide based on all the facts how I should proceed in my treatment. As Alan Donagan puts it, "In duping another by lying to him, you deprive him of the opportunity of exercising his judgment on the best evidence available to him" (Donagan, 1977a, p. 89). In light of the necessity of information for consent, this paradigm for the understanding of the ethics of truth telling is promising. It is more restrictive than consequentialism, and its restrictions track a significant aspect of why we think lies are wrong.

The autonomy approach does allow leeway in a number of circumstances. First, since agents may sometimes relinquish some degree or other of their autonomy, agents might voluntarily relinquish their right not to be lied to. So, one might argue that because the state's duty to pursue the common good requires the relinquishment of various forms of autonomy, citizens implicitly give up their right to have no lies told to them by agents of the state.

Second, since agents can forfeit in various ways their right to autonomy, agents might in these ways also forfeit their rights not to be lied to. Consider those who are aggressing against others, intending, perhaps, to kill an innocent person. Since such an agent forfeits his right to not be physically restrained, perhaps he also forfeits his right to not be lied to. Lying to the SS member who comes to your house seeking Jews is permissible on an autonomist approach to lying. Similar sorts of considerations govern the dispensing of truth.[4]

As with consequentialism, it might be that even if a stronger case can be made against lying, still, autonomy considerations might play a role in the ethics of truth telling. It might be wrong for agents of the state to lie to you in pursuit of their ends, even in pursuing the ends of (e.g., criminal) inquiry. But while an aggressing agent might not, for reasons given below, forfeit his right not to be lied to, he might certainly forfeit his right to be told, positively, the truth. Surely one ought not to tell the SS agent where the Jews are hiding, nor has he any right to that truth, even if one is also morally prohibited from lying about it.

The autonomist conception has roots in Kantian considerations. So does the third paradigm, which draws our attention to the communicative function of language, and the order of communication that is established between all rational agents in virtue of a common language. This order, it is suggested, is ruptured by lies. Alasdair MacIntyre quotes Mary Geach: "'A lie is a cheating move in the language game of truth-telling'" and goes on to describe the position in more detail: "To tell a lie is wrong as such, just because it is a flouting of truth, and it is an offense primarily not against those particular others to whom the particular lie has been told, but against human rationality, everyone's rationality, including the liar's own rationality" (MacIntyre, 1995, p. 315).

On this paradigm, the ethics of lying is quite strict, since seemingly any lie ruptures the communicative order of language. Kant believed the restriction to be absolute. However, if this is the primary objection to lying, then there will be instances in which some form of non-truth telling will be permitted, not because of an exception as such, but because it will be possible to lie without intending the rupture, or the violation of truth, but only for the sake of some good, such as saving an innocent person's life. For why should one take oneself to be violating that order, which seems ultimately to be an order of justice, rather than accepting a certain amount of damage to it as a side effect of one's life-saving activity? MacIntyre, for example, asks why it should be impermissible to lie to save a Jew's life, but permissible to shoot an assailant.

On the fourth paradigm, lying is universally prohibited; the essential justification for the prohibition lies in the inevitable damage to an agent's integrity. It should be pointed out that this paradigm is entirely consistent with the third, and is often expressed with the third, e.g., by Aquinas. But on this paradigm, a lie always divides one's inner self from one's outer self by communicating (externally) something at odds with what one (internally) takes to be the case. This is essential to the nature of a lie; thus all lies inevitably violate the basic good of integrity or authenticity, in a way that they might not inevitably violate the order of justice in communication.[5]

Both the third and the fourth paradigms continue, however, to draw a distinction between lying and truth telling, and both can hold that in certain circumstances it will be wrong positively to offer the truth, whether because of the gravity of the consequences, or because the speaker's hearers are not entitled to the truth on some matter. So aspects of the consequentialist and autonomist paradigms may be incorporated into the third and fourth views.

One might object that nothing really has been shown to be wrong with the autonomist view, which did, after all, return more permissive verdicts on lying than the integrity view. In an important sense, this is true: the autonomist view does explain part of what is wrong with many lies. The problem is that those lies also involve damage to an agent's integrity, and that aspect of a lie's wrongness continues to be present even in lies that do not violate another agent's autonomy. If we recognize that the liar who violates another's autonomy also violates his own integrity, and further recognize that this gives an undefeated reason for that agent not to lie, then it is difficult to see how any lie could be justified without recourse to straightforwardly consequentialist considerations. But since consequentialism is a failure as a moral theory, such considerations cannot be brought in here. Thus the prohibition on lying is absolute, without exception, as a considerable part of the Western moral tradition has held.

## LYING IN INQUIRY

In addressing the question of lying in inquiry, it makes sense to look first at lies in the context of medical and scientific research, then at lies in the pursuit of other forms of inquiry. There are two reasons for this. First, the discussion of lying in medicine and science overlaps much of the discussion of informed consent. The need for informed consent rules out much lying. Second, I will return to the issue of lying in the sciences and other academic areas later in this book in the discussion of the internal, truth-centered ethics of inquiry. There I shall argue that in addition to any general norms that lying in inquiry might involve, lying among medical researchers, scientists, and academics constitutes a significant breach of the internal ethics of those disciplines.

Here, it is enough to point out that lying is uncommon neither in the pursuit of knowledge, nor in the dissemination of knowledge or pseudo-knowledge.

To give examples of the first: the famous experiments of Milgram on subjects who believed they were giving electric shocks to agents who failed correctly to answer test questions involved lies to the subjects (Milgram, 1974). Patients were lied to in the Tuskegee experiments (Jones, 1993). Subjects of anthropological and sociological studies have been lied to about the identities and occupations of the researchers. Scenarios have been staged by social scientists in public to test the reactions of passersby. And the use of deception in sociological and psychological experiments on human subjects in a laboratory setting appears to be not uncommon, and is permitted, if certain conditions are met, by the American Psychological Association, and the American Sociological Association (Baumrind, 1985; S. Bok, 1989; Clarke, 1999).

In the dissemination of knowledge and pseudo-knowledge, scientists and other scholars have been accused of plagiarism from others, of suppressing the contributions of graduate students and assistants, of spinning or ignoring data, and, in the most extreme cases, of making up results and putting them forth to the scientific community as knowledge. The case of Hwang Woo-Suk, the Baltimore affair, plagiarism by historians, and the Bellisiles case, in recent years, seem prominent instances.[6]

All such forms of deception are obviously impermissible. The question seems more difficult, however, where non-scientific inquiry is concerned. First, much inquiry in these areas has a largely instrumental character. Although scientific research brings with it many resultant benefits, scientists are often committed to pursuing the truth about nature for its own sake, as well as for its benefits. But police, espionage workers, and journalists all pursue information and knowledge primarily for the sake of the benefits of such knowledge. Moreover, as we have seen, those agents who work for the state are immune from some considerations that govern private citizens as regards the obtaining of information. So it might seem that lying for the sake of achieving important social ends, such as the protection of the state from terrorists, or the capture of criminals, would be similarly excused.

Further, these forms of inquiry really are, in ways that do not always extend to scientific inquiry, furthered by lying. Part of this is because these forms of inquiry deal so extensively with human beings, rather than impersonal nature. Human beings more willingly part with information to those they like, or trust, or believe to share the same goals and ideals; so spies, for example, typically insinuate themselves into the lives of others by feigning these sorts of sympathies. On the other hand, people also respond to threats and warnings; so the police will threaten actions that they know they are not entitled to perform in attempts to frighten suspects or others into providing needed information. And, of course, people will not provide information to those they believe are collecting it to use against them; so spies, police, and journalists all have lied, in varying degrees, about their own identity.

Consider the practice, common to both the police and the profession of journalism, of going "undercover." Journalists for TV shows pose as customers, or as job applicants, to gain inside information on a company's suspect practices.[7] Police pose as drug dealers, or criminals to get inside criminal organizations.[8] These activities involve extensive patterns of deceit.

This leads to further reasons why there will be more resistance to ethical criticisms in these areas. For one thing, those investigated are typically suspected of having already violated the public trust—so perhaps they are not entitled to the truth anymore. For another, these forms of investigation have become deeply entrenched parts of our culture, to the extent that we naturally tend to overlook the ways in which they involve lying. For example, traditional Catholic doctrine restricts most, if not all, lies (*Catechism of the Catholic Church*, 2003), and Augustine condemned lying to infiltrate oneself into a heretical sect. Yet there seems to be no real Catholic opposition to undercover police work or espionage; and there are devout Catholics in both the FBI and the CIA. Such professions are in an uneasy tension with the Augustinian tradition, yet the tension generally goes unrecognized.

Moreover, lying seems to be an established part of the cultures of work and personal life in our society; we readily accept, for example, that people lie at work, to their bosses or their subordinates. Students who cheat on exams say that they are simply imitating what they see from other parts of society. If so, it should come as less of a surprise that lying is tolerated and even expected in those forms of work that involve criminal investigation, or are in the service of other aspects of the public good (MacIntyre, 1995, pp. 319–22).

Nonetheless, there are good reasons to think that all such lying is morally impermissible, not only for private citizens, but for all moral agents. The integrity of a public officer is not protected by his status when he lies: inevitably the liar intends to accomplish his purposes precisely by issuing a public communication at odds with what he genuinely believes to be the case. So the liar always erodes his own integrity, even though only as a means. Moreover, the second and third paradigms are also of importance here. To lie to suspected criminals does seem to offend against the public order of communication—in fact, to lie to wrongdoers or suspected wrongdoers seems to re-create the playing field on their terms, rather than on upright terms. Lying to wrongdoers is a way of giving in to them.

Finally, while it is true that in some cases those who are spied on are already known to be planning, or have planned, significant acts of violence against others, still, lies are used by journalists and police investigators to obtain information from many who are only suspected of wrongdoing, and to obtain information about those suspects from others who are not even suspected (Levy, 2002). It is self-serving to claim that such suspects have forfeited their rights to honest communication prior to the determination of whether they really are guilty. Much lying by police and journalists should therefore be considered impermissible even on the autonomist paradigm.

The consequences of such a view are, however, extreme. On my view, all undercover work is morally impermissible, whether carried out by police, journalists, or spies. Much espionage, in fact, at least as it has traditionally been carried out, involves lying, or inducing others, such as informants, to lie to obtain the trust of others. But not all aspects of espionage involve lying. The various uses of technology to listen in on conversations, to intercept electronic communications, or to take pictures from high in the air seem, assuming procedural safeguards for the sake of privacy, to be permissible, as do some forms of "open source" espionage. Given the arguments of this chapter, these approaches are precisely where the future of espionage and police investigative work should lie.

The past two chapters have ranged broadly over a variety of contexts of inquiry, and an equal variety of moral difficulties. It is time now to narrow our focus somewhat, to address in more detail some of the most pressing issues of biomedical inquiry and investigative activity of our time. These are, first, the ethics of human embryo experimentation; second, the issue of animal experimentation; third, the use of torture; and fourth, research into human enhancement possibilities. In the next three chapters, I show that the basic goods approach can shed light on all these issues.

# 5 The Ethics of Human Embryo Research

There is no more disputed area of the ethics of biomedical research than that regarding the creation, use, and destruction of human embryos. Many scientists and others are convinced that the key to curing a variety of serious diseases lies within such embryos, both from the knowledge to be gained from their study, and from the therapies to be developed using embryonic stem cells. On the other hand, try though some may, it has been impossible to separate the ethics (and politics) of stem cell research and other research involving human embryos, such as cloning research, from the nation's larger debates about abortion and respect for human life.

Successful resolution of the ethical issues regarding human embryonic research will not settle all the normative questions in these areas, for some argue that moral considerations should play no role in the politics of these matters. In Chapters 8 and 9, I shall return to these and other matters to settle the question of whether the ethical positions I defend in this chapter form the proper basis for political objections or permissions.

## WHAT IS THE HUMAN EMBRYO?[1]

What is the human embryo, and what respect is it due? These questions are related to the following: what are you and I, and why are we deserving of moral respect? The commonsense and philosophical answers to these questions often overlap: we deserve respect because we are persons, beings who can think, will, and act rationally. In terms of the ethical framework outlined in this book, we may say that because we are such beings, we may participate in basic goods, and that such goods must, in us, be respected, as opportunities for us to flourish. Thus, the notion of "respect for human persons," which some philosophers claim to find elusive or opaque, is to be understood in terms of the requirement on agents to act for the sake of ideal integral human fulfillment.

Linking the requirement of respect to our nature as persons, however, creates difficulties for thinking about both our nature, and the nature of early human embryos, as well as comatose, seriously retarded, or even sleeping human beings. First, "person" both does and does not seem to be an accurate way of answering the question "What am I?" On the one hand, it does seem apt, for our capacities to think, will, and act mark us off radically from other beings that can do none of these things. But it can seem inapt for reasons articulated in recent work on the metaphysics of personal identity.

This work is indebted to a revival of the Aristotelian distinction between substance and accident. As David Wiggins points out, everything that exists is a "this such," and it is the concept under which a thing falls as a this such, rather than concepts that indicate what it is doing, or what color it is, and so on, that tells us *what* the thing is (Wiggins, 1980, p. 15). For at least some things that we ordinarily characterize as particulars, the concept under which they fall as particulars will be their substance concept. This concept tells us what the thing in question most truly is, and, as Eric Olson writes, it is this concept that "determines persistence conditions that necessarily apply to all (and perhaps only) things of that kind" (Olson, 1997a, p. 28).

The language of substance may not be equally amenable to all, but everyone involved in the debates at the heart of this chapter should have an interest in understanding what you and I and things of our sort are most fundamentally, because this understanding will determine when we come to be, as well as when we cease to be. But what most defenders of abortion, and many philosophers of personal identity, have held, implicitly or explicitly, until recently, is that you and I are essentially persons. "Person" was understood to involve such properties as psychological continuity or connectedness; from this it was inferred that no person existed prior to the presence of such psychological properties.[2] From this it was concluded that embryos and fetuses, lacking the relevant psychological properties, are not persons, and are not entitled to the respect ordinarily due persons.[3]

There are many problems with this view. For example, this would mean that you and I were the same kind of *substance* as intelligent Martians, angels, and perhaps members of the Trinity. But Olson has raised the most damning criticism. He points out that on the received view, you and I were never fetuses, for you and I are essentially persons, and substances of the person sort do not come to exist until the onset of psychological traits. But fetuses themselves belong to a substance class—they are particulars of the substance sort "human animal." And this raises problems for the view that you and I are essentially persons. What has happened to that other substance, the human animal? Does it continue to exist in the same space as the human person? Did it cease to exist with the coming to be of the human person? If the former, how can it not share exactly all of the person's properties, and if so, why is *it* not also a person? If the latter, is there now no longer a human *animal* in the space that I occupy? None of the options seems metaphysically acceptable (Olson, 1997a, Chapter 4).

The solution is that you and I are essentially human animals; thus you and I were once fetuses, and, at least plausibly, embryos and zygotes as well. But if you and I are not essentially persons, but animals, what sort of concept is the concept "person," and when and how do we become persons? The difficulty is to do two things: to answer the question "What are you and I?" by naming the substance kind to which we belong, and to then show what the relationship is between existing as members of our substance kind and being persons deserving of moral respect.

The course of the discussion through the rest of this chapter will be as follows. I will explain first how we can think of ourselves as *both* persons and animals. The key here is to consider the peculiarly temporal nature of animal life. Because of this temporality, animal natures cannot be understood by a view of what the animal is or does at a particular time, but only by viewing the animal's existence through time. I argue that if we consider what sorts of animals we are, keeping in mind the fact that animal lives are temporal, then our personhood makes good sense.

I shall then argue that embryos (and fetuses) are the same sorts of beings as you and I, and thus persons deserving of the same moral respect as you and I. Among the ways in which we are to be respected, as was seen in Chapter 2, is in respect for our bodily integrity. If such respect means anything, it means not being destroyed in the course of another's research. So embryo research, if it threatens the lives of those embryos at all, is morally impermissible.

Recently, however, philosophers have objected to this position by focusing on the question of whether that embryo is an *individual* or not. For if it is not an individual, then it is not an individual human being, and hence not a person. The ability of the embryo to twin is central to the argument that the embryo is not an individual. I shall argue that this crucial objection to the claim that embryos are deserving of the same moral respect due to other members of the human species fails.


## ANIMALS AND PERSONS

Why is it so difficult for some to conceive of our animal nature as compatible with our being persons? Lynn Rudder Baker suggests that it is implausible to think of animals as meeting the criteria for personhood, which include the ability to reason and will:

> If . . . we are most fundamentally animals, *then our uniquely characteristic abilities do not stem from our being the kind of entities that we are.* This is so because on the Animalist View, what we are most fundamentally—human organisms—can exist and persist without [psychological states]. Having a first person perspective, on the Animalist view, is irrelevant to the kind of being that we most fundamentally are. (Baker, 2000, p. 164, emphasis added)

Baker claims that this is a deep "reason to reject any Animalist criterion" of personal identity. Again, "[A]n animalist criterion of personal identity over time simply leaves out these person-making features. On the Animalist view, 'psychology is completely irrelevant to personal identity'" (Baker, 2000, p. 124, quoting Olson, 1997b, p. 97). Baker concludes that our pretheoretical notion of what personhood involves cannot be honored if we insist upon our essential animality.

But Animalism *can* honor this pretheoretical notion. It is, in fact, only because of a kind of temporal displacement in our manner of looking at the human animal that we can fail to see that the human animal fits this pretheoretical description. To see this, we need to look at a crucial misunderstanding of Baker's regarding the nature of the fetus. Once we see that being a person is, quite literally, natural to a human fetus, it will be relatively easy to work backwards to the claim that it is also perfectly natural for a human embryo to be a person.

My basic claim regarding the human fetus is that one's understanding of the nature—the intrinsic nature—of the fetus should lead one to conclude that as part of its normal development, it will grow into a being with psychological states. While not independent of other beings for its development, the fetus is self-actualizing in ways that artifacts such as flags and statues are not, and its self-actualization leads to the having of certain sorts of psychological states.

This will be missed if we fail to view the fetus in its fully temporal existence. If we take a snapshot of the fetus at some particular stage of development, we will assign it essential properties based entirely on what it has at the moment of the snapshot. It will seem, if viewed early enough, not to be sapient, or even sentient. But this is an inappropriate perspective for determining the nature of an animal. Tigers are essentially carnivorous, and, as such, have certain types of teeth and claws. We would hardly say that a tiger cub, not yet fully developed, was for that reason not a tiger. By contrast, a piece of cloth that has not yet been made into a flag is in no way a flag.

Of course, Baker, like all who distinguish the "I" who is a person from the coincident human animal, accepts that the fetus is identical with the later adult *animal* on precisely such grounds as these—the large difference in capacities and features between the fetus and the adult human animal does not incline her to deny that they are the same, identical being. What she denies is (a) that "I" am identical to the fetus, or the animal; and (b) that persons are identical to animals or fetuses.

The distinction between "I" and "persons" is important for Baker to make in arguing against some animalists, such as Olson, because Olson thinks that, while I am essentially an animal, I am not essentially a person. "Person," on Olson's account, is a phased sortal, like teacher or spouse; an animal can become a person and cease to be a person. To this extent, Baker and Olson agree. But Baker thinks that I am essentially a person; Olson, that I am essentially an animal. I want to argue, however, that I am essentially an animal; and that this animal is, by its nature, a person. "Person" is not a substance term, but rather a term that applies to something in virtue of that something's substance, and at all times that that something is that substance. So a much closer relationship obtains between the human animal and the human person than either Baker or Olson.

To show this requires that I show the connection between animals and persons, given that persons, on Baker's account, necessarily have mental states and animals do not. My argument proceeds in two steps.

First step: sleeping spells. What does it mean to say that persons necessarily have mental states? It cannot mean that necessarily, if $x$ is a person at t, then $x$ has mental states at t. Consider Sleeping Beauty, cast into a dreamless sleep. Only if Prince finds her, and kisses her, will she awake before the death of her body. However, if Prince is waylaid by robbers and killed, then Sleeping Beauty will never wake again. Her mental states are at an end, even though she might live organically for many years. Suppose, then, that Prince *is* killed; is Sleeping Beauty then no longer a person?

This answer is absurd—if Prince is not killed, Sleeping Beauty will be restored to full mental flourishing, and hence will be a person. If so, she could not have failed to be a person prior to Prince's kiss. But whether Sleeping Beauty is a person or not can hardly be a function of whether some *other* person is dead or not. So if she is a person, while in a dreamless sleep, on the version of the story in which Prince survives, then she is a person on the version of the story where Prince dies. And if this is so, then there is a time at which Sleeping Beauty is a person, but does not have mental states.

Baker herself acknowledges, as most deniers of personhood to embryos also do, that occurrent mental states are not necessary to be a person. A "capacity" for such states is sufficient. This is an ambiguous notion, but it is clear, I think, that Baker could not hold that Sleeping Beauty has the relevant capacity, for Baker holds that a fetus that has been aborted or miscarried was not a person immediately before its demise. But if we suppose that Sleeping Beauty's spell is permanent, but for Prince's kiss, then the two cases are structurally the same. The fact of the matter is that neither entity will ever have mental states; but we have reason for ascribing a genuine *capacity* for mental states to each. So if Sleeping Beauty is a person in virtue of what would happen, counterfactually, if she were kissed, then the fetus is a person in virtue of what would happen, counterfactually, if it were not aborted. Indeed, the case is stronger for the fetus. In Sleeping Beauty's case, something special must be *done* in order for Sleeping Beauty to have mental states in the future; but in the case of the fetus, what needs to be done to assure future mental states is precisely nothing. Leave the fetus alone, and it will develop into a being with mental states on its own.

So if a certain type of capacity is necessary for being a person, then both Sleeping Beauty and the fetus must have that capacity. This is brought out by contrast with entities that are like Sleeping Beauty and the about-to-be-aborted fetus inasmuch as they will never have mental states, but unlike them in that they truly have no capacity for mental states: entities like balls of wax, or tin cans, or sea slugs. Unlike these, Sleeping Beauty and the fetus do have a capacity for possible mental states even though in fact they will never have them. What more can we say, though, about this relation to possible mental states?

The second step of my argument is this: What we should say is that Sleeping Beauty is a member of an animal species that is such that its members, by their nature, develop to the point of having mental states. Animals of this species are such as to develop into beings with mental states—necessarily, by nature—even if some member, or many members, do not in fact so develop. Such development is a function of their species-nature. Similarly, it is a function of the nature of tigers to have sharp teeth, and this generates the proper sort of statement about tigers: they are such as to have sharp teeth. Michael Thompson has called this sort of claim an Aristotelian Categorical; its truth cannot be appreciated by looking at a snapshot of the organism's life. One must look at the broader, i.e., temporal, context (Thompson, 1996). We should understand "human persons necessarily have mental states" as an instance of the Aristotelian Categorical, true of individuals of the human species.

Keeping the larger context in mind, we can hold that persons do necessarily have mental states, and have reason and will, but understand this to mean that persons are individuals of a rational species (see Boethius, 1918). Moreover, *Homo sapiens* is one such rational species, so individuals of that species are persons, and necessarily so. That they lack, at some time or times, mental states does not militate against their personhood. Nor, if I am necessarily a person, does this militate against my once having been a fetus.

Thus, Animalism, with a sensible view of personhood, and a temporal look at the human organism, puts the relationship between being a human being and being a person on sound footing. It answers Baker's representative claim about the underlying failure of Animalism—that it makes psychology irrelevant to personal identity. It is true that the soundest guide to the identification of a person through time is by repeated identification of something as the same organism, and not by identification of some relationship between psychological states. But the animal life by which we do identify ourselves through time is also a personal life—one such as to develop psychological features in time.

It follows that all human animals are human persons, and due the respect accorded to persons. They may not be intentionally harmed or killed or otherwise manipulated. Any view that attempts to make either the person I am different from the coincident animal, or that views personhood as a status that some human animals achieve and that many eventually lose, is false.

This latter view, the view of philosophers such as Judith Jarvis Thomson, Eric Olson, and David Boonin, lacks plausibility next to the picture I have drawn of the relationship between human animals and human persons (Thomson, 1995; Olson,1997a; Boonin, 2003). It is true that it is not subject to the metaphysical difficulties of the substance view of personhood.

But it arises from the same unwillingness to look at the nature of the human animal temporally, and thus this inability to see how personal traits are natural to the human animal.

The deep problem with such views is that when we cease to look at such personal traits as natural, then personhood itself becomes, inevitably, arbitrary: a matter of convention, degree, or choice. Each of the authors mentioned, and many others besides, have favored views of when the human animal achieves the status of personhood: when the primitive streak forms, when the brain forms, when the fetus is viable, when the fetus or child is self-conscious, and so on. Each such approach singles out some valuable trait or characteristic among many others and attributes to it supreme significance in matters of life and death. But each such trait is arbitrary next to the competing others, in the same way that it is arbitrary whether we assign driver's licenses at age sixteen, seventeen, or eighteen. Such arbitrariness is unavoidable in certain pragmatic decisions. But it should be avoided in our assessment of who deserves to live, and who does not. It is more adequate, both theoretically and morally, to view personhood as a condition natural to human beings, rather than as a status to be achieved.

The crucial question, then, for the ethics of embryonic research is: When does the human animal begin? Here, there is disagreement among philosophers otherwise committed to the Animalist thesis. Eric Olson, for example, following Norman Ford, argues that the embryo becomes a human animal only about sixteen days after fertilization. His reason for this cut-off is that prior to the specialization of cells, more or less completed by this point, twinning is possible. Thus Ford writes, and Olson quotes,

> Prior to this stage, we do not have a living individual human body, but a mass of pre-programmed loosely organized developing cells and heterogeneous tissues until their "clock" mechanisms become synchronized and triggered to harmoniously organize, differentiate and grow as heterogeneous parts of a single whole human organism. (Ford, 1988, p. 175; quoted by Olson 1997a, p. 91)

This argument is of crucial importance to the stem cell and cloning for research disputes. It has not, however, been especially convincing to human embryologists who, when working precisely as scientists, and not as advocates for some form of disputed research, agree with remarkable unanimity that a human animal begins at fertilization.[4]

At the one-celled stage of the embryo, sperm from the male has fertilized the woman's egg; male and female chromosomes from each have lined up at syngamy, and a new, genetically distinct, individual human organism exists with a single, diploid nucleus (Larsen, 1997, pp. 1–3). This organism is continuous in a variety of ways with the later embryo, the fetus, and the newborn: physically, vitally, genetically. If we wish to ask, in the way suggested in this chapter, when does a being begin that will naturally develop into a human being with the ability to think and will, then the answer is: at fertilization.

The following questions, then, must be addressed. First, why should the possibility of twinning be thought to defeat the claim that the early embryo is a human being? Second, if that embryo is a human being, is it legitimate to destroy it for research purposes? Finally, the following difficulty must be addressed. There are at present many hundreds of thousands of embryos cryopreserved from previous assisted reproduction interventions. These early embryos will eventually die, and there is little that can be done for them. Even if it is in itself morally impermissible to research on human subjects in a way that will lead to their demise, does not the inevitability of their demise argue in favor of their use? Such an argument has been put forth in recent years, even by some otherwise committed to the sanctity of human life. It must be addressed as well.

## TWINNING

Why should twinning be thought to militate against the humanity of the early embryo? One crucial consideration in the argument concerns the individuality of that embryo. Recall the Aristotelian suggestion, that everything that exists does so as a this such. So any particular substance will be a member of some class, but it will also be an individual in its own right. This consideration is important in considering whether certain sorts of entities that appear to be substances really are. For if something genuinely is a this such—a substance—then it should be the case that it has determinate identity conditions, even if it is not always possible to identify them, or to identify whether they are satisfied or not. That is, there should always be a definite yes or no answer to the question: is this the same substance as that (was).

This condition is not met by some things that for more or less pragmatic and social reasons are given names and treated as if they were genuine individuals. For example, a pile of trash is not really a substance. Its beginnings and its endings are vague and a matter of convention, as are its physical boundaries. When large bits of the pile are replaced, there need be no definite yes or no answer to the question "Is this the same pile of trash as the one that was here yesterday?"

There are other arguments for not treating the pile of trash as a genuine substance. The pile of trash does not have its own causal powers. Although it stinks, and thus causes the wrinkling of noses in its vicinity, and attracts flies, the causal powers of the trash seem entirely reducible to the causal powers of its parts, and ultimately to its smallest parts. This is not true of organisms: that this is a dog, or a cat, or a human being, enters necessarily into our explanation of why this is chasing a rabbit, or a mouse, or a high-paying job. No explanation merely, or entirely, in terms of the nature of its parts will suffice.

Trenton Merricks and Peter van Inwagen have extended these considerations to argue that *none* of the ordinary artifacts that we find around us daily are, after all, genuine individual substances (Van Inwagen, 1990; Merricks, 2003). Merricks and Van Inwagen conclude that such objects are not really entities after all: there are no baseballs, no statues, no flags, merely simples arranged baseball-wise, statue-wise and flag-wise. In essence, their arguments work by showing that everything that is not an individual substance is ultimately no more than a heap, any one of which might be more or less important to us in our social life, but all of which are ontologically on par with one another.[5]

Substances are thus "natural wholes which are subjects of concrete predicates" (Braine, 1992, p. 258). As a natural whole, a substance has a definite beginning and ending, and it plays a necessary explanatory role in certain causal stories. Of course some groups of persons play such a role as well, and thus philosophers typically hold that an individual substance cannot be composed of other individual substances—individual substances are ontologically basic (Chappell, 1997).

Why, then, does the embryo's capacity for twinning render it unfit to be an individual substance? Which specific criterion does it fail to meet? And what is its status supposed to be in the time period in which "it" is not yet a human animal?

One proposal is that precisely because of the early embryo's capacity for twinning, it cannot be an individual. But if not an individual, then not a substance, and hence not a human animal. This argument seeks to show that because of what the embryo can do, it cannot be an individual; similarly, if some supposed entity was capable of shaking hands and going two separate ways, it too would not be an individual substance. The argument is conceptual; it depends upon what it *means* to be an individual.

A second argument relies on a Lockean claim, plausible in itself, about what is responsible for the persistence of some particular organic substance. Peter van Inwagen summarizes the claim:

> If an organism exists at a certain moment, then it exists whenever and wherever—and only when and only where—the event that is its life at that moment is occurring; more exactly, if the activity of the $x$s at $t_1$ constitutes a life, and the activity of the $y$s at $t_2$ constitutes a life, then the organism that the $x$s compose at $t_1$ is the organism that the $y$s compose at $t_2$ if and only if the life constituted by the activity of the $x$s at $t_1$ is the life constituted by the activity of the $y$s at $t_2$. (Van Inwagen, 1990, p. 145)

Now a one-celled zygote has a life; it is a single organism. And an embryo at, say, three weeks has a life; it too is a single organism. But Van Inwagen claims that the two-celled "organism," and similar collections of cells, do not have a shared life:

They adhere to each other, but we have seen that that is no reason to suppose that two objects compose anything. The zygote was a single, unified organism, the vast assemblage of metabolic processes that were its life having been directed by the activity of nucleic acid in its nucleus. No such statement can be made about the two-cell embryo. No event, I should say, is its life. The space it occupies is merely an arena in which two lives, hardly interacting, take place. . . . (Van Inwagen, 1990, pp. 153–4)

This argument is biological, not conceptual; it depends upon a claim about what the life of the embryo is in fact like.

The biological issue has priority over the conceptual issue. Surely, it is theoretically imperative first to look at whether the purported entity in question—the early human embryo—seems to have one life, or to be a collection of several lives; for if it is best characterized biologically as a single organism, then this should determine the answer to the conceptual question: can a biologically unified substance divide into two independent substances?

Indeed, there are good biological reasons for thinking that the early human embryo is a single biological organism (Howsepian, 1992; Johnson, 1995; Lee, 2001; George and Tollefsen, 2008), and good conceptual reasons for thinking that any interpretation of the biological data that renders the intermediate stages of the embryo a mere "virtual object," or a mere "collection of adhering cells," is itself in deep difficulties. From the biological standpoint, we typically recognize that the parts of some aggregate fail to compose a whole because they do not have clearly established boundaries, or because their mutual labors are insufficiently coordinated, or because the primary focus of unified action seems to be at a more focused point than the collection as a whole. Patrick Lee, summarizing recent embryological work on the very early embryo points out that none of these are true of that entity:

> Recent embryology has shown that the process from day 1 to day 14 is complex, organized, and coordinated from within the embryo itself. On day 2 or 3 compaction occurs, which is the process in which the cells change their shapes and align themselves closely together. And at the two-cell stage already the embryo is producing the glyco-protein that will later guide that compaction process. Again, at the 12- or 15-cell stage, which would be day 4, the visible differentiation between the inner cell mass and the trophoblast appears. Indeed, recent studies of the development of mouse embryos have shown that the sperm entry point into the oocyte influences how the zygote will divide, and which cell (even at the two-cell stage) will give rise to the embryoblast (the embryo proper) or the trophoblast (the chorion and the embryonic portion of the placenta). In other words, from day 1 onward it is clear that this is multi-cellular organism, internally coordinating its various activities toward the next more mature stage of the human organism as a whole. (Lee, 2001, pp. 11–12)

The multicellular embryo between days one and fourteen thus seems biologically to be a unified organism, and not a mere collection of one-celled organisms bound together.

Contributing to this appearance is the fact that the very physical boundaries of the embryo are stable, and determined from within its own nature. Some suggest that the zona pellucida is merely an external limit, like the plastic wrap surrounding a collection of marbles. But from the earliest stage, it resists, like the skin of the developed organism, external difficulties in the environment, as when it prevents the blastocyst from implanting in the fallopian tubes. Meanwhile, the internal communication between cells is quite different, occurring over so-called "gap-junctions," differentiating the embryo from a mere collection of individual organisms.

If biology trumps metaphysical speculation about individuals, then the evidence indicates that the early embryo is an individual substance of the human sort. Indeed, speaking of the embryo in this way is natural even to those who deny that it is an individual. Thus Ronald Green, a prominent critic of the individuality of the early embryo, nonetheless frequently calls it an "entity," and even an "organism" (Green, 2001).

A similar phenomenon is apparent in Barry Smith and Berit Brogaard's summary of embryonic development in their article "Sixteen Days." As they show, the process begins with fertilization, after which there are a number of cell divisions that take place within the physical boundaries of the zona pullicida. Some subsequent steps in the progress towards gastrulation, in which cell folds form the predecessor structures for a variety of bodily parts and organs, and neurulation, in which the initial structures of the nervous system are generated, include implantation, which is prior to gastrulation, and the formation of the morula.

This description as a whole gives the unmistakable impression, apart from other salient features, of a single entity acting with purpose: develop body parts, and implant in the uterus *in order to* begin to take in nutrition and establish firmer and more rigorous boundaries, *in order to* continue to grow and develop. Thus, when we look at the embryo's temporal progress, we see a single self-directed entity, the nature of whose self-direction is species specific: the course of events outlined by embryologists is the characteristic course of activity of the early human embryo in much the same way that it is characteristic of the adult dog to chase rabbits. What is the alternative? Only that the hundreds, and eventually thousands, of cells that are present prior to and during gastrulation and neurulation, each have their own species-specific nature that causes them to bring about, each individually, a massively complex state of affairs that has not been coordinated by a single agent.

Such a possibility violates Ockham's razor: why think that the many do what appears to be done by one? The simpler view is best: the embryo is, from the one-celled stage, a single, whole organism, functioning as a biological unity, to bring about its own more advanced stages of development. It is, in other words, a human being.

Earlier, I characterized the two issues concerning individuality as biological and conceptual. Biologically, we have seen than the early embryo has the characteristic structural and behavioral features of a single organism. What of the conceptual question: can something capable of dividing into two really be one? I suggest that in light of the biological evidence, the conceptual puzzle should cease to perplex: that something *does* happen from time to time shows that it is possible, and twinning is a fact of early human embryology. Since it is more sensible to hold that the embryo is a single organism—a single entity—then it follows that it *is* possible, at least in some circumstances, for one entity to divide into two. But since this was already known—we can divide sticks, and even flatworms—this fact should not even strike us as surprising. So we are again led to the very natural conclusion that the human embryo, from conception, through its first few weeks, and into its fetal stages is a single human being, numerically identical to the child, adolescent, and adult it will later, if all goes well, become.

## INEVITABLE DEMISE

Some philosophers and politicians have suggested that even if early embryos are human beings, and hence human persons, it is nonetheless morally permissible to experiment on those embryos that would otherwise be destroyed. Since their use promises great good, and they will be destroyed anyway, it seems reasonable to some that they be used, rather than simply wasted.

Of course, if early embryos are human persons, then the first response to the surplus of embryos is to recognize the grave moral deficiency of scientific or medical processes that create surplus embryos (Sandel, 2007). It is contrary to every concern for the human fulfillment of these persons that they be created merely to be put "on ice," for the use of others. The very notion of being a surplus "person" should call to mind the various other historical circumstances in which human beings were treated in such menial and overtly economic ways.

But still, what about extra embryos? There are many of them, and they are doing no good, and their demise is inevitable. If they are going to die anyway, why should their deaths not do some good? Indeed, won't we end up killing them one way or another? I offer two responses to these objections.

The first concerns so-called "embryo adoption." Many infertile couples desire children, and would be willing to adopt children in the embryonic stage; moreover, even fertile couples might so adopt as an act of mercy towards those who otherwise would not live past their earliest stages.[6] If this is, as it seems, morally permissible, then every effort should be made to establish adoption programs for these extremely disadvantaged human beings.

Unfortunately, it is unlikely that embryo adoption could meet the needs of the vast number of cryogenically preserved embryos. Where adoption is unlikely and the biological parents have effectively abandoned their children, the embryos seem doomed. Is there a way in which such embryos might best, and in a way consistent with the basic human goods, meet their fate? I suggest that we view them in a way parallel to those who are in need of an organ transplant that they are unlikely to get, but who are presently receiving life-preserving treatment. If they had the organ, they would survive, but they won't, in fact, receive it, and their treatment is thus extraordinary—it offers no hope of improved prognosis, and it keeps them alive at great costs, of various sorts.

In such circumstances, it is not killing to remove the extraordinary treatment, where the intention is not to kill, but to mitigate the sorts of costs being incurred. Similarly, if efforts to find donor wombs for homeless embryos has failed (analogous to the failure to find the necessary life-supporting organ in the transplant case), and the biological parents will not take responsibility for the embryos' welfare, then they could be removed from the cryogenic life support, not with the intention of killing, but with a view to mitigating the costs, for the embryos, and for society, incurred by their preservation.

Many people will be unsatisfied with this. Arthur Caplan, for example, has suggested that "even if you believe that an embryo is a person, however, and should not be used in any research that would cause its destruction, you must still consider the promise that the therapies from embryonic stem cells hold for those who are paralyzed, burned, dying of liver and pancreas failure, brain injured and suffering from many, many other diseases and injuries" (Caplan, 1998).

Such reasoning is utilitarian: we must do what is necessary to achieve the greatest amount of good, even if it requires sacrificing the rights of the few. But consider all the good that could be achieved through experimental research on the elderly, or dying infants or children. Would we be so quick to be swayed by the promise of great benefits so as to be willing to kill such subjects of research? It is true that refusal to violate straightforward ethical requirements, such as the moral absolute that one not intentionally kill the innocent, can have a cost. Some advocates of research into adult stem cells have perhaps not fully acknowledged the possibility that these cells might not have all the potential that embryonic stem cells will have. Perhaps there are great cures residing in embryonic stem cell research; indeed, in Chapter 9, I will argue that the likelihood of this possibility creates important political considerations for such research. Nonetheless, we should resolutely refuse to sacrifice our ethical ideals for the sake of scientific progress.

## CONCLUSION

We should therefore accept the following. First, the human embryo, even from its earliest zygotic, or one-celled stage, is a single individual of the human species. Human beings do not generally come to be at some later stage in the embryo's existence.[7] Second, you and I are human beings as well; and it is in virtue of our membership in the human species that we are persons, entitled to moral respect, i.e., respect for the human goods insofar as they are and can be instantiated in us. Third, to kill a human being is to disrespect a person, by directly violating the good of human life in his or her person. Thus intentional killing of a human being is always and everywhere morally impermissible. Fourth, and finally, to perform a lethal experiment on an early human embryo, even at the zygotic or near zygotic stages, is to kill a human being, thus, to kill a human person, and therefore to violate an exceptionless moral principle. All lethal experimentation on human embryos, as well as any experimentation that would result in less than fatal but permanent damage, that is not intended for the primary benefit of the embryo itself is therefore morally wrong. The ethics of embryonic research is thus strikingly simple at its core, yet it resonates with the tradition of medicine with which the ethics of inquiry is continuous: first, do no harm.

# 6 Animal Research and Animal Rights

I turn now to research on and using animals. While the position I shall argue for is considerably more permissive than the position of animal rights advocates, and considerably more permissive than my position on human embryo research, I shall nonetheless argue for some kinds of moral restrictions not always acknowledged by defenders of animal experimentation and research.

Some animal research is fairly non-interventionist, as when a scientist studies animals in their natural habitats.[1] Other forms involve not just interventions into the lives of animals, but sometimes cause their deaths. Animal research is done for a number of reasons, of which the most important are the following three, all of which potentially can involve both interventionist and non-interventionist research.

First, some scientists are interested in animals and their lives purely for the sake of knowledge about those animals. When we speak of animal research, we often implicitly assume that we are discussing research the purpose of which is ultimately to be found in some practical benefit, but it is perfectly intelligible that some scientists wish to know about the nature of this or that animal, or to know more intricate biological or chemical truths about animals. Some animal embryologists are motivated, for example, simply by the desire to know more about mouse, or dog, or cat embryology.

Second, a considerable part of animal research is primarily for the sake of satisfying market concerns. Testing perfumes, for example, or other cosmetics, is done neither for the sake of knowledge as a good in itself, nor for health benefits as such, but rather with a view to producing a more saleable product. Of course, such research can overlap in intention with other sorts.

Finally, animal research exists as part of the larger framework of biomedical research. Such investigation aims at producing new vaccines, therapies, or enhancements for human beings, or at refining already existing ones. Most researchers believe that some experiments must be performed on animals before they may be performed on human beings. Such research is often, although not inevitably, interventionist, and frequently threatens the well-being of the animal. It, and the market-driven research alluded to in the previous paragraph, are frequent targets of criticism from animal rights advocates.

Animal advocacy—the defense of animals against the interventions of scientists and other researchers—comprises a more or less limited set of positions. Among the most prominent defenders of more stringent restrictions on animal research are the following.

First, there are utilitarian defenders of animals, such as Peter Singer. On Singer's view, equal consideration for the interests of all sentient creatures grounds a sound treatment of non-human animals. These interests are understood in terms of the creature's ability to experience pain and pleasure. In discussing a similar position of Jeremy Bentham's Singer writes:

> Bentham points to the capacity for suffering as the vital characteristic that gives a being the right to equal consideration. The capacity for suffering—or more strictly, for suffering and/or enjoyment or happiness—is not just another characteristic like the capacity for language or higher mathematics . . . If a being suffers, there can be no moral justification for refusing to take that suffering into consideration. No matter what the nature of the being, the principle of equality requires that the suffering be counted equally with the like suffering—insofar as rough comparisons can be made—of any other being. (Singer, 2003, p. 34)

At the same time, Singer holds that sapient beings that have an achieved capacity for reason and self-awareness have lives of greater worth than beings without such a capacity. So, on the one hand, sentient non-human animals must be brought within the "sphere of moral concern," but on the other, human beings who have not achieved self-awareness and reason are of less value than fully normal adult human beings and some adult non-human animals.

The consequences for animal research are significant, for if animal interests are to be accorded weight in our moral calculus, much infliction of pain in research is immoral; on the other hand, at least some lethal research on very young human beings, such as embryos and fetuses, or even perhaps on retarded human beings, will be preferable to similar animal research involving animals of greater awareness.

Although Singer uses the phrase animal rights, as a utilitarian, he cannot be truly said to acknowledge *any* rights. Tom Regan, by contrast, is concerned to show that at least some animals have rights in the same way that human beings do. For Regan, rights are not grounded in a capacity for reason or choice, but in the fact that some being or other is the subject of a life. "Each of us is the experiencing subject of a life, a conscious creature having an individual welfare that has importance to us whatever our usefulness to others" (Regan, 2005, p. 149). Beings with such individual welfares that are of importance to them are said by Regan to have inherent value, and all inherent value is equal. Thus, the right to life of a dog or cat is the very same right to life that an adult human being has.

Regan draws the obvious conclusion regarding animal research, a conclusion stronger than any that Singer's utilitarianism can sustain. The animal rights position is, says Regan, committed to "the total abolition of the use of animals in science" (Regan, 2005, p. 144). Regan is aware that this will have consequences for the progress of science, but in the face of rights, he argues, scientific progress must stand aside: rights take precedence.

These two views are the most prominent of those philosophical views on the ethical treatment of animals that have consequences for animal research. Let me add two further views, however, one for its similarity to certain arguments to be made in later chapters, the other because it provides a helpful way of introducing the basic goods approach into the discussion. The first position, but not the second, could be held by those who disagree with the claim that it is intrinsically wrong to harm animals for research purposes.

Charles K. Fink has argued that researchers and the Western world generally must face up to the terms of the following choice: should we spend billions of dollars on research that will involve untold amounts of harm to animals, but that promises only speculative and future benefits for human beings, or should we spend that money on humanitarian projects that will have as their immediate consequence the saving of many human lives and significant benefits in terms of human welfare? Fink writes: "In a much better world than our own, no one would seriously consider spending millions of dollars in space exploration when thousands of children die each day from starvation; and no one would consider spending millions on animal research when every day thousands of people die from treatable diseases" (Fink, 2000, p. 218; cf. Ryder, 1975). Generalized, such questions raise serious difficulties in both the politics of inquiry and the internal ethics of inquiry. Politically, reasonable decisions must be made about the extent and nature of funding for research projects of various sorts, in the face of widespread human misery. Ethically, there are difficult questions that must be faced by all inquirers about the reasonableness of their chosen areas of study, and the resources that those areas require.

A fourth view is important because of its philosophical likeness to the basic goods view. Tim Chappell has defended a similar view, alike in beginning from a consideration of basic goods, and structurally similar in its derivation of moral norms. Faced with the basic goods, which include, for Chappell, goods such as life, knowledge, aesthetic experience, accomplishment, and pleasure, practical reason issues three demands: that one promote the goods, that one not violate the goods, and that one respect the goods (Chappell, 1997).

But Chappell's view is neither as strictly eudaimonistic, nor as deeply anthropocentric as the view discussed in Chapter 1. On the view I defend, the basic goods are basic *human* goods, and they are good because they promise human well-being—they offer *us* the opportunity of human flourishing. On Chappell's view, the goods are more deeply objective, not linked essentially to the welfare of human persons, and thus not necessarily promising human well-being or flourishing. In consequence, the good of animals and of nature may constitute the ground of genuine reasons for human action, without those goods offering or promising anything specifically human to the agents who pursue them (Chappell, 2004).

But why should goods that are not human goods give *humans* reasons for action? A reason is a consideration in light of which action is intelligible, and action is intelligible to the agent in virtue of its perceived desirability. On the basic human goods view, desirability is explicable precisely in terms of the notion of human well-being, and this is completely intelligible: humans are deeply lacking in various ways, deeply needy in various ways, deeply incomplete in various ways, and the basic goods underwrite the promise made by certain available ways of action to end our lack, satisfy our needs, and complete us, towards all of which ends we are naturally inclined. Desirability and anthropocentricity thus go hand in hand.

Non-anthropocentric accounts of the goods leave the desirability of the good mysterious, both theoretically and practically. Of what relevance to me is the good of some entity if that good is not essentially related to my fulfillment? Such a question is equally raised in any ethics that grounds reasons in desires: why should your desires, which are different from mine, matter to me when they do not intersect with my desires? But the basic human goods approach is not desire based, and the good of others is not independent of my well-being and flourishing.

Patrick Lee argues similarly:

> Could that which makes options X, Y and Z appealing be the perfection of something alien to me? Could it be a value independent of me, or the fulfillment of duty viewed as independent of my fulfillment? To say "yes" to these questions would be incoherent. Any tendency toward an object which is *not* my fulfillment, in some way or other, would not come from within me, that is, from my nature, which just is an orientation toward actualization in one direction rather than another. Were I naturally inclined toward the fulfillment of something completely outside me, then that inclination would make me naturally an extrinsic instrument of something else—and nothing can be just an extrinsic instrument, since it must have some inherent nature of its own. (Lee, 2001b, p. 138)

The goods of persons are not independent of my good. As Lee writes, ultimate reasons for action are "fulfillments for me and for those persons with whom I am in communion" (Lee, 2001b, p. 138). In fact, the notion of being a reason for action and the possibility of persons in communion are deeply interrelated: the possibility of genuine communion is underwritten by the possibility of shared goods, and the goods of persons are genuine reasons only because they are shared, i.e., underwrite genuine communion. With beings with whom a shared pursuit of goods is impossible, there is no possible communion, and no shared reasons: such beings exist outside our moral community.

Non-human animals seem to be exactly that sort of being. With such animals, there is no communion: they cannot, in principle, pursue goods with us, and they manifestly do not share with us even the types of many goods that are humanly important, such as knowledge, friendship, and integrity. Our reasons for action are not their reasons for action for they have no reasons, existing rather in a space of instinct and desire (McDowell, 1994). They exist, therefore, outside our moral community.

So the difference between a eudaimonist, anthropocentric account of the basic goods and the more objectivist non-eudaimonist conception has consequences for our treatment of animals. The basic goods are not pursuable for the sake of those animals themselves. A good like human life, which makes negative demands on us as regards actions such as killing, and positive demands with respect to actions such as those of the Good Samaritan, makes no direct demands on us in relation to animals. Although it is absolutely impermissible intentionally to kill another human being, no such prohibition exists regarding animals.

It is clear, then, why merely being the subject of a life is likewise insufficient to ground animal rights. To say that a being has a right is to express, from the point of view of that being, the moral demands upon other beings that are in communion with that being. But animals are outside of our communion, since they do not share reasons for action with us. That they have, in some analogous sense, interests may be true as an expression of the fact that they have natures, and natures incline towards their own completions—animals seek to remain alive, to reproduce after their species' fashion, to eat, rest, and live in the way appropriate to their species life. But to have an interest in this sense falls short of being within a space of reasons for actions with other beings such that rights are a possibility.

Finally, that non-human animals have a capacity for feeling pain and pleasure, while relevant to the question of how they should be treated, is insufficient to ground the claim that their interest in pleasure and avoiding pain counts equally with our own. The concept of counting equally is itself one that is conceptually linked to the notion of being in communion with: it is with those beings with whom communion is possible that we must recognize a fundamental equality of worth, or, by lack of that recognition, rupture the communion itself. There is indeed a genuine insight among those who advocate animal rights, namely, that our regular instrumentalization of animals is incompatible with any form of community between humans and animals; but it is the inevitable lack of communion that justifies the instrumentalization; and the lack of communion is itself a consequence of a lack of shared goods.

I conclude, then, that the three strongest positions in favor of a radical rethinking of our obligations to non-human animals fail, and the failure of all three stems from the same source: the goods that are reasons for human

action are necessarily human goods that animals do not share. They therefore do not exist in the sorts of communion with us from which direct moral
obligations flow.

But this does not mean that humans have no obligations in respect of
animals. Historically, among those who have denied direct moral obligations to non-human animals, two related considerations have generated an
argument for indirect duties to animals (Wilson, 2002).

The first of the two considerations relevant to the indirect duty view
holds that humans who abuse animals are thereby more inclined to be cruel
to other human beings. The second holds that misuse of animals, in particular, cruelty to animals, is degrading to the humans who misuse them. Kant
and Aquinas subscribe to both claims, and to the conclusion that there is,
therefore, an obligation not to be cruel to animals. Kant writes:

> [W]e have duties towards animals because thus we cultivate the corre-
> sponding duties to human beings. If a man shoots his dog because the
> animal is no longer capable of service, he does not fail in his duty to the
> dog, for the dog cannot judge, but his act is inhuman and damages in
> himself that humanity which it is his duty to show toward mankind. If
> he is not to stifle his human feeling, he must practice kindness towards
> animals, for he who is cruel to animals becomes hard in his dealing with
> men. (Kant, 1997, p. 240)

The notion of "cruelty" here extends beyond simply shooting one's dog
to causing gratuitous or unnecessary pain. We should notice the dual role
that pain can play in an organism's physical and mental integrity; excessive
pain can make it impossible for an animal, human or otherwise, to function.
But pain also plays a beneficial role in an organism's life, alerting the organism to danger and threats to its physical integrity. If an organism failed to
feel any pain its life would quickly end, as it would cease to have the appropriate avoidance reactions to threat and danger.

Pain has this dual role both in the lives of human beings and in the
lives of non-human animals. It threatens to disrupt an organism's physical
and mental integrity, but also, under appropriate circumstances, it serves
as a warning against other, often serious, threats to that integrity.[2] Now
for human beings threats to the various forms of our integrity are threats
against a person, and against a person's basic goods, but this is not the case
with animals. Unlike the case of torture, where, as I shall argue in the next
chapter, threats to an agent's integrity are an illegitimate means to what
might in some cases be a legitimate end, the deliberate infliction of pain on
an animal is not necessarily an illegitimate means. Rather, its legitimacy or
not should be determined by the legitimacy of the end.

This, in turn, provides a ground for understanding the notion of cruelty
to animals. Where we are cruel to humans every time we deliberately impair
their physical and mental integrity for some end, we are cruel to animals

only when we deliberately impair their physical and mental integrity for trivial, or base, or no ends, beyond the end of seeing them suffer.

This should give us some purchase on the Kantian claim that cruelty to animals is degrading to the agents who inflict it. To see this, I shall introduce the concept of an obstacle to action. If I am considering going to a party, and I will have to drive half an hour to get there, then the fact that I am feeling tired is an obstacle to my going. Similarly, unless I am of a sterling character, if I am considering parting with great sums of money to aid others, desire for money will pose an obstacle to me; as will feelings of antipathy when coming to the aid of someone I dislike. Fear is an obstacle in many cases, as can be contrary desire, or disgust. An obstacle to action just is some factor that blocks action, as providing an emotional push or pull away from the action in question.

The concept of an obstacle to action is not the concept as such of a *reason,* much less a decisive reason, against an action. There can be obstacles to actions one ought to perform—an emotional repugnance, for example, to doing something for *that* person, to whom one is obliged to provide aid. And there can be reasons against wrongful choices without those reasons providing obstacles, because they are not themselves, nor are they attended by, emotional repulsions. An obstacle to action is the block thrown in our way by the emotional and passionate side of our nature.

Now consider an agent's relationship to any means, in relation to which there is an obstacle, to an end that he considers trivial. In proportion as the end seems trivial, the obstacle will tend to be more effective, and indeed, may become transformed into a reason. If there is no, or little reason to do something towards which I have an aversion, then the fact that I have an aversion can become a good reason not to do the thing: not to do it will preserve my integrity, by maintaining unity between action and feeling. If I have no reason to do something, the fact of an obstacle seems to render the action pointless—it is transformed into a defeating reason against the action in question. For example, if I am offered an opportunity to eat something I find repulsive, I might overcome the obstacle for the sake of some serious and worthy end: to show respect for my hosts, for example. But if I am given no reason for eating, or only trivial reasons ("I dare you"), then the repugnance I feel at the food will possibly be transformed into a genuine reason not to eat.

The infliction of damage to something, and in particular the infliction of damage to something that is like us in virtue of its having a mental and physical life, typically generates an obstacle to the doing of anything. Damaging something, anything, in itself provides no positive reason for action, but is something towards which there seems to be a natural resistance. And the more significant the entity damaged, the greater the obstacle: it would be difficult to overcome the natural repugnance to damage the Mona Lisa even for very significant reasons, and very few would be particularly interested in destroying even a chair or desk for no reason at all.[3]

That there are such generalizable obstacles to action seems clear: laziness is typical, as is disgust at certain situations. It is a moral question as to what an appropriate response to these typical obstacles should be, and in this case, we are considering the fact of a generalizable obstacle to the infliction of damage, an obstacle typically more pronounced when we are concerned with living beings, than with non-living, and higher order living beings, than with lower order. What, then, does it say about someone who is able to overcome this natural obstacle for trivial, or base, or no good reasons?[4]

Such an ability would evince at least an insufficient desire not to inflict damage, and possibly a willingness to inflict damage for its own sake—otherwise, what could account for action, given the paucity of other reasons for action? Such an agent either makes it the case, or demonstrates, by his lack of obstacles, or his ability to overcome them, that damage and harm themselves are taken to provide sufficient reasons for action in these cases. Such an agent makes for himself a reason—damage and destruction—something that is no real reason at all, and, indeed, is typically an obstacle to us in action.

For example, an agent is given a plastic ball in one hand, and a small animal, such as a hamster, in another, and is encouraged to crush either for the sake of an experiment. There is a natural repugnance to the thought of crushing a small animal, and, in this case, no real reason to. An agent who nevertheless crushes the hamster thus makes the infliction of damage an end, or part of an end, in itself.

This is indeed to degrade oneself: it is to accept as a reason for action something that is not a human reason for action, not a human good at all. Moreover, this seems likely to generate a disposition to cruelty to persons, for insofar as one has made destructiveness and damage themselves into quasi-reasons for action, base goods that one finds desirable, and the obstacles to which one has overcome, then the humanity of others will seem an increasingly minor consideration; indeed, some who are cruel to the non-human might find it *more* attractive to be cruel to humans, insofar as the obstacle to be overcome would be greater. Cruelty to animals—the infliction of damage or destruction for trivial, base, or no reasons—thus is both degrading, and likely to generate further dispositions to cruelty.

These considerations would hold true of agents who were willing to damage or destroy *anything* for trivial, base, or no reasons. Our willingness and ability to overcome our emotional repulsions to acts of destruction is itself debasing and corrupting of character. But the fact is, our natural revulsion is greater when holding the hamster in one hand, and a ball in the other, to squeezing the life out of the hamster for no reason.[5] The moral question is then whether this greater revulsion can be intelligibly defended. If so, there must be some way of articulating the superior value of animals over artifacts. So I propose to supplement the considerations given so far with two further reasons for thinking damage and destruction of animals without sufficient reason wrong.

The first is that all entities are naturally good precisely insofar as they exist. But animals have a superior form of existence than do artifacts, as we saw in the previous chapter: animals have natures; they are full-fledged entities, with beginnings and endings, unlike artifacts, which have arbitrary boundaries, at both their beginnings and endings. Moreover, their development is a function of their own nature. Organisms are wonderfully complex—they have a fullness of being lacking to even very complex super-computers and airplanes, and they develop themselves into their natural complex state from relatively modest beginnings. They are thus possessed of a degree of realness that corresponds to a general judgment concerning their natural goodness: animals are of more value, naturally, than artifacts, and their wanton destruction is the wanton destruction of good beings.

From a theological standpoint, this means that the wanton destruction of animals is an offense against the goodness of God's creation and hence against God (Grisez, 1993, p. 786). One who is cruel to animals thus offends not only against himself, but against the source of the animal's being. So the intuition that animals are of greater value than artifacts and non-living entities, even though they have no rights, is reasonable, and justifies our increased repugnance at their wanton destruction.

Our natural repugnances where animals and nature are concerned do not stop here, however. Few can enter a factory farm where cattle stand row upon row in their own feces, or enter the facilities where cattle or chickens are mechanically slaughtered, without feeling emotionally distressed and repulsed. The feeling is similar in some ways to our feelings upon looking at a bit of once beautiful land that has been strip-mined; for the natural world, of which animals are a significant, but not the only part, is itself a reality of extraordinary complexity and indeed beauty. This beauty is of considerable value to us, and is unlike the value that animals and natural resources have to us instrumentally; for nature and animals are of instrumental value to us through our intervention, but they are of great beauty considered as natural, and to the extent that they are unmolested by us. Even when nature, and animals, are used by us in ways that are reasonable, the fact of our intervention intrudes upon our sense of their natural beauty, to a greater or lesser degree. No one could fail to recognize a degree of human intervention in an organic farm, or a well-planned zoo, but these jar us less than a factory farm, or a series of small, enclosed cages.

In consequence, I believe that there is a further moral objection to certain kinds of treatment of animals, seen most frequently perhaps in factory farms, some zoos, and abattoirs, but also in research laboratories, that overly mechanize animal existence. Even when this is done for good reasons, the procedure robs the natural world of a beauty that it has for us in its independence from us. And this beauty can in part be maintained even when animals are being used, by keeping them in reasonably natural conditions, providing them access to con-specifics, and refusing to make mechanization of animal life, on the farm or in the lab, into something like an end in itself.

It follows that even when there are good reasons to engage in animal research, it is necessary also to attend to the means used; no harmful treatment of an animal may be justified for trivial, base, or no good reasons, but even when there are good reasons, there is also a reason for resisting the temptation to make our laboratories into something functionally resembling concentration camps. While this would not satisfy those who believe that comparing abattoirs to Nazi death camps is a fully satisfactory analogy, such as Elizabeth Costello in J. M. Coetzee's *The Lives of Animals,* it will nonetheless make the shared animal and human world at once more natural and more human (Coetzee, 2001).

But are there good reasons for engaging in sometimes destructive research on animals? Do those reasons encompass benefits that are non-essential to human well-being such as improvements in cosmetics, or benefits that are not instrumentally beneficial, such as knowledge for its own sake? These questions must be addressed for the argument regarding animal research to be complete.

The easiest cases are those in which animal research is deemed necessary to further research that will eventually be helpful to human beings: the testing of therapeutic drugs for toxicity and side effects, or the testing of vaccines, for example. Much AIDS research is, and must be carried out on animals before it is carried out on persons. Similarly, medical procedures may be tested on animals to see whether they are feasible.[6]

As C. S. Lewis writes, however, if such research is permissible, then it is a duty: a proper concern for those with whom we are in genuine communion requires that some degree of health-related research be carried out, and this research is more safely and more effectively pursued if animal experimentation is permitted. It would thus be inefficient, or riskily harmful to human persons, to refuse to experiment on animals, either unduly slowing down work, or subjecting human subjects to greater threats (Lewis, 1998).

As animal rights activists sometimes point out, many of the benefits are, at the initial stages of research at least, merely speculative: it is impossible to know beyond a shadow of a doubt that this or that research will be successful, a point true generally of research on human subjects as well. This is not a license to do anything, but it does require that the possibility of blind alleys be recognized and permitted, as these are ultimately unavoidable. In consequence, animal experimentation may, and often must, be done when it promises health-related benefits to humans.

Second, there is research that is performed on animals, though some of this sort is also non-interventionist, that is done primarily for the sake of knowledge itself—not for benefits that will accrue in the field of human medicine, for example, but simply to know more about the animals themselves. Here a distinction may be drawn that will highlight the difference between trivial and non-trivial research. In the previous chapter, I used the expression "species life" in discussing the relationship between the human embryo and its eventually developing certain skills and abilities. The phrase was taken from Michael Thompson, who used it in the context of discussing so-called "Aristotelian categoricals"—propositions true of natural beings in a way particularly appropriate to them. "Bobcats mate in the spring," is not true of every bobcat, nor is it necessarily true that a majority of bobcats mate in the spring. But it is of the nature of bobcats that they mate in the spring, and this kind of knowledge is the object of a study of the bobcat nature (Thompson, 1996).

Does the species life of the bobcat encompass more than its macro-level activities, and more than what is expressible primarily in terms of Aristotelian categoricals? I see no reason to think it does not: facts of bobcat digestion, reproduction, blood circulation, motion, and so on are facts that require not simply external study of the bobcat in its natural environment, but interventionist study into the biological, chemical, and physical workings of the bobcat; moreover, many of these facts are expressible in the language of law-like generalizations more familiar to philosophers of science than Aristotelian categoricals. But properly conducted scientific research into the micro-aspects of animals teaches us about the nature of the animal in question. The high school dissection of a frog, and its subsequent study aims, for example, at being a study of part of the frog's species life, as does a study of frogs in their natural habitats.

But consider the high school student who wants to know what the frog will do if he sticks it "like this." Or what would happen to the frog's heart if given a great electric shock. Or how much frog skin, or bones, can resist vigorous pulling and crushing. Such "experiments" are not inquiries into the frog's species life, even though their outcome is knowledge about frogs. Of course, it is not impossible that something beneficial to humans will be learned in the course of these studies, but this is not the point of the "experiments." Rather they seem primarily to be exercises in overcoming our natural aversion to destruction for trivial or perhaps non-existent reasons, and in consequence, morally impermissible, whether carried out by schoolboys, or scientists in labs.[7]

Here, a distinction can generate a difference between animal research, even destructive research, for the sake of knowledge itself that is morally acceptable, and research that is not. If the object of inquiry is knowledge for its own sake, then it should be knowledge directed at an understanding, whether at the macro or micro level, of the animal's species life. To the extent that research diverges from this goal, the motives must seem questionable and insufficient to justify damage and destruction to animals.

What, finally, of animal research that is directed neither towards knowledge for its own sake, nor towards findings of great health-related benefit? Such research includes testing of cosmetics on animals for toxicity, for example, or testing the safety of recreational products. Is it acceptable to damage or destroy animals for the sake of research driven primarily by consumer concerns?

The line between this category of research and what we could more broadly call welfare-related research is not always clear. Suppose that airbags or seat belts could most effectively be tested with chimpanzees; although safer cars are a consumer-driven need, safer cars also greatly contribute to general welfare. Similarly, animals are routinely used to test the toxicity, and the capacity for eye irritation, of cleaners, detergents, and other household products. Such products serve more than a merely "cosmetic" purpose.

Even apart from such considerations, however, there are difficulties in separating out research that does and research that does not contribute to human welfare by looking merely to health concerns versus "entertainment" or "cosmetic" concerns, for entertainment and cosmetics can themselves contribute to human welfare. Human beings can legitimately desire to improve their appearance, and play, rest, and recreation play an essential part in maintaining a harmonious life. Food is both essential to health, but also contributes to sociality and rest. Research that contributes to these goals should not be thought of as merely trivial or pointless.

On the other hand, there is reason to question whether the Western world in general, and apart from considerations of animal experimentation and research, has become altogether too consumerist and desire driven. Many companies thrive primarily because of their ability to generate new desires, or desires for novelties that constitute no genuine improvement over what was already given (Clark, 1989; Barber, 2006). Criticism of this consumerist mentality is not new; but it is in this context that questions concerning adequate reasons for market-driven animal research should be addressed. To the extent that some such research turns out to be grounded in trivial or base reasons, this will be a result of a wider corruption of our social world, and not strictly linked to the issue of animal research at all. Much non-animal research—into useless gizmos and manipulative advertising strategies to generate desires for these gizmos—would stand equally condemned. Correspondingly, to the extent that the market, and the various forces driving the market, are responding to genuine human needs and legitimate desires, then even destructive research on animals seems permissible, and preferable to any other approach that would increase risk for human persons.

On the basis of these various criteria, it would appear that much of what is currently done using animals is morally permissible. I have abstracted in this chapter from questions concerning the legitimacy of state funding of such research; moreover, I have touched also upon issues that will be readdressed in Chapter 11 concerning the legitimacy of one's choices of how to focus one's inquiries, particularly as those inquiries form part of the structure of one's vocational commitments. But the general conclusion is clear: it is morally permissible and often morally obligatory to experiment on animals when this is necessary for human welfare, legitimate to experiment on animals for the sake of knowledge about the animals themselves, and often legitimate, subject to the findings of a larger cultural critique, to experiment on animals for the development of commercial products. At the same time, effort must be made to ensure that such experiments are not performed for base, trivial, or non-reasons, and that where possible, the integrity of nature, including animal nature, be accorded respect as the source of a great deal of what we find beautiful.

# 7 Coercion, Torture, Enhancement, and the Inviolability of the Person

Previous chapters of this book have been concerned with the nature of the human person, and person centered restrictions on biomedical and scientific inquiry. In Chapter 5, I argued that you and I are human animals. However, because of our personal nature, we are capable of acting for reasons, reasons identified as basic human goods, basic forms of human well-being and flourishing. In Chapter 2, I discussed two forms of integrity, bodily and personal. The normative importance of bodily integrity was reinforced through the discussion of our animal nature: because we are animals, attacks on our body are attacks on *us*. The nature and importance of personal integrity emerged in Chapter 2 from the recognition that our practical nature is complex, structured along a number of axes: emotion, reason, and will. I explored the normative implications of this recognition in Chapter 4 in the discussion of lying. Even Chapter 6, on animal research, was also about human persons. Animals, I argued, do not stand in a relation of community to human beings, for they do not share reasons—human goods—with us.

The various discussions of our nature—a nature that is animal, yet more than animal, given by the body yet formed and directed by practical reason—make possible now a discussion of two types of inquiry not usually addressed together. In this chapter, I assess the moral legitimacy of coercion, or force, as a tool of inquiry. This question moves us outside the domain of biomedical and scientific research; yet it is clearly continuous with the discussions of the previous chapters. I then turn to the question of human enhancement. Scientists, philosophers, and others have recently speculated about the possibility of changing human nature, whether through genetic enhancement, robot technology, or otherwise, and this has prompted moral reflection on the ethical permissibility of such changes. Since such change will not be possible save through much research, is inquiry into these techniques of enhancement morally permissible?

What both issues have in common is this: adequate answers to moral questions about these issues require an adequate understanding of the nature of the human person. It is for this reason that, having defended a number of claims about our nature, I now turn to these two vexed issues.

## TORTURE AND COERCION

Torture, force, and coercion can be used in non-inquiry-related contexts. Yet it is precisely insofar as it is part of the ethics of investigation that the morality of torture is an open question. No civilized country uses torture as a form of punishment, or to wreak vengeance on, or to instill fear in, its enemies.[1] It is only insofar as torture offers us the hope of important information that there is an important ethical question to be addressed.[2] The use of coercion, physical and otherwise, is also sometimes used by law enforcement officials in the context of attempting to get information about the suspect's possible criminal activity. This too falls within the scope of the ethics of inquiry.

The question of what constitutes torture, and whether it may be permissible under some circumstances, has become a more pressing issue recently. After the scandal at Abu Ghraib prison, in Iraq, questions were raised as to whether the activities there—putting prisoners on leashes, forcing them to remain naked, enforced masturbation, and so on—rose to the level of torture, or whether they were merely "abuse." Further questions were raised by the suggestion that these "abuses" may have been promoted by senior officials as necessary to attain crucial information in the war on the Iraqi insurgency. Policies involving torture or something like it seem to have been promoted at Guantanamo Bay; and the practice of rendition of terror suspects to countries with records of human rights abuses in interrogation has also come to light (Knight, 2005). Further, officials of the Bush administration carried on high-level discussions concerning whether the president was legally prohibited from authorizing the use of torture for interrogational purposes, as part of the war on terror (Feldman, 2005).

This has made more urgent the theoretical question of whether torture might be acceptable under certain rare but extreme circumstances. Some countries and persons have adopted an ambiguous position on these matters. The Israel Supreme Court, for example, ruled in 1999 that torture, and indeed any significant form of coercion as a tool of interrogation, was prohibited, even in so called "ticking bomb" cases. Yet it also cited the "traditional common-law defense of necessity," according to Alan Dershowitz, and "left open the possibility that a member of the security service who honestly believed that rough interrogation was the only means available to save lives in immanent danger could raise this defense" (Dershowitz, 2004, p. 263). Dershowitz himself has suggested that torture, since it is inevitably used as an instrument of interrogation, even by countries who entirely foreswear its use, should at least be legally regulated, so as to be used only in approved circumstances (Dershowitz, 2002, 2004).

Others have straightforwardly argued that coercion and torture are morally justified. The political commentator Cal Thomas has said, "The only way to protect ourselves is to extract information they might have by any means necessary. This war won't be won if we impose on ourselves restrictions that the terrorists do not impose on themselves" (Thomas, 2005, p. 19). Bush administration lawyers initially held that the Geneva convention did not apply to Al Qaeda suspects. They also adopted an extremely narrow definition of torture, requiring the intentional inflic-tion of pain "equivalent in intensity to the pain accompanying serious physical injury such as organ failure, impairment of bodily function, or even death."[3] The overall justification for adoption of such measures is the demands of national security. Such justifications are often straightfor-wardly consequentialist: if the stakes are high enough, and the good to be gained, or the evil to be avoided, serious enough, then torture might be justified.

From a more nuanced theoretical perspective, Michael Walzer and Jean Bethke Elshtain have also offered quasi-justifications for torture. Walzer writes that "dirty hands" are inevitable for any serious politician. Torture is always morally wrong, but in cases of necessity, an upright politician must accept the moral burden of dirty hands as part of his responsibility for the political good (Walzer, 1973). Elshtain takes a similar view, with the addition of the hope of Christian forgiveness. Envisaging a situation in which torture is required to save several hundred children from a bombing she writes:

> Ask yourself who you would want in a position of judgment at that point. A person of such stringent moral and legal rectitude that he or she would not consider torture because violating his or her conscience is the most morally serious thing a person can do? Or a person, aware of the stakes and the possible deaths of hundreds of children, who acts in the light of harsh necessity and orders the prisoner tortured? The irony, of course, is that the leader who demurs in the name of living up to a moral code we probably share with him, or her, becomes directly complicit in the deaths of hundreds of innocents. Parents, grandparents, and siblings of those children will probably curse his or her name, and they are right to do so. (Elshtain, 2004, p. 83)

Elshtain writes that the politician who authorizes the torture can subsequently "stand before God as a guilty person and seek forgiveness" (Elshtain, 2004, p. 83). So for Elshtain, as for Walzer, torture remains morally wrong, even when it is necessary, and when it is something that a moral agent *must* do.

These discussions raise several questions. What sorts of activities con-stitute torture, and, is it absolutely impermissible to torture other human persons, even when the obtaining of critical information is possible? What are the boundaries separating torture from other forms of "abuse" or "degrading treatment," and do these boundaries mark an important moral distinction? And, even when torture is morally impermissible, are there still circumstances in which one must dirty one's hands, or voluntarily stand guilty before God, as Walzer and Elshtain, respectively, suggest?

Such questions highlight the similarity between terror and torture. Certainly, terror and torture are impermissible if done for either wrongful or insufficiently serious motives. Thus, no one would justify torture or terror in service of wicked ends, such as Nazi domination, or of insignificant ends, such as to resolve a minor dispute over territory. But both terror and torture have their defenders when the stakes are high, and no other means seems available.

Terror and torture are further similar in that the restrictions on each seem rooted in the same concerns for the bodily life and health of human persons, which may not be directly attacked. Moral restrictions on terror bombing, for example, are a straightforward application of the norm against intentionally taking the life of non-attackers; the terrorist attempts to achieve his ends precisely through such an attack. He intends to achieve otherwise unattainable political ends through the threat, and carrying out of the threat, to kill non-attackers.

But our life is an organic, animal life. Attacks on our body are directly attacks on us. When you cut out my eye, or cut off my hand, you do not deprive me of something that is mine; rather, you damage me in your attack on my bodily integrity. So the general norm forbidding intentional killing of persons is reasonably extended to forbid intentional damage to the organic lives of persons.

This norm is part of the foundation of the restriction against torture. Cutting out an eye to induce a suspect to provide information is an intentional harm to a person, and morally wrong. Infliction of such damage to extract information is therefore morally wrong. But to focus exclusively on the threat to physical damage seems too narrow. The human person is a very special sort of organism, for it has a complex mental life, a complex moral life, and a complex spiritual life, all potentially, and normatively to be unified as the life of one person.

It is true that chopping off a limb imperils the physical unity of the human person, but so do the infliction of serious physical pain, infliction of social humiliation, and the frustration of moral and spiritual needs, imperil the overall unity of the person as the unique sort of organism it is. The threat and infliction of serious pain can compromise our ability to think and act reasonably; being treated like animals or slaves compromises our personal dignity; and being coerced to act or speak in ways contrary to our commitments threatens our moral integrity. All of these forms of behavior towards others, as part of an attempt to punish, or to obtain information, or assistance, or a conversion, are, like deliberately chopping off an arm, or blinding, morally wrong.

Yet this does not mean that the infliction of pain as such is morally impermissible. Rather than being an intrinsic evil, pain serves an important function in the life of all organisms. Through pain an organism is alerted to threats to its well-being. That pain can legitimately serve this instrumental role in the natural order of things suggests that it might also play a legitimate role in the moral order. Pain is used by parents as a deterrent on small children, as when a child is spanked after running into the street, or as punishment for misbehavior. Pain is used by some ascetics to discipline the body. A slap might be administered to someone suffering hysterics, or from inattention in a serious situation.

Similarly, a slap or some other administration of pain might be used in an interrogation to calm, or restrain, or focus a suspect. Perhaps it could even be used to provide a disincentive for silence. The infliction of pain itself for such purposes is not torture. Rather, just as the cutting off of an arm to induce a suspect to talk is an intentional damaging of a person's bodily integrity, and thus morally wrong, the infliction of pain in interrogation is torture, and wrong, when it is part of an intentional effort to damage an agent's physical or mental integrity, by bringing them to a point of such pain that they are incapable of physically functioning, or of making their own decisions, or of maintaining freely, or freely changing, their moral (or immoral) commitments. *Torture* through the use of pain, like torture through the use of amputation, or social or religious humiliation, is an attempt to "break down" the person, intentionally to inflict harm on the person. This is what is always morally impermissible, whatever the ends, and what distinguishes the legitimate infliction of pain from torture.[4]

Torture, then, should be defined as the deliberate attempt to do damage to the integrity, broadly construed, of another human being for some further purpose.[5] Such purposes include punishment, deterrence, and sadism. But torture also includes the deliberate attempt to damage the integrity of a human being for the purpose of extracting or obtaining important information. What makes something torture is thus not the end, but the means, a means that is by its nature contrary to a basic human good.

Torture so defined is wrong even when the torture victim is himself an evildoer or a threat. But it is important to distinguish between the threat utilized in torture and the sort of force that it is permissible for law enforcement officers or military combatants to use. Law enforcement officers, by the arguments earlier in this book, are accorded more leeway in the use of force to restrain or subdue, not because they are permitted directly to harm other agents, but because they are charged with protecting the common good, and can, therefore, accept more significant side effects without unfairness than can ordinary civilians. So force that would be unacceptable for a civilian to use, force that causes damage, and even, on occasion, death, can acceptably be used by law enforcement officials or military personnel.

This justification does not require, however, that such agents be permitted deliberately to kill or harm to achieve some end. No doubt most police officers and military personnel are taught precisely to kill those whom they see as a threat. But it seems that if this is accepted as normative, then indeed torture *will* be morally acceptable under certain circumstances for those publicly authorized.

However, while the police officer certainly uses force, and thus frequently causes harm, or damage, in subduing the subject, and may fire at, and thus harm, someone committing an armed robbery or some other dangerous crime, still, if acting appropriately, he ought not to harm to subdue his subject, or intentionally kill to stop the robbery. The use of force, even lethal force, is applied to restrain or stop, while injury or even death is sometimes accepted as a side effect. Similarly, the police officer might inflict pain in a number of permissible ways: as a side effect of the use of force, or as a means of bringing the suspect to attention or compliance. Even the use of a stun gun seems morally permissible as an instance of this, and preferable to the infliction of harm.

By contrast with the permissible uses of force and pain, in torturing another the intention is precisely to inflict or threaten damage to the integrity, whether physical, moral, mental, or spiritual, of the subject. Damage to the well-being of the subject is the means chosen to bring about the desired end, and thus the action is ruled out morally as involving an illicit intention. If this analysis is correct, there are never any circumstances under which torture may be morally used.

This seems adequately to distinguish the boundaries separating torture from legitimate coercion and use of force or pain. Violent suspects may be physically restrained, and may be physically forced to remain in place while answering questions. Pain may be used instrumentally for limited objectives, including as an inducement for some forms of behavior. But any attempt to induce them to answer questions by threats to their integrity, broadly understood, is illicit.

This boundary would have significant consequences if strictly applied. For it seems plausible that prisoners, military and criminal, are frequently forced to endure physically or mentally threatening circumstances to induce them to talk. Thus dogs are brought into the interrogation room to help question Middle Eastern subjects who are afraid of dogs, or bogus threats are made concerning the well-being of a subject's family members, or subjects are made to remain sleepless, or unclothed, or hot or cold, or are hit or yelled at, not because such measures are necessary to restrain them, or physically place them in the interrogation room, or even to bring them to attention, but to induce them to answer questions by breaking down their resistance. Many of these techniques are not considered "torture." Some, such as sleep deprivation, are defended as ordinary. But all are immoral ways of prosecuting an investigation, even in emergency or ticking-time-bomb situations, if they are intended as part of a project to break down the person, to disrupt their unity as a physical, mental, and spiritual being.

Still, are they all forms of *torture*? In the memo for Alberto Gonzales cited above, Jay Bybee stresses that under the Convention Against Torture and Other Cruel, Inhuman and Degrading Treatment or Punishment statute, torture is constituted only by "acts inflicting, and that are specifically intended to inflict, sever pain or suffering, whether mental or physical." Bybee then concludes that "certain acts may be cruel, inhuman, or degrading, but still not produce pain and suffering of the requisite intensity to fall with . . . [the] proscription against torture" (Bybee, 2002).

Bybee's intent here seems to be to legitimate the use of "cruel, inhuman or degrading" tactics that fall short of torture, since such acts are not criminally liable under the relevant statute. And there does seem to be an intuitive distinction to be drawn between taking humiliating photographs or placing women's underwear over the head of a detainee, and inserting needles under the fingertips, or shocking the genitals. My account above, one might object, fails to respect that difference.[6]

The objection asserts a difference in kind between torture and these other forms of abuse. The difference in kind is supposed to explain our differences in attitude towards "mere abuse" and torture. But such a difference in kind is unnecessary. To say that torture is a greater wrong in this context than abuse requires attention to the relationship between a norm and the human goods that the norm protects. Various norms protect aspects of human persons by restricting certain kinds of actions or attitudes that would be destructive of those goods, or enjoining actions or attitudes that would promote the good: the injunction against murder protects the good of life in one way, while the positive injunction to eat well and get some exercise protects it in another. But where the same good and the same norm are concerned, one violation may be more destructive of the good than another. So, to drink to excess on occasion violates norms regarding the proper treatment of one's bodily and mental health; to become a heroin addict violates the same norms, but is vastly more destructive to the goods those norms protect. In consequence, heroin addiction is a greater failure of responsibility than alcoholism.

The relationship between torture for interrogative purposes and abusive, inhumane, degrading, and cruel treatment for the same purposes is similar. Torture is morally worse than abusive treatment, not because it violates a different moral norm but because the damage to human goods done by the torturer is more extreme. But both the torturer and the interrogator who merely abuses his prisoners violate the same norm, the norm against directly attacking the integrity—physical, moral, mental, or spiritual—of another human being. In consequence, it is no justification for an attack on the integrity of a subject to plead that the attack in question fell below the standard of torture.

Finally, we must address the Walzer–Elshtain view. If torture and even "abuse" are morally forbidden, does that mean that any particular agent, when faced with the "need" for torture, must therefore refuse to engage in torture? Would it not be better for such an agent to accept dirty hands, or commit a grave sin, knowing that he can then stand before God in contrition, asking for forgiveness?

Some confusions must be cleared up. The first is that the agent who opts not to torture does so from some extreme form of moralistic or legalistic rule following, and a concern not to sully his purity. Agents do have such concerns; but such concerns are second-order concerns that depend upon first-order moral reasons not to torture. It is because torture involves an intentional destruction of human goods that it is wrong, and *this* is why the "pure" agent refuses to torture. It is because torture is independently wrong that an agent's moral integrity is compromised by choosing to torture.

The second is that the agent who does not torture "becomes directly complicit in the deaths of hundreds of innocents" (Elshtain, 2004, p. 83). The agent who does not torture is in no way "complicit" in the deaths of the innocents. He has made no choice to kill them, nor has he established the conditions under which they are at risk. Moreover, the one sufficient condition for their lives being saved—that the suspect talks—remains entirely in the hands of the suspect: he is free to speak, and save their lives. When such a choice remains entirely in the hands of the suspect, it is not appropriate to speak to the non-torturing agent as the one responsible for the deaths of the children.

Finally, it is necessary to question the coherence of the sin now, repent later strategy. This requires the following oddly disjointed form of consciousness: the torturer must intend both knowingly to do wrong and to repent for that wrongdoing. But one cannot genuinely intend to repent unless one already meets the conditions morally necessary for such repentance: unwillingness to repeat the act, and regret at having ever done it. But these conditions, if truly met, would result in not doing the act at all. There is a great difference between feeling revulsion, even moral revulsion, at what one is doing, and the condition of repentance. One can be disgusted, even morally disgusted at what one is doing, but one cannot be repenting of what one is doing as one does it.

When mistakes about complicity in the deaths of innocents have been cleared up, Walzer's "dirty hands" view also suffers, for the dirty-hands view must assume that if the agent does not torture the suspect, he is then guilty of a moral wrong, just as the torturer is guilty. That is, the dirty-hands view must assume that the politician presented with the need for torture is in a genuine moral dilemma: damned if he does and damned if he does not.[7] Walzer's particular avenue to this conclusion runs through a premise about the responsibility of a political leader for the good of the polity. Political leaders and governments do, as I will argue in the next chapter, have a responsibility to promote the common good. But if the non-torturing agent is not "complicit" in the deaths caused by the terrorist, then it is difficult to see how his adherence to the norms of morality can also be described as dirtying his hands; his responsibility to the common good does not take precedence over, but is rather governed by the basic goods and the norms of morality. So again, torture is wrong for this agent, *and* is something he must not do.

In the end, there are really only two options regarding the morality of torture for interrogational purposes; for if torture is something that must be done, then its performance is something morally demanded, rather than morally wrong, but somehow still necessary. And if it is morally demanded, then this is because of straightforwardly consequentialist calculations about the demands of the greater good. But consequentialism has been rejected, in this book, in favor of a basic goods view, a view that does, unlike consequentialism, generate both options and constraints. That an absolute rejection of torture is one of the constraints of a morality based on the goods might seem an unfortunate lesson. But it is neither incoherent, nor a mark of fetishistic rule following; the norm is rooted in the nature of the human being, and the relationship between that nature and the basic goods. It is fundamentally humanist.

## HUMAN ENHANCEMENT ISSUES AND THE TECHNOLOGIES OF THE FUTURE

The second topic of this chapter concerns inquiry into human enhancement and changes in human nature. Various types of research—in genetics, nanotechnology, artificial intelligence, and robotics (GNR)[8], for example—are currently under way to provide enhancements to that nature. Some such technologies raise questions that go beyond the issue of enhancement; research into military technologies, for example, has always raised significant moral questions. However, I will primarily focus the relationship between such technologies and human nature, and only briefly say something about the wider range of moral questions regarding technological inquiry.

In a way, human enhancement constitutes a separate issue in bioethics, and not one in the ethics of inquiry: questions about the permissible and the impermissible in regards to human enhancement may be taken up directly: is this or that form of enhancement morally acceptable or not? For example, it is not an issue of the ethics of inquiry whether it is morally permissible for a high school student to take Ritalin for the sake of improved performance on his SATs, or whether embryo screening to prevent some genetic disease is acceptable.

This is true generally of almost every question in enhancement ethics. Each type of enhancement, potential or actual, may be taken up one by one and assessed: Is it permissible to introduce foreign DNA into human genes to promote or discourage this or that trait? Is human growth hormone acceptably administered to the merely short (Fukuyama, 2002; The President's Council on Bioethics, 2003; Elliott, 2003; Sandel, 2004)? But the ethics of human enhancement intersects with the ethics of inquiry precisely because many of the conceivable types of enhancement are not at present possible: the relevant knowledge must be obtained, the relevant techniques developed. Here the ethics of inquiry is implicated, as well as the ire of those who think that ethical (or political) considerations should play no role in scientific research.

The tension is illustrated in a disagreement between Bill Joy, one of the chief architects of Sun Microsystems, and James Watson, co-discoverer of the double helix structure of DNA with Francis Crick. As Jon Gertner wrote in the *New York Times Magazine,*

> Joy had singled out James Watson . . . as a scientist who rejects Joy's arguments for weighing benefits against bad outcomes. Watson has indeed said that it makes little sense to stop research on account of unspecified risks or "evil." In the name of science and discovery, he says, we are ethically obliged to go forward. "That position has to be wrong," Joy insists. In his view, we are ethically bound to slow down. (Gertner, 2004, p. 36; see also Joy, 2000)

We have already seen that Watson's position taken on its own makes little sense: research is no different from any other human activity in being subject to moral norms. But there are special difficulties in this area, worries on the part of those wary of new biotechnical and enhancement research, and responses on the part of the defenders of research.

On the objectors' side, two sorts of worries predominate. The first is concern for unforeseen consequences, and malevolent uses of new technologies. Scientists in the lab might design a new virus, a new weapons system, or a new agricultural technology, the consequences of which, in each case, could be disastrous, whether by accident or human design. A new virus might cause the spread of a deadly plague; a new weapon might be stolen by terrorists; a new technology might have unforeseen but highly destructive consequences for the environment. Human enhancements might contribute to increased social stratification, an "arms race" for intelligence, or an overwhelmingly elderly or insufficiently reproductive population, or might cause considerable shifts in social structures such as the family.

The second, and for this chapter more significant, objection concerns the nature of the human being, and what new discoveries and techniques could portend for that nature. Francis Fukuyama, a former member of the President's Council on Bioethics, has titled a recent book *Our Posthuman Future,* indicating his worry that the fruit of such research will be a change in our very humanity, a worry shared by his fellow Council member Charles Krauthammer (Fukuyama, 2002; Krauthammer, 2001). Such metamorphosis must be considered a future contingent at best, yet present-day research, on such views, brings us closer to the possibility minute by minute.

Defenders of research may take the indefensible position of James Watson, but even a more moderate defender of current research has several other possible responses.

The first is to point out that for almost every ill consequence that can be imagined from any *particular* discovery, one can usually imagine a corresponding benefit: designed viruses might help us to design vaccines, new weapons might make the world safer, and new agricultural technologies might end world hunger. In fact, much of the research of concern to objectors such as Joy or Fukuyama is directed to good ends; so the worries are essentially no different from the worries that we should have about misuse of the technologies we already possess, and there is, therefore, no more reason to worry about unforeseen consequences in the arena of developing technologies than in any other field.

Second, the defender can point out that in addition to the unknown negative side effects and the hoped for benefits, there may also be unknown positive side effects. If it is legitimate to argue against utilitarianism on the ground that we simply cannot know the long-range consequences of our actions, then it is illegitimate to focus on largely unknown negative consequences of the new technologies. So someone might have argued, at the turn of the twentieth century, that the automobile would be responsible for untold numbers of deaths, as it has been; but it is probably impossible to calculate all the ways in which the automobile has been of benefit in addition to those ways that would have been more or less predictable at the time of its invention.

Defenders of the new technologies can also respond to the Fukuyama–Krauthammer sorts of concerns about changes in human nature head on. More radically, they can embrace the possibilities of significant changes in human nature, viewing it as one more step of Darwinian evolution, though in this case, a step deliberately brought about (Silver, 1997). In its most radical embodiment, this proposal is part of the philosophic, social, and political agenda of the so-called "transhumanist" movement (Ramez, 2004).[9]

This response must be addressed on its own terms: Is it genuinely worrisome and morally problematic to contemplate significant changes to human nature? Could we not improve on human nature as we know it, and if so, might we not have an obligation to pursue such a possibility? Moreover, there are possible goals that fall short of radical change in nature, but that would involve some change that would seem inevitably to be for the better: if we could eliminate genetic tendencies to crime, or to alcoholism, for example, we would not have changed human nature as such, but we would certainly have radically altered its parameters, and some would argue, for the better.

This last question raises the second avenue of response, less radical than the wholehearted embracing of the opportunity to change human nature. There is a relatively murky line between enhancing our nature and changing it. Suppose that it becomes possible to download information into mechanically enhanced brains, so as to lead to increased memory, or superior intelligence, or even virtual experiences. Would such a circumstance constitute a change in human nature? If so, how would it differ from the use of prosthetic limbs, or even contact lenses? Even if we take our nature as a moral given, defenders of the new technologies could say, this still leaves a considerable amount of room for experimentation, ultimately with a view to introducing significant, but not nature-altering, changes in our identity.

Two points about our human nature are of special importance in addressing these questions. The first is that our nature is in part a practical nature: it is a nature specified by our practical possibilities, in particular, by those basic goods that constitute the horizon of our possible flourishing. This practical nature in turn has a dual aspect. On the one hand, our good, though of vast depth and breadth, is not infinitely plastic. Although any particular human good—life, knowledge, play, for example—each offers a vast number of ways of pursuit, promotion, and participation, nevertheless, the core list of the basic goods is finite, relatively small, and permanent. But the status of life as a basic human good is inflexibly essential to our nature.

The other aspect of our practical nature, beyond the essentially fixed horizon of possibilities, is that these possibilities must be brought about for us by our own action. It is true that some of these goods are beneficial for us regardless of our choices. We are simply better off for being alive, whether we have deliberately acted to sustain or promote our life, or not. Nonetheless, our *given* nature is largely one of capacities, which require our action to be brought to actuality. Our life must be a life of deliberation, choice, commitment, and action if it is to be a good and flourishing life. We do not want our lives to be lives of merely passive benefit, of induced experiences, but lives of action, lives of which we are agents and authors.

Thus the first two-sided point: our nature is practical, involving a necessary relation to a finite set of goods, and requiring action on our part to participate in those goods and flourish as selves. The second point, familiar now from Chapter 5, is that our nature is also an animal nature: we are not human spirits, essentially disembodied, but are human animals, notable for being spiritual animals in a way that other mammals are not, but animals nonetheless. This aspect of our being is tied up with the first in a wide variety of ways: it is our bodily life that is a good in itself, not simply the life of our soul. It is through our senses that we come to know, through our physical communion with others that we play, marry, raise children, and so on. Art is experienced through our bodily senses; integrity is a matter not just of doing, thinking, or willing one thing, but of feeling in accordance with the dictates of reason. In short, our animal nature pervades our practical nature, and vice versa.

In consequence, there are three ways in which enhancement and other technologies could threaten us in respect of our nature. They could threaten the relationship between us and the finite set of goods that offer our fulfillment as human persons; they could threaten our ability practically to pursue those goods, and to participate in those goods through our own creative activity; and they could show disregard for the particularity of our animal nature, a disregard that would likely have consequences in regard to our relationship to the goods as well.

Consider, for example, research aimed at making us asexually reproductive. Current technologies such as in vitro fertilization, and, to a greater extent, reproductive cloning, already have brought us part of the way towards such a state of affairs. The aim of such research is to remove from the sphere of sex, marriage, and family the act of creation of children, and indeed, to remove it from any necessarily interpersonal context at all (Silver, 1997). Forward-looking thinkers such as Ray Kurzweil predict that within 100 years, our species will no longer reproduce sexually; sex will become recreational, and indeed, mostly virtual. Procreation, meanwhile, will be essentially medical/technical.

Now, although such a situation might be taken by some to be a good thing, it is a different and a lesser thing than traditional procreation in the context of a marriage, for two reasons. First, sex and marriage are other-related, interpersonal realities. Our human fulfillment and well-being essentially require relation to others, particularly in such goods as friendship, marriage, and family. To narrow our reproductive world in this self-focused way, by becoming asexual procreators, is reductive of our possibilities for well-being, by removing us from those others with whom we would have had the potential for interpersonal communion. Cloning is akin to mastur-bating for children, a lonely and solipsistic business; a world in which all reproduction had become disjoined from sex would be similarly depersonal-ized, as Kurzweil's visions of virtual sex between avatars makes clear.

Second, this reduction is especially apparent in the relationship to the created children that are the fruit of a technical process, rather than of a loving, human relationship. Children created through technical means are ultimately, in the eyes of their creators, artifacts, products of their will and design, rather than persons. Parents-to-be hope for children, rather than plan them (they can, of course, plan *for* them); but cloners will be the design-ers and manufacturers of their children. Cloning parents, by adopting this relationship, alienate themselves from their children. So the relationship of cloners to their children is stunted, leaving again a lesser scope in the rela-tionship to basic goods. Once more, what would be true in cloning would be true on a greater scale were the envisaged changes in human reproduction to become part of our nature.

Such considerations form the groundwork for argument against research aimed at limiting our species' dependence on sexual reproduction; the state of affairs envisaged in such research is one intrinsically limiting of the goods available to us in action. And in so limiting these goods, the envisaged future, in which reproduction is severed from sex, constitutes a genuine threat to our well-being, a threat most vividly seen in imaginative thought experiments such as that of Aldous Huxley, in *Brave New World*.

A related threat to one of the basic goods is also welcomed as desirable by some futurists such as Kurzweil. An important fact about both our practical and our animal natures is the separateness of persons. No person is a part of another, and there are definite limits to the extent that persons can share in experiences, choices, and actions. On the one hand, such boundaries limit the extent to which certain goods are available to us, such as friendship. Yet, on the other hand, these boundaries are also necessary for that good. For in the absence of boundaries, it is impossible to make the choices to share, to communicate, to give of one's self to another (and to withhold from yet others) that are necessary to make relationships of any sort possible.

Kurzweil anticipates a merger of biological and technological intelligence that will essentially break down such barriers, which, he says

> . . . are just a limitation of biological intelligence. The unbridgeable distinction of biological intelligence is not a plus. "Silicon" intelligence can have it both ways. Computers don't need to pool their intelligence and resources. They can remain "individuals" if they wish. Silicon intelligence can even have it both ways by merging and retaining individuality—at the same time. As humans, we try to merge with others also, but our ability to accomplish this is fleeting. (Kurzweil, 2005, p. 376)

The merger of biological and silicon intelligences that Kurzweil foresees here seems to threaten the conditions under which friendship is possible, conditions that might seem like "limitations," but are essential to the basic human good of friendship.

The second threat mentioned above was also to our practical nature, namely, the threat against our abilities to participate actively in our own well-being, in the making of our own lives and choices. Various enhancers currently pose just such a risk when taken, not to alleviate a condition that itself poses a threat to our activity, but to substitute for the labor of making ourselves more disciplined, harder working, more in control of our emotions, more capable in our relationships to others, more able to hit a baseball or run a race, and so on. The use of Prozac and Ritalin, not by those who are sick, but by those who simply wish to perform better, or the use of steroids by athletes, among other things, makes us increasingly passive in our pursuit of well-being (PCB, 2003, Chapters 3 and 6). Robert Nozick's famous "experience machine" thought experiment brings out just such a threat.

Nozick's thought experiment centers on a machine that promises the experience of a fully meaningful life (Nozick, 1968, p. 43). Plug yourself into the machine, and you will be provided the experience of creating great art, pursuing valuable relationships, and thinking great thoughts. Nozick's intuition, shared by most philosophers, is that plugging in would be undesirable, regardless of what form of life we would therein experience. For ultimately, what the machine offers, with regard to any of the various aspects of a meaningful life, is mere appearances; but what human beings desire, what matters, is what is available to us through genuine action.

What characterizes the difference between the experience of some activity and the reality? Some capacity of the human being must be actualized in genuine action that is not actualized in the mere experience of performing that action. In the experience machine, what is missing is any act of the will. The experience machine renders us utterly passive. We are unable to act, while the machine acts on us. Since there is an experiential aspect even to acts of the will, the machine will, in the course of providing us with the experience of a meaningful life, provide us also with the experience of genuine activity. But confronted with the experience machine, we distinguish between willing something and the experience of willing something, performing an action, and experiencing that performance. What emerges is that experience that is not grounded in the reality provides only the illusion of the truly desired reality (Finnis, 1984, pp. 37–42; Tollefsen, 2003a).

The experience machine should help us to get a handle on what is disturbing about the use of Ritalin or Prozac in the healthy. To the extent that, as Nozick's thought example revealed, our active self-constitution is what we want, rather than merely external satisfactions, or successes, use of drugs and other enhancers to accomplish what we should accomplish through our own labor is actually unenhancing.

Two caveats are necessary. First, many of these enhancers have other legitimate uses—to treat depression or hyperactivity, or to provide therapy to those suffering from muscular disorders, for example. Here is a good instance of a case in which, although potential negative side effects exist, and might have been foreseen, the fact of those negative side effects alone does not show that the research that brought about these developments should never have been carried out. But, by the same token, if there are drugs or techniques being developed that serve no such therapeutic purpose, but would only serve simultaneously to bring us greater success in some area, while making us more passive in respect of that success, then research into these types of enhancement seems threatening to our actively practical nature.

An obvious objection to this raises the second caveat. Ritalin, Prozac, memory aids, steroids, and so on are far from removing every aspect of our control of our lives, even in some limited domain, from us. Although the healthy student who takes Ritalin to do better on his exams does both provide himself with an advantage and borrow that advantage from an external source, it is still the case that whatever knowledge is displayed by the student is largely his own. He has not completely surrendered his active participation in his own self-constitution.

There are, however, aspirations on the part of some to more or less completely bypass such activity. It will be helpful to divide the discussion at this point into a consideration of two different sorts of goods in relation to which we might become artificially passive.

Consider, for example, drugs or surgical techniques that could be developed that would make us professional-class athletes, without the need for workouts, diets, and weight-lifting, or memory downloads that would provide us with knowledge of places we had never been, or fields we had never studied. Agents who took such drugs or received such implants would in fact be healthier and more knowledgeable than those who had not. So, such agents would indeed be better off than their less advantaged peers. Life and knowledge are substantive goods—our participation in such goods contributes to our well-being even apart from our having chosen so to participate.

By contrast, consider the good of friendship. Suppose that technologies became available that would create in two people the belief that they were friends, or would virtually create a world for an agent in which she was happily married. Such technologies are variants on Nozick's experience machine. Similar technologies would enable us to download virtues, or even biographies, constructed according to our desires. If we wished to be braver or more temperate, we could download a character change, becoming virtuous without pain; who could object to such a manner of becoming better? Perhaps we dislike not simply our character, but the entire life that has brought it to be as it is. We could then download a new identity, in the so-called narrative sense, a new story-history about ourselves that we would now take to be real. Or perhaps we are unhappy with our integrity: our feelings, choices, and reasons for action might often fail to cohere. Reconfiguration of our identity might solve precisely this problem (Kurzweil, 1999, 2005).

Such scenarios seem farfetched. But they are variations of the images provided by some proponents of new genetic technologies to rid the world of crime by genetically making all children "good," or more social and altruistic, less aggressive and self-centered. And while there seems little reason to think such drugs, techniques, and so on are around the corner, there is certainly research oriented to the discovery of precisely these sorts of technologies, techniques, drugs, and so on. Perhaps such research is a colossal waste of time; is it also morally suspect?

What we should note about goods such as friendship, virtue, good character, integrity, and the like is that all require, in order to be genuine, acts of the will. True friendship cannot be downloaded, uploaded, or installed, for true friends make mutual commitments to one another's goods, and no genuine commitment can be made by anyone except the agents in question. Two people can be forced to marry, but they can never be made to love one another. So unlike the cases involving goods like knowledge or health, when techniques or drugs become available that will make us more virtuous, that will create virtual friends, that will eliminate crime, that will create new biographies for us, and so on, these techniques will in no sense make us better off with respect to the goods being sought. They will bypass those goods altogether by removing a necessary condition for their reality, human choices, and commitments.

Any such "enhancement" thus poses a very serious threat to our well-being, and to our practical nature. Nor do there seem to be any legitimate uses of such technologies that would not involve exactly the same "moral bypass," a side run round our ability practically to constitute our own selves. Such technologies would therefore, I conclude, be morally wrong. So all research aimed at discovering ways to download character traits, biographies, or to genetically eliminate crime or hostility, insofar as these are not unwilled consequences of pathologies, should likewise be viewed as morally misguided. The prospect of a world in which everyone acts morally is a promising prospect only if it is genuinely a world in which everyone acts.

What, though, about the substantive goods, which really do make us better off even when we participate in them through no choice of our own? Here too we should see a significant value to our own self-constituting activity. Although it is good to be healthy, or knowledgeable, whether we have actively pursued health or knowledge or not, it is more desirable to have become healthy, or knowledgeable through our own activity. Health and knowledge do not simply benefit us in the obvious way, namely by making us healthy and knowledgeable, they also help to define who we are. The body-builder or long-distance trainer has defined herself in a certain way as a healthy person; the philosopher has similarly defined herself as a seeker of wisdom. Such self-definition as a person for whom one or another of the goods are significant is possible only because we choose, actively, to pursue these goods, to cultivate them, and own our participation in them. All this would be lost if there were a pill for bodily strength, or wisdom, or ability.

Here, though, we can see possible therapeutic uses to drugs or surgical techniques aimed at health or perhaps knowledge. Bodies and minds grow ill and decay, and some of this sickness and decay is premature. It is reasonable to hope for cures for muscle wastage or Alzheimer's, but critical to remember the importance of self-constitution even here. So while research in such areas cannot be ruled out altogether, there must be concern for the uses to which new enhancers are put, and a determination to steer research as much as possible to the genuinely therapeutic. As a general rule, I would suggest, such research stays on safer ground insofar as it is concerned with the protection and restoration of our *capacities,* rather than with providing us directly with that which someone with functioning capacities and an active will could achieve.

Finally, what of changes to our bodily existence? Can lines be drawn here to protect our animal identity? Two points should be clear. First, some changes in our bodies would be such as to rupture our relationship to certain basic goods. So if, pursuant to the goal of making us asexually reproductive, changes were systematically introduced in the human body to make us no longer differentiated sexually as male and female, this would radically rupture our relationship to the goods of marriage and procreation. Or, suppose that our bodily senses were gradually eliminated in favor of computer navigation systems implanted in our brain. This might increase our ability to respond in common in certain situations, for example, among soldiers in war.[10] But would this also radically diminish our capacity for enjoyment of the arts of music or painting? To sacrifice these capacities for new abilities of a purely instrumental value would seem a violation of the goods of the person.

Second, some bodily changes could no doubt make it more difficult for us to be self-constituting agents. While the ability to make choices is not a bodily-based ability—no mere animal could make choices, but only a spiritual animal—it is an ability deeply conditioned by the existence and experience of our animal body. Changes in the brain, or perhaps even other parts of the body, might erode this necessary condition of freedom and reason and render us less able to act autonomously, and in certain respects, in a more merely animal manner. Imagine a change that made us *more* susceptible to physical pleasure than we are already. Such a change might be considered attractive in our hedonistic society. But such a change would make temperate choices more difficult, and would reduce our scope for truly human action.

But these threats—to our relationship to certain goods, and to our ability to judge and choose—I would argue, are the *only* real threats to our human identity. Insofar as bodily changes could be brought about that would not negatively bear on either our relationship to the basic goods, or our ability to actively pursue them, such changes would not constitute *any* genuine change in human nature. For our human nature is determined by our being animals for whom *this* precise list of goods is constitutive of well-being, which well-being can be pursued in action following free and deliberate choice. So long as we remain animals, benefited by these goods, and capable of constituting our selves through the pursuit of these goods, we remain the same species.

Suppose that, not by artificial means, but by the pressures of evolution, we grew a third leg. Would this constitute a change in human nature? It would not. Nor would the development of some new organ, or the enhancement of some organ, in such a way as to radically change our physical abilities: if we grew gills, or something analogous, and were able to stay underwater for hours at a stretch, this would not constitute a change in our nature. Moreover, some such changes might genuinely result in new opportunities to pursue human goods in creative ways.

If natural selection could change us without essentially changing our natures, would it therefore be morally permissible to deliberately bring about such changes in our animal bodies? Is research into at least some such possibilities morally permissible precisely because it would not be impermissible to utilize the fruits of such research? Such research might, within certain bounds, be acceptable. And the boundaries are those already established in this book: no research that involves damage or destruction to human persons, including human embryos; no research oriented towards drugs or techniques that would change our essential relationship to the finite set of basic goods put forth in Chapter 1, or that would reduce our ability actively to participate in those goods. And of course, no research that would violate any of the principles put forth in Chapter 2, requiring, for example, informed consent, or that would otherwise be considered irresponsible research. These boundaries might, or they might not, constitute such a considerable hedge around research into changes in our animal bodies.

It is worth noting, however, that some, at least, of the research that is envisaged as necessary to make possible enhancements to human nature, will require experimentation on human embryos. Of the three planks of the predicted revolution in human nature, genetics certainly, and possibly both nanotechnology and robotics, will be wholly successful only if their integration into our current biological existence is furthered by knowledge primarily available through human embryonic research. But if we are human beings, who begin as embryos, then such research, much of which is destructive of the embryo, and all of which, clearly, takes place without the embryo's consent, is immoral.

This moral boundary, however, is contingent; it might well become possible to rely on computer models and animal experimentation to obtain the knowledge we seek, without the necessity of invasive and destructive embryo experimentation. But for the moment, the boundary seems such an obstacle to research into changes to our animal bodies that this sort of research should be considered morally impossible.

There is one final principle in need of articulation in this context, but of wider application, the so-called Precautionary Principle. According to this principle, it is incumbent upon those engaged in new research into, e.g., biotechnology, and also upon those charged with regulating such research and subsequent development, to be safe rather than sorry. The presumption is *against* the safety of new technologies, such that their safety must be proved before they can be used. This principle corresponds to the final type of objection that I mentioned at the beginning of the discussion of enhancement, namely, the objection from possible bad consequences.

This principle draws our attention to what should be an obvious set of normative considerations for anything that we do: we must sufficiently consider the consequences of our actions to ensure that we do not bring about great evils by accident, through carelessness, or through lack of consideration of the natural proclivities of human beings. So the principle and the concerns underlying it are of wider application than simply to enhancement issues, and this is why I close this chapter with a brief discussion of it.

Some moral wrongs come about, not through intention and design, but because of inattention, disregard, and recklessness. The mountain climber who leads his charges up the slopes despite evidence of a coming storm does not intend their harm, but can be blamed for failing to care enough for their well-being to recognize obvious threats to it. Similarly, the sloppy mountain climber risks his life and the life of others, again, not intentionally, but through lack of due concern. And only a fool, seemingly, would lead a group to the summit of a mountain if he was aware that they were each of them in a high-stakes competition to get to the top first, and that in the past, under similar circumstances, some of these climbers had deliberately neglected aid to other climbers, or in other ways obstructed them. Add to these considerations the fact that thin air at the highest elevations makes reasonable decisions all the more difficult, and you have good reason for thinking that the climber who leads such a group is failing to consider, or simply ignoring, some obvious facts about human nature (Krakauer, 1999).

Similarly, scientists who work on toxic substances, or infectious agents, or genetic alterations of crops or organisms, or military weaponry, whether biological, chemical, or nuclear, and those who oversee such scientists, all have a variety of responsibilities with respect to general human safety and well-being. If a lethal virus is not properly cared for and "escapes" the lab, or if a genetically modified crop overruns various other species, or eventually is found to cause disease in humans, or if a weapon system of incredible destructive capacity is invented, then we may ask whether scientists and their overseers have taken sufficient care, and anticipated adequately the human condition, in their work. May the scientists who worked on the nuclear bomb be entirely absolved from working to create a weapon that arguably may never be (and has never been) ethically used, simply because the decision to use it was not theirs? It seems not (Douglas, 2003).

Nor is it a compelling argument to suggest that if scientist X does not develop such and such, then scientist Y will, at any rate. My concern in this book is with the context of individual and group decisions regarding inquiry, and our responsibility in such decisions is to ourselves do the right thing; and then, no doubt, make sure that no one else is doing some very wrong thing. That someone else *might* do something immorally dangerous is not a reason for me to do it, but it might be a good reason to attempt to stop the other fellow.

Such a concern with due care for the consequences is a principle of the ethics of inquiry that is somewhat at the border of the external and internal ethics of inquiry. All human action requires due care for the consequences, including, in many cases, the consequences that will result from the expectable behaviors of others. But it is also a matter of concern to the inquirer herself, considered as an inquirer, that her work be "foursquare and beyond reproach." Scientific, and other systematic knowledge, is a great good intrinsically and instrumentally, and of great benefit to human beings. The morally sensitive scientist should wish to preserve this status, and thus should take due care that her work not be the cause of the potentially untold amount of human misery that science can also be capable of bringing about.

Is the Precautionary Principle, stated as above, too strong? What due concern rules out cannot be risk as such, or there would be *no* mountain-climbing ventures. What must be ruled out is undue risk, and here, again, we must have recourse to the notion of fairness. When I am insufficiently careful in cutting vegetables, I risk my own well-being, but when I am insufficiently careful on the road, I risk not only myself, but others. Similarly, biotechnology, weaponry, artificial intelligence, and a host of other developments, put others, not simply their developer, at risk. When are such risks fair?

The relevant considerations include the following: Have all the foreseeable risks been adequately assessed? Are those at potential risk also potentially to benefit? Is the potential benefit significant enough relative to the potential harms and the likelihood of harms? Is it significant enough compared to the disadvantages of doing something else? And finally, have those who create the risks done everything reasonable to prevent the risks from taking place? Every new bit of scientific advance, no doubt, in some direct or indirect way creates risk, and a policy of eliminating all risk is certainly too strict. But inquirers, scientific and otherwise, have in many past cases been careless and unconcerned for human well-being when evaluated against this set of questions.

## CONCLUSION

This chapter concludes my discussion of the external ethics of inquiry as such. But the external approach is not yet complete, because the ethical considerations canvassed in these past few chapters need supplementation by a consideration of explicitly political concerns. For it is not in all cases clear that returning an ethical verdict one way or another on some form of inquiry will have political consequences. So it is to the relationship between research and inquiry, and the nature of law, the state, and politics, that I turn next.

# 8  The Scientific Profession and the State

What, normatively, is the relationship between my, or indeed anyone's, ethical findings in the ethics of inquiry, and a reasonable political approach to the permitting, regulating, forbidding, and funding and of research, investigation, and inquiry? Such questions are particularly salient where scientific research, including biomedical research, is concerned. But related questions exist about non-scientific forms of inquiry, such as the inquiries of journalists. Even inquiry in the humanities can be considered from a political standpoint; is such inquiry of any worth to the state, and should the state support, or ignore, such inquiry? In this chapter and the next, I ask what forms of *scientific* research governments may, may not, and perhaps must support and fund. In Chapter 10, I consider first what relationship the state should have to inquiry in the humanities. Is the research of philosophers, literary theorists, and classicists reasonably supported by the state, or is this an insufficiently practical-minded waste of public monies? I then consider what relationship the state should have to journalistic inquiry.

In this chapter, I first discuss the nature of science with a view to answering one particular question: in what ways are scientific inquiries public and in what ways are they not? Insofar as something is not public, I will, following customary usage, call it private.

In the second part of this chapter, I discuss at a general level the relation between public and private in political terms: what political norms govern the public, and what govern the private? This will serve as a prolegomenon to the discussion in Chapter 9 on the politics of scientific inquiry. There I will ask: how are reasonable political norms brought to bear on science and scientific inquiry?

## SCIENCE AS A PROFESSION

I will argue that science is public in three crucial ways: in regard to its procedures, in regard to its findings and derived benefits, and in regard to its expressive capacity. This will require that I first say something about what I mean by science. Not any form of inquiry should be called scientific. No one thinks journalists are scientists, and very few, if any, think philosophers are. Following other philosophers, such as David Resnick, I hold that science is a profession. I shall thus begin by giving an account of what I mean by a profession, and then use this account to identify what particular kind of profession the scientist belongs to.

My approach to the nature of the professions generally may be called an internalist approach: crucial to understanding any profession will be an understanding of its peculiar point.[1] To clarify what it means to say that any profession has its peculiar point, I will rely on Alasdair MacIntyre's well-known concept of a "practice." I will return to the importance of this concept for understanding the nature of inquiry in Chapter 11.

A practice is:

> . . . any coherent and complex form of socially established cooperative human activity through which goods internal to that form of activity are realized in the course of trying to achieve those standards of excellence which are appropriate to, and partially definitive of, that form of activity, with the result that human powers to achieve excellence, and human conceptions of the ends and goods involved, are systematically extended. (MacIntyre, 1984, p. 187)

As we will see in Chapter 11, practices are, for MacIntyre, the contexts in which the virtues are needed and developed. Here, it is more to my purposes to understand more clearly what is meant by a practice.

Consider the game of basketball, as an everyday instance of a practice. In the absence of a certain social setting, and certain social decisions, there would be no basketball—it is socially established. But once the appropriate social context has been established, the game of basketball creates the possibility for people to realize a certain kind of good—play—in an entirely new way, a way internal to the game itself, and perhaps most fully appreciated by those who play the game. Further, the good of basketball is both complex and coherent, unlike the pastime of shooting set shots, and this makes possible a continuing development of possibilities for excellence among players.

Moreover, and again because of the complexity of the game, excellence of achievement in basketball will typically open up new avenues for pursuing that same game, and its goods, and hence new ways of being excellent. A player's excellence at basketball—the excellence of a Michael Jordan, for example—can reveal new aspects of the game previously unappreciated, or even non-existent, thus generating new opportunities for excellence by other players.

Basketball is social not just in its origins, but in its nature: it is a genuinely cooperative form of human activity, at least when played well. The level of complexity and skill required for the players to be able systematically to extend the available forms of excellence of performance requires that the game be played neither alone nor individualistically. Basketball requires shared activity with others to be good. Moreover, as a practice that exists not just across a number of individuals but through time, there is a quasi-cooperation between basketball's players today, and the players of yesterday, from whom today's players inherit their opportunities, and the players of tomorrow, who will in turn be the heirs of today's players.

Any profession can be understood first in terms of the practice that underwrites it, and hence of the goods internal to that practice. But it is not the case either that every practice is a profession, or that professions are no more than practices. What is responsible for transforming a practice into a profession is twofold. First, the practice in question should bear upon the social, or common, good in important and widely recognized ways. Second, in response to this recognition, the practice must become, whether deliberately or through custom, embedded in an institutional context in order that its social benefits may be more easily achieved, promoted, and distributed.

To make this point, it is necessary to say something about the way practices bear on the common good. This notion of the common good will be increasingly important in this chapter, in particular in the third section of the nature and function of the state.

A community, as I understand it here, exists precisely so that its individual members may flourish as human beings, including flourishing as human-beings-in-community. It follows from this that a community does its job, and prospers, to the extent that it has provided the conditions under which its members may prosper. For some communities, both the form of flourishing and its conditions will be fairly rigorously specified, as in a community of Christian monks. In other communities, such as the political community, the contribution to flourishing will be more instrumental and somewhat less specified in its details.

At very broad levels of community—the communities of states or peoples—it will be necessary to foster an environment in which various kinds of practices may flourish. But with many practices, communities need not contribute directly to the conditions necessary for the successful promotion of this or that practice. Consider chess, which is an example favored by MacIntyre. Good general forms of community, such as a flourishing state, are communities within which it is possible for smaller communities of chess players to form, but the larger forms of community need take no particular interest in the practice of chess.

Some practices, however, engage with the good of the community in ways that go beyond the goods of chess. Such practices are structured around internal goods that themselves provide conditions necessary for, or greatly contributory to, the well-being of many, or even all, members of the larger community. So in the excellence of performance and achievement of these goods, not only are the practitioners benefited, but the community is benefited from the nature of the goods pursued in these instances. Medicine provides a case in point. When medicine is practiced well, it provides potentially wide-ranging benefits for the community. Similarly, failure in medicine has a negative impact on a community significantly unlike the social consequences of poorly played chess.

In consequence, a community might decide that social structures were needed by which the practice in question might be encouraged, and transmitted, by which its benefits might be coordinated and distributed, and by which its practitioners might be rewarded or punished. Thus certain practices, such as medicine, might, for social reasons, come to be situated in certain kinds of institution. It is this institutional embeddedness that constitutes a large part of the difference between a practice and a profession, and that explains many features of professional life and professional ethics.

Some believe that the professions are currently in a period of crisis, and that professionals of various sorts—doctors, lawyers, athletes—are more concerned with social prestige, power, money, and so on than with the goods internal to the practices of these professions. Lawyers, on a popular view, are narrowly concerned for victory at any cost, even if this requires the humiliation of an innocent witness; journalists will invade private lives for the sake of better ratings; doctors are too concerned to see as many patients as possible to satisfy their HMOs, and fail to listen to and care properly for, their patients. In each of these cases, various sorts of pressures exerted by the institutions within which a practice has been situated give rise to motivations and temptations out of sync with the internal goods of those professions.

This tension is a consequence of the very purposes that the institutional context is meant to serve: the obtaining and providing of the external goods, such as money and other empowerments necessary to keep a practice going and to ensure its capacity to provide its benefits to those in need. There is always a tension between the internal and the external goods of any institutionalized practice, and this is never clearer than in the case of a profession.

Moreover, as institutions typically function in a way structured by technique, habit, ritual, and bureaucracy, it can become the case that life within these formal structures overtakes life within the more open-ended, less technical, sphere of the practice. Professionals sometimes merely go through the motions, behave habitually, suffer burnout and anxiety, and so on.

The picture of the professions given here coheres with a number of commonly held views about the professions. In discussions of the nature of professions, the following characteristics recur, all of which are applicable to the scientific profession.

First, professions are thought to have some more or less structured set of entrance requirements. Correlative to this is the expectation that a profession sets certain educational requirements for its members, and is often in the business of providing for the education of its entering members. This is true of contemporary science. Before the days in which science was a profession, it was possible to be self educated in science and self-trained in what technique existed. Today, no one would be considered a scientist who had not achieved a Ph.D. or M.D. at a reputable university.

Second, professionals are thought to possess skills and knowledge not held at large by the non-professional public; this is true of scientists both at a general level and at the more specific level of particular fields of scientific study.

Third, professions are thought to be distinguished from many other forms of occupation, and to be important, because of their contribution to the public or social good. To enter into a profession is to enter into a life of service—hence both the frustration with professionals who seem primarily motivated by self-serving ambitions, and the common association of one's profession with one's vocation.

Fourth, for related reasons, professionals are held in esteem by non-professionals. Finally, professionals are expected to be self-regulating to some degree, with a degree of autonomy in both decisions and operations. They are expected to maintain their own disciplinary control over their members, although not necessarily exclusive disciplinary control. Such self-regulation need not take the form of written codes, but where there are such codes, their creation and administration is largely an internal matter.

If science, then, is a profession, it should meet in one way or another all of these criteria; moreover, our understanding of the nature of science should be easily integrated into the discussion of professions as institutionally embedded practices of a certain sort. It seems that these marks *do* characterize science, and that science is an institutionally embedded practice of the correct sort.

It need not be the case that scientific practice is embedded in some one particular institution. No practice seems to be of precisely this sort: medicine exists, for example, within a more and sometimes less structured web of institutions: hospitals, clinics, universities, the AMA, the federal and state governments, insurance companies, and so on. Science is similarly multiply situated. Nor is it necessarily the case that institutionalization was accomplished all at once, or in an explicitly deliberative way. The institutional setting of science, like that of medicine, has developed, and is developing, in something like an organic way, without being the result of some master plan of some individual or group of individuals. But the important point is that science, like medicine, has become so situated across such a wide range of overlapping and interlocking institutions, for the reasons mentioned: in order that important social goods may be adequately promoted and distributed, and in order that those pursuing and providing these goods may be rewarded, encouraged, and, as necessary, punished.

## SCIENCE IS PUBLIC

Science, then, like medicine, law, and journalism, is a genuine profession. This helps us to see why science is inevitably public across three important axes. It is public in respect of its results and the goods derived from these results, in respect of its method, and in respect of its expressive power.

Consider first the issue of the benefits that science provides. Any practice, to become a profession, must provide benefits of the right sort not just to its practitioners, but potentially to the much wider society, as does medicine. This, after all, is the justification for integrating the practice into the relevant web of institutions: by so integrating the practice, the relevant benefits may be more effectively distributed across the wider community. The knowledge provided by science is, in two respects, of benefit in precisely this way.

First, scientific knowledge, as a general and systematic understanding of nature, is valuable in itself. The fact that science provides a general and systematic understanding of nature elevates it above piecemeal and local understandings—it has human significance because it teaches all of us, systematically, about the world in which we live. That this is widely seen as a social benefit may be seen in the pride that nations take in their sciences, or that the Western world takes generally in its scientific track record. By contrast, the Soviet Union was deficient not just because of its various political and moral failings but also inasmuch as it suffered from tainted science.

Some degree of scientific knowledge, moreover, is thought to be of importance not just to future scientists, but to all children, as part of an adequate education. If science were to disappear from the curriculum of primary and secondary education, our social world would for that very reason be significantly impoverished. This aspect of the benefits provided by science is relevant to its professionalization: general scientific knowledge is a social good whose distribution is made possible by, and no doubt is partly responsible for, the professionalization of science (Resnick, 1998, p. 39).

A second form of benefit provided by scientific knowledge turns on its instrumental value. Scientific technology has provided us with an abundance of benefits, including advances in health care, agriculture, architecture, and engineering, to name a few. It has provided us with inventions such as computers, automobiles, and airplanes, and techniques such as open-heart surgery, genetic alteration of plants, and the fission of atoms. Much of the modern world is built on a technological foundation laid down by modern science.

Both these types of goods are deeply social, and public. Unlike a good game of chess, which primarily benefits those who play it, society at large benefits from the general scientific knowledge of the past few hundred years, and society at large benefits from the technological advances made possible by such science. Even someone who learned no science in school or perhaps never went to school is still likely to be benefited in many ways by modern technology.

The benefits of science are so deeply public that they are often unavoidable. Everyone's life is touched by the advances of science and it is virtually inconceivable to imagine life otherwise. One could no sooner refuse all the benefits of science than one could refuse all the benefits of law enforcement. One's general safety rests, in innumerable ways, on the fact that others are doing their job—it would be impossible to opt out of those benefits, for even if one refused to call the police in the event of a burglary, the fact that one was not being regularly burgled would itself be attributable to the existence and adequacy of local law enforcement. Similarly, even if one were to opt out of the benefits of, say, vaccinations, as some do, nonetheless such an agent would benefit from the fact that so many others had been vaccinated. This is especially true of the technological side of scientific progress, but our lives are also affected by the fact that we live in a scientifically enlightened age: we have more opportunities for knowledge and understanding than ever before, and have a richer picture of our world available to us than was ever previously possible.

This does not mean that every gain made by science, whether in advancing our theoretical knowledge of the world, or our instrumental capacities to deal with it, is equally beneficial, or equally widespread. Indeed, that some of the possible aims of scientific investigation are trivial and insignificant should be important to a scientist's critical self-assessment of her own projects. That the instrumental benefits of some technological advance would be of aid only to a few, perhaps a privileged few, should be a crucial consideration in the determination of what kinds of projects should receive state assistance. But the general point stands: in virtue of both sorts of benefits that science provides, it should be considered deeply public, and this is central to its evolution into a genuine profession.

The second way in which science is deeply public is as regards its methods. Scientists rely on a method of inquiry, largely, although not exclusively, modeled around hypothesis, prediction, and experiment, that is deeply social. Scientists work together to design and carry out experiments, promulgate the results of their research, and then rely on the work of others both to test their findings, and to pick up where they left off in the advancement of understanding. Scientists share their findings, pass them on from generation to generation, and together constitute a tribunal before which each new block in the architecture of understanding must come under scrutiny before being accepted.

Such cooperation is not accidental to science. Science is not the only form of inquiry, and it is not the only form of social inquiry. But science is especially cooperative and especially public in its method. Hardly anyone could profitably pursue philosophy in isolation from all other philosophers: at the least, an awareness of other philosophers in history is necessary. An awareness of other living and recent philosophers and their work also is of inevitable benefit. But a philosopher could retreat to his study, and produce work that would not see the light of day for years and, under such circumstances, possibly succeed to a considerable extent as a philosopher. This path is no longer open to scientists: it is only insofar as they subject their work to the critical scrutiny of others that they are responsible as scientists.

David Resnick has pointed out that, among the developments leading to the professionalization of science were both the invention of the printing press and the spread of the university (Resnick, 1998, p. 37). These made possible a radical progress in the social context within which science could be carried out. A scientist's findings were now available to other scientists for criticism and development; today, science apart from its methodological sociality is, like a science whose benefits were private, unthinkable. Further, without the benefits of the work done by other scientists, both in the past and at present, an aspiring scientist would have little hope of success: a division of labor, like the sharing and mutual criticism of results, has become part of the nature of science.

Moreover, the experimental method itself is public in important ways beyond the need for subsequent promulgation and criticism. For these aspects of science's public nature are made possible by the initial publicity of experiments themselves: in principle, an experiment is a public putting to the test of a hypothesis itself made publicly. The power of science in generating knowledge depends in part upon its special ability to make its ideas public via an experiment: the experiment gives a publicly recognized meaning to the ideas, and a public assessment, in a public space, of their validity (Peirce, 1957b). In fields of inquiry where this ability to make public is not present, such as philosophy or literary theory, there is not only a great difficulty, if not an impossibility, in generating a consensus, the achievement of which is so striking in science, but even great difficulties in achieving understanding of what a particular thinker is saying, or what a particular view entails. This does not mean that the humanities should necessarily be made more scientific, but recognition of these aspects of science certainly led thinkers such as Dewey or Peirce to advocate movement in that direction (Peirce, 1957a, 1957b; Dewey, 1957).

Finally, science is deeply public because it both expresses the broader culture within which it exists, and shapes that culture. In part, this is a consequence of the previously mentioned points. Consider, for example, the way in which a practice becomes a profession: certain goods are deemed of sufficient social significance that steps must be taken to ensure their adequate promotion, protection, and distribution. Institutional structures are established, or perhaps, as is more likely, emerge through time, to ensure that this is done. But is it a priori the case that some particular set of goods, and some corresponding set of practices, will be such as to demand this sort of institutionalization?

The answer seems to be: yes and no. Some goods are inevitably such as to demand recognition of their great social significance. Thus medicine is easily seen to be of considerable importance. On the other hand in some societies, for various reasons, it might be deemed more important, or equally important, that some form of play or art be considered the ground for professionalization.

Such considerations bring out several points. First, genuine professions must ultimately be rooted in intrinsic human goods: life (medicine), knowledge (science), play (professional sports), or just society (the law, and probably journalism). But with regard to each of these goods, there will be a variety of possible manifestations, a variety of possible ways of participating in them. In some cultures, some of these ways might be given prominence over others for a variety of reasons. At times, and in certain places, the professionalization of medicine might make less sense than the professionalization of law, or sport, because of insufficient understanding and technology. Rome, for example, achieved a much more significant professionalization of the law than of medicine. In other cultures, some other practice might come to be the locus of the culture's sense of identity and self-esteem. By professionalization of that practice, the culture establishes more firmly that identity.

By its very professionalization of a practice, then, a culture expresses its value commitments, as well as its historical identity and its condition of development. A culture that strongly emphasizes the medical profession defines and expresses itself differently than a culture that, for whatever reason, gives greater emphasis to the professionalization of sport. And this holds as well for science.

First, by its professionalization of science at all, a culture, such as the culture of Western Europe at a particular time, expresses itself in a particular way as committed to theoretical knowledge of nature. Such a commitment is far from inevitable: a culture might so spiritualistically understand nature that it deems it sacrilege to investigate it empirically. A culture could reject science as associated with a set of related values towards which the culture was antagonistic. Finally, it is conceivable that from some deep perversity of will a culture could turn its back on the systematic understanding of the world and become a society of "know-nothings."

Second, by a culture's scientific emphasis, e.g., its choices of projects and defined interests, and by its ranking of science next to other professions, the culture further identifies and expresses itself. And third, by the manner in which it carries out its science, a culture again defines and expresses itself. Thus, there would seem to be a different expressive capacity in the choice to fund and vigorously pursue space research, versus the choice to fund and vigorously pursue health research, to pursue projects more or projects less instrumentally valuable, and to pursue projects in more or less morally appropriate ways. Some worry that our own scientific culture is becoming increasingly utilitarian, and that this utilitarian strain is spreading to encompass other forms of learning and inquiry such as philosophy and literature. A culture whose science and knowledge was significantly, or solely, in the service of technological benefits, and hostile to the growth of understanding for its own sake would be critically different from a culture of the liberal arts, whose science was consistent with this commitment.

That a culture's moral character expresses itself in its scientific conduct is equally clear: the barbarism of national socialism and the ideological blindness of communism appeared as much in the science of Nazi Germany and the Soviet Union as anywhere else. A general climate of racism in the southern United States was not unrelated to the experiments at Tuskegee. And our current culture of status and money has arguably its own consequences for honesty and integrity in science.[2]

The relationship between science and culture is, in fact, a two-way relationship; for not only does the science express the culture, including the moral culture, of a society, it establishes, fixes, and focuses that culture. A society not initially overtly racist could become increasingly so by its tolerance of racist science, and similarly for almost any other form of ethically suspect science. Had there been no outcry over the experiments in Tuskegee, America would by that fact probably have become *more* racist. Similarly, those experiments and others in which no form of consent was sought from participants offered America an opportunity to become more or less paternalistic; finally, some believe that the course of scientific and especially medical culture since the rise of a strong requirement of informed consent has shaped and been shaped by the West's increasing individualism (Pellegrino and Thomasma, 1988). So the culture of science and the larger culture would appear to be mutually reinforcing in virtue of science's expressive power.

Professionalized science is thus an extremely public reality. Perhaps some scientists, in defending the immunity of science from ethical and political considerations, think of science as private in the way that sex is. Of course, sex has public consequences, but it nevertheless requires a zone of privacy if the intimacy that makes it meaningful is to be preserved. But a more appropriate analogy is the family, which is considerably more public an institution than the activity of sex. Families contribute, by their health or decay, to the health and decay of society. They contribute to the continued existence of the polis. And by their rearing and education, including their moral formation of children, they build up the culture of the succeeding generation of a society in crucial ways. Thus, while there is room for disagreement about the extent to which the family is an appropriate object of concern on the part of a society, including political society, there is widespread agreement that the family is a legitimate object of public concern.

Science, then, is both deeply public and of deep social significance. In this chapter, however, my concern is not simply with science in itself, but with its relationship to the state: in what ways must, may, or may not the state promote, regulate, fund, prohibit, and so on the course of science? Discussion of the public nature of science brings us partway to an answer to such questions. To complete an answer requires now some discussion of the nature of the state, its purposes, and its limits.

## THE STATE AND THE COMMON GOOD

The concept of a, or the, common good has considerably wider application than simply in a political context. The purpose of this section will be to limn some of this wider context with a view to seeing what a specifically *political* common good is and is not. Three errors, however, must be avoided: to think of the political common good as too similar to that of smaller communities, such as the family, that pursue a common intrinsic good; to think of the common good as a mere aggregate of welfare or utility, to be pursued by the state in the most efficient way possible; and to see it as divorced in its significance from the discussion throughout this book of the basic goods and genuine human well-being. The first misunderstanding will be addressed shortly; the last will be the focus, in particular, of a later section. Of the second, the peculiarly utilitarian view of the political good, this conception stands or falls, and hence falls, with consequentialism generally: there is no "greatest good," nor does the state have a mandate to trample rights, or abuse persons in the name of some fictitious "greater good."

As John Finnis, to whom the discussion in this section owes much, points out, the basic goods are the ultimate foundation of the notion of a common good (Finnis, 1980, Chapter VI; Finnis, 1998, Chapters IV and VII). The basic goods are common in the sense that the same set of goods are good for every human agent: life is thus a good common to all human beings, and to be respected in all human beings, including oneself. This way in which the goods are common underlies another. By being goods for all, the basic goods provide the foundation for the possibility of a common pursuit of goods. It is this notion of a common pursuit of goods that is at the core of the notion of a common good.

What does it mean to pursue a good or goods "in common"? What is a shared pursuit of a good or goods? There are various ways of dividing up a taxonomy of goods that may be pursued in common, but three are of critical importance: states of affairs or goals may be pursued in common; values, or basic goods may be pursued in common; and instrumentalities necessary to the pursuit of either states of affairs or values can be pursued in common.

Consider two builders working on a house. Both share in the pursuit of some common good: the completion of the house, itself an identifiable state of affairs, a goal. Any time two or more people are similarly engaged in a project for the sake of a shared outcome, they share a common good. But why are they working together? Possible answers to this question might indicate more or less deeply shared common goods; for while it is possible that each builder has his own ends, his own external purposes, it is also possible that they share not just the goal of completing work on the house, but a further reason for pursuing that goal. They might both be committed, for example, to providing shelter to a family in need, out of a generalized concern for that family's life and well-being. Their common action is rooted in a common basic, or intrinsic good, not merely in an end state or goal, namely, the good of human life. By contrast, if each is occupied primarily for the sake of getting a paycheck, then their common good does not extend past the distinct outcome that both desire.

Finally, whether their common good is simply the house, or whether it also extends past that outcome to some shared value, our builders will no doubt also have an interest in the necessities required for building a house together: coordinated activity, a common supply of tools and other equipment, an established routine. Such instrumentalities are neither the concrete goal being pursued, nor the ultimate good, but nonetheless constitute a common good for these agents, without which their other goods will not be achieved. From considerations of similar sorts of cases, Finnis's definition of the common good emerges:

> In each case, therefore, "the common good" [refers] to the factor or set of factors (whether a value, a concrete operational objective, or the conditions for realizing a value or attaining an objective) which, as considerations in someone's practical reasoning, would make sense of or give reason for his collaboration with others and would likewise, from their point of view, give reason for their collaboration with each other and with him. (Finnis, 1980, p. 154)

Yet another case needs to be considered. Our builders might be collaborating, in addition to all the other reasons, also for the sake of each other's well-being, good, or flourishing. The concern that each has does not merely go through the other to whatever other goods are at stake, but also rests in the other: A wants for B what B wants, precisely because B wants it, and vice versa. As Finnis says, "The good that is common between friends is not simply the good of two successfully achieved coinciding projects or objectives; it is the common good of mutual self-constitution, self-fulfillment, self-realization" (Finnis, 1980, p. 141).

So A may wish the project to succeed not only for the sake of the project itself, but because it is what B wants; and vice versa. Both A and B might wish to be part of the project itself as a way of working together, at having a common context in which to pursue their friendship. So the goods pursued within a friendship, and within the acts constituting that friendship, might be quite complex.

An essential point to make here is that friendship, which Finnis calls "the most communal" form of community, is such that its common good is always a basic good, namely, the basic good of friendship itself, and may also have in various contexts other basic goods as the common good of the actions performed together by the friends. Such a characterization of friendship must be kept in mind when distinguishing the common good peculiar to the state from other common goods; for while every common pursuit of a good constitutes a form of community, the temptation should be resisted to think that the community appropriate to the state should be this "most communal" relationship of friendship, or something analogous to it in pursuing an intrinsic good.

Where, then, does the state, and the common good of the state, enter into things? By the analysis given so far, a great number of social realities emerge as realities whose shape is a consequence of their shared pursuit of common good(s): families, churches, business associations, clubs, schools, hospitals. Of these, the family is, from one point of view, the most important: arguably, it instantiates a basic good itself, and provides the necessary framework within which all individuals get their start in life, including the formation and education necessary for a subsequently successful pursuit of well-being and virtue. Why is there a need for a further common good at all, and how does this further common good differ from others? Cannot this set of communities occupy a shared space without the need for some other overarching community? No; there are three ways in which the sum of such existing communities, with their sometimes overlapping, sometimes competing, common goods, would be inadequate relative to the needs of their members, if they existed without the benefit of the state.

First, and most obviously, each and all of these communities and their members might come under threat: from individuals, from one another, or from external communities. So individuals, and groups, are threatened by robbers and murderers, frauds and charlatans. Groups compete for space, for resources, and for sway over their members, external groups see the possibility for expansion, and all are tempted to take what they need or want by force or guile. There is thus a standing need for protection and defense against the wicked, and, as we saw in Chapter 3, for punishment, none of which can be effectively, or fairly pursued by any one of the groups in question.

Second, even if the communities in question are comprised of men and women of the best possible intentions, there is a need for a fair system of coordination. How can a number of even non-competing groups get along successfully if there are not common procedural methods for settling disputes or questions arising between them, commonly held rules to prevent disputes or questions, and generally a common form of life accepted as authoritative for all, the following of which will generally prevent members and groups from "bumping into" one another, and colliding in the social scrum? Further, no one group will ever be self-sufficient, so trade and exchange between groups is to be expected; but how in a coherent and fair fashion will this exchange of goods, necessary to achieve self-sufficiency, be carried out? There is thus a need for a conclusive and just solution to a variety of coordination problems.

Finally, some individuals, insufficiently rooted in small communities, or in weak communities, or disadvantaged by birth or accident of history or the wickedness of others, have greater needs in various respects than others. Ill health does not always strike those able to pay for care, or rooted in communities willing to care for them. Not all are born in circumstances that would otherwise contribute to an adequate education, and subsequently adequate opportunities for employment. No doubt other individuals and groups, sometimes clearly defined, at other times not, have obligations to those in need; but not all will always be willing to meet such obligations, and in many cases it will be unclear who has the obligations or how they are best met. There is thus a need for a "safety net," for those unable to care for themselves and with no one proximate to care for them.

In the absence of a solution to these various needs, the lives of men, while not, perhaps, nasty, brutish, and short, are nonetheless inadequately organized to make possible a successful pursuit of the basic goods, and of general well-being, in the lives of human persons. "So," as Finnis writes,

> . . . there emerges the desirability of a "complete community", an all-round association in which would be coordinated the initiatives and activities of individuals, of families, and of the vast network of intermediate associations. The point of this all-round association would be to secure the whole ensemble of material and other conditions, including forms of collaboration, that tend to favor, facilitate, and foster the realization by each individual of his or her personal development. (Finnis, 1980, p. 147)

It is precisely here that the first of the possible misinterpretations of the political common good can arise; for the political common good can now be seen as the all round flourishing and well-being of the state's citizens. But the all-round flourishing of any human agent is robustly moral: it includes, for example, all-round virtue, deep and lasting commitment to genuine goods, robust relationships of friendship, a good will, an adequate relationship to the divine, and so on. Is the state, as a community whose common good includes the all-round flourishing of its members, committed to making its citizens good, to promoting their virtue in every possible way, to ensuring that they worship adequately, have the right friends, and so on? Are the concerns of the state in relationship to its citizens the same sort of concern that a virtuous friend has to her friend, or a parent has to a child, or a church has to its members? Is the state's commitment to all-round flourishing a commitment to *make* its citizens flourish?

It is not. Here we must again credit Finnis, and Germain Grisez, for their recent discussions of the essentially instrumental and limited character of the political common good, and, in Finnis's case in particular, for a rereading of Aquinas that reveals his sensitivity to the moral limits of the state. Finnis moreover highlights the way in which, for Aquinas, this specifically political common good is called by Aquinas the "public good." So the discussion here will eventually tie in with the discussion earlier in this chapter of the public nature of science.

To call the political common good "public" here draws attention to two points, one implicit in the justification for the state and its laws, and one rooted in facts about what the natural limits of a state are. As we saw, the whole point of a state, and law, is as a supplement. Individuals, families, and, secondarily, various other associations all pursue human well-being and flourishing. Individuals directly instantiate in their lives the various basic goods. So, arguably, do families. But individuals, families, and other associations were seen to be inadequate for a fully sufficient pursuit of those goods, not because there were other intrinsic goods that required some other reality to be instantiated, but because individuals and families, especially, needed other realities to assist *them,* the individuals and families, in achieving *their* goods. Following Finnis, and Aquinas, we can summarize what is needed in two words: justice and peace (Finnis, 1998, p. 227).

But both justice and peace are in this context essentially public: they concern dealings *between* persons, rather than concerns, pursuits, or activities of individuals that do not have any, or have only little, bearing on the lives of others. So a first gloss on the "public" good that states pursue is that it concerns the acts of its citizens insofar as they bear, in regards to justice and peace, on one another.

Secondly, but not unrelatedly, the state has no competence over the inner life of its subjects. Human persons are agents engaged in self-constitution, as we have seen repeatedly, and this self-constitution extends not simply to their external acts, but to their innermost intentions and feelings. But the state is simply unable to demand of its citizens that they act from this or that intention, with this or that feeling. So a second gloss on the "public" good that states pursue is that it concerns not simply interpersonal acts but also primarily external acts of its citizens.

Moreover, as we have seen in numerous contexts, it is part of the good of individuals that they be self-determining in their own pursuit of the good. Some goods require that those participating in them have chosen them. Even substantive goods, like life and knowledge, are critical to an agent's constitution of her own identity in a way that requires that the agent in question make the relevant choices in relation to the pursuit of these goods. So the "lack of competence" of the state over an agent's inner life includes those of her choices that are critically self-determining, subject to the caveat related to the first sense of 'public"—that these self-determining choices not adversely affect the agent's public relation to others in ways that would disrupt peace or violate justice.

What we see, then, is a kind of ambiguity in the phrase "all-inclusive common good." This common good would include the all-round flourishing in action and virtue of all the citizens of a state, and this is what is desired by those citizens in their willing oriented-ness towards the state and its laws—it is what they hope to obtain thereby. But this does not mean that the state should seek to make itself sufficient for that all-round flourishing; it is merely necessary for it. Thus Finnis writes,

> Public good is a part or aspect of the all-inclusive common good. It is the part which provides an indispensable context and support for those parts or aspects of the common good which are private (especially individual and familial good). It thus supplements, subserves, and supervises these private aspects, but without superseding them, and without taking overall charge of, or responsibility for, them. (Finnis, 1998, p. 237)

As Finnis points out, recognition of this truth is related to Aquinas's "partial anticipation of the principle of subsidiarity: 'it is contrary to the proper character of the state's governance to impede people from acting according to their responsibilities'" (Finnis, 1998, p. 237). This principle is the reflection of the insight above that one aspect of the state's lack of competence is as regards its relation to the self-determining choices and activities of its members.

The specifically political common good, then, is public, limited, and, ultimately, instrumental. Politics and the sphere of the political is not the attempt directly to instantiate a basic good, but rather the attempt to make more possible the ability of the citizens of the state themselves to instantiate, participate in, pursue, both individually and together, the basic goods that constitute the horizon of human flourishing.

Failure to recognize this instrumental character is not without significant consequences in the ethics of inquiry; for the failure to recognize these features of the limits of the state is typically attended by one of three metaphorical understandings of the state: the state as a form of friendship akin to the friendship of a family, the state as a parent, to whom citizens are related as children, or the state as an organism. Sometimes all three potentially dangerous metaphors are found together, as in Plato and Aristotle. Before turning in the next chapter to the relationship between a proper understanding of the state, and the ethics and politics of inquiry, it is worth saying something about how these metaphors can warp the politics of inquiry in harmful ways.

Three particular types of harm, related to one another, potentially accompany this family of metaphors, and all are instantiations of more general failures in the relationship between the state and its citizens. The general failings are of the following types: first, states that understand themselves according to one or all of these images or metaphors are inclined to subordinate individual good to the good of the state. This subordination need not trade in fictions such as the utilitarian fiction of an aggregate greatest good. But the subordination is similar in making the good of a particular kind of whole—the state—more important than the good of its parts. Second, states that understand themselves in these ways typically assume a greater understanding of individual well-being, and responsibility for it, than is reasonable. Third, such states can be tempted to subordinate scientific truth, and the truth of other forms of inquiry, to their own self-understood well-being.

The first inclination, to subordinate the good of the parts to the good of the whole, follows closely from the image of the state as organism. In an organism, the good of the parts really is the good of the parts as parts of the whole. Hands, hearts, and eyes have no good separated from the organism and a whole; they are good precisely insofar as they contribute to the good of the whole. So a severed hand is not really a hand, and an eye that is harmful to the body should, if it cannot be healed, be removed.

Generally speaking, then, an organic conception of the state is at risk to hold that individuals are good and to be respected only insofar as they are parts of the state, and only insofar as they contribute to the overall well-being of the state. So individuals who are non-contributors might be looked upon as cancers or parasites to be disposed of at the command of the ruler. Worse, as the person commands the hand, and even sometimes sacrifices her hand, for her overall well-being, so the state might command, and sometimes sacrifice the individual for the overall well-being of the state.

In the context of scientific inquiry, this could result in the out and out use of citizens in scientific experimentation in ways that would violate the principles laid down in Chapters 2 through 7. We might also consider here Plato's radical revision in *Republic* V of the nature of the procreation of children on the model of animal husbandry. It would take a number of generations before the principles of eugenics were adequately understood. In that time, citizens of the state would be available for research into the principles of procreation, for the good of the state, as envisaged by Plato, would depend upon this. Similarly, and historically, the mentally retarded and terminally ill were considered under Nazi ideology to be a drag on the system. Many were not simply eliminated, however, but were made the objects of scientific experiment so as not to be utterly useless to the state.

The second temptation of states dominated by these images is an unacceptable paternalism, which may again be seen, in the context of the ethics of inquiry, in Plato's *Republic*. For Plato, the rule of the state extended over almost every aspect of the citizen's life, including the choice of whether and what to inquire into. Only the Guardian class would be educated into philosophy and allowed to pursue speculative inquiries. And only the mature Guardian class would comprise individuals capable of making decisions about who the future members of that class were to be.

Similar circumstances still obtain. To speak anecdotally, I was, in my first year of graduate school in philosophy, friends with a Chinese citizen, also a graduate student in philosophy. His true interest, he told me, was literature, but in consequence of the state-administered tests, the Chinese government had determined him best suited for philosophy and had arranged his education accordingly. Similar cases may be found in other states based on Marxist-Leninist ideology.

The third temptation can also be seen in the history of science and other academic disciplines in Marxist-Leninist states, such as the former Soviet Union, and is at least potentially present in the *Republic*, although with slightly different emphasis. Plato was sufficiently concerned with the truth that he recognized that suppression of truth in service of the good of the state was a form of lying, even if a noble form. But in the former Soviet Union, falsehood passed for truth, as, for example, in the agricultural sciences, and in the humanities as well. Where the state sees itself as prior to, more important than, or superior to the individual, it seems that it is tempted to construe the fruits of intellectual discovery in a way that suits itself (Soyfer, Gruliow, and Gruliow, 1994).

In sum, we must steer away from understanding the notion of the common good of a state—the political common good—in terms of the images discussed, just as we must steer away from understanding it in terms of the notion of a utilitarian aggregate. The strictly political common good is limited and instrumental, even if of surpassing breadth and considerable authority. Only by keeping this in mind can the dignity of persons, in general, and as involved in inquiry, be preserved.

We must now return to the question of the relationship between the overall picture of the political common good that I have presented, and the description of science put forth earlier in this chapter.

# 9 Science and the Sovereignty of the State

Science is public as regards its results and benefits, as regards its method, and as regards its expressive power. In all three respects, science may, therefore, under certain circumstances, be subject to the power of the state. Under some circumstances, the state will be able to regulate, and under some circumstances, to promote, scientific inquiry.

In the next three sections, I will establish several normative considerations governing the state's relationship to institutional science, corresponding to these three ways in which science is public. I will also draw attention to one critical respect in which science is not subject to the concerns of the state, namely, as regards the content of its findings. Throughout, a recurring theme will be the disputed issue of human embryonic research. I will give several reasons for thinking that state regulation of such research is entirely appropriate. I will close the chapter with an argument that assumes, however, a background of continuing disagreement over the morality of this research.

## THE STATE AND THE BENEFITS OF SCIENCE

Consider the public nature of the benefits of science. Scientific knowledge is intrinsically good, and, because it also provides a systematic understanding of the world in which we live, it is of itself beneficial to a society in which it is found, in two ways. A group, whether political, or subpolitical, just is better off to the extent that it is generally scientifically informed, rather than not, and to the extent that there exists within it important scientific knowledge, even when that specific knowledge is not widespread. Not everyone, or even many people, can know theoretical physics, but a society is better off if some people know and understand theoretical physics. Second, the consequences of scientific knowledge, i.e., the various forms of scientific technology, are likewise of important, albeit instrumental, benefit. The following normative suggestions follow from this.

First, insofar as scientific inquiry is of public value, it is generally something that the state can and should promote. The state is responsible for providing conditions necessary for its citizens to flourish, and to pursue their well-being in reasonable ways. This typically cannot be done in widespread ignorance of the ways of the world, and it is usually better done given a background knowledge of the world. A society in which the sciences are left to languish, in which scientists receive no encouragement, much less financial support, will not thrive for two reasons: it will, as a society, lack knowledge that is intrinsically good, and it will lack the various benefits to be gained from such knowledge.

These benefits are so significant that it is reasonable to hold that a state has some obligation (a) to provide funding for at least some scientific inquiry if that inquiry cannot be better funded privately, and (b) to fund mechanisms for the distribution of scientific benefits, including scientific knowledge. The situation with science is somewhat analogous to medicine, and somewhat disanalogous to, say, religion. Both medicine and religion are of great benefit to the citizens of a state; both must be supported if citizens are to flourish. To a point, both may be supported and promoted by a state without this involving direct financial contributions: a state can make known its commitment, for example, to religious liberty, and can further make it known that it views this as a liberty by which its citizens may pursue something of critical human importance, rather than a liberty by which they may engage in slightly nutty behavior. Similarly, the medical profession can be well or poorly affected by the state's non-economic support; states can support or fail to support healthy lifestyles, for example, by making it more or less difficult to smoke, by encouraging a healthy diet, by regulating bogus claims to "quick fixes," and so on.

But medicine and medical research are increasingly expensive. In consequence, successful medical research, and successful distribution of medical benefits, may require not just moral support, and indirect financial support, but direct financial assistance from the state: subsidies for medical research and treatment, state-sponsored hospitals and clinics, or possibly a state-sponsored insurance scheme, for example.

Religion, by contrast, while equally important, and in need of state support, is less in need of direct financial support. Religious organizations may benefit from tax-exempt status and receive other favored treatments; but direct state funding of a religious organization is often unnecessary, and sometimes threatening. When an institution becomes too dependent upon state money, there is a concern that the state will begin to influence the institution in illegitimate ways.

Scientific inquiry and research is more on par, in these respects, with medicine than with religion. Scientific inquiry is often expensive, and there are additional expenses in distributing the knowledge and its benefits. So if it is not possible or efficient for important aspects of scientific research to attain private or corporate or university funding, then it may be that in such cases a state has an obligation to provide money in support of science, for example, by the provision of grant monies, the funding of public universities, and so on. Such support has been a significant part of the U.S. budget since the middle part of the twentieth century.[1]

This argument does not yet provide an adequate discrimination of what types of scientific inquiry in particular should be so supported. The principles governing decisions to fund science may be understood by recognizing the limits, not just of the obligation, but even of the permissibility of state funding, even for otherwise legitimate projects. There is no *general* right to have one's particular projects of inquiry funded, any more than to have, say, one's particular artistic projects publicly funded. Rather, as far as particular projects of inquiry go, something like the norm articulated by Germain Grisez in relation to the funding of artistic projects will be applicable. Grisez writes,

> Arguments for continuing the NEA should confront a single issue: For whom is the art the U.S. government subsidizes intended? The nation's common good is the only principle that can justify any appropriation. How does this subsidy promote the common good? Attempts to answer this question must not beg it by supposing that the satisfaction of every group's legitimate interests pertains to the nation's common good, which includes only the satisfaction of those legitimate interests that are both widely shared and best satisfied by cooperation at the national level. (Grisez, 1997, p. 841)

Just as the common good underwrites the state's responsibility to take an interest in scientific research, and perhaps even to fund it, so does that common good operate as the necessary limit to unreasonable use of state funds to promote particular scientific projects. Crucial to Grisez's account are the final two criteria: legitimate interests that are (a) widely shared and (b) best satisfied by cooperation at the national level.

Application of these criteria can be seen by considering the case of reproductive cloning. One common justification for such research is that it will help develop reproductive technologies that will be of assistance to couples unable to conceive. This, in turn, has been used to justify a demand for tremendous expenditures of money.

In the general discussion of cloning research carried out by the President's Council on Bioethics, commission member Mary Ann Glendon raised a number of points about these justifications that apparently received little consideration. Glendon pointed to the great cost of such procedures, the uncertain outcome for those who use them, and the assumption, which she questioned, that most people who use these procedures are infertile couples (Glendon, 2002). These considerations raise the following question: is it just to spend money on this sort of research when it will evidently be of benefit only to a very few, and when there are other concerns of more pressing social weight? The numbers of those who suffer from infertility are relatively few; and any reproductive technologies likely to be developed from embryonic cloning research are likely, in view of current technologies, to be prohibitively expensive to all but a few of those needing them. In light of this, we must ask whether public money might be more effectively spent on other projects of more importance to the common good. Indeed, it is reasonable to ask whether this is a fair or just expenditure of even private money.[2]

Other projects of less intrinsic moral dubiety, but that seem similarly limited as regards their relation to the public good, might include the super-conducting super-collider, or space exploration. It is beyond the scope of this chapter to discuss these cases in detail, but it is essential, if such research is to be justified, that it be shown how their pursuit will substantially relate to the common good in the right ways; for even though society is made generally well-off by the fruits of science alone, the common good pursued by the state must necessarily be of greater significance than this, lest every project of intrinsic worth be owed public funding. The justification for such funding must thus move to an account of the way in which the specific benefits of the proposed research will be widely distributed and appreciated, and the reasons why these benefits would not be better achieved privately. Space exploration provides an example of this latter consideration. In the not-to-distant future, those who most deeply wish to study space and pursue its exploration will be able to attain private financial backing from those who view space exploration as a promising investment (see "Lift Off For Enterprise," 2004). Given the prohibitive costs of space exploration, and the need for financial resources in many other areas, this might be a case in which privatization is ultimately what is morally called for.

Does this mean that the general value of scientific knowledge plays no positive role in a state's funding considerations, and that technological development trumps pure research when considerations of state funding are at stake? I do not think so. True, because of the limited role of the state, there is a strong case to be made that specific projects should meet a high threshold of utility to be fundable. But four considerations should be kept in mind. First, general scientific knowledge remains a potential benefit for all. The state should ascertain that scientific education is widespread and equally available to all citizens; state money can reasonably be spent in undertaking such a mission.

Second, certain projects of pure research are of great intrinsic importance. Some forms of scientific inquiry promise significant contributions to our overall knowledge of our world and our place in it. There should be room, when possible, for such inquiries in a state's funding for science. Third, it is frequently not possible to tell what relationship will hold between some area of pure research and some area of useful technology. Fourth, as we will see below, it can be part of a society's expressed identity that it maintain a commitment to pure scientific research. So, by the common-good approach, technology is given a certain edge over pure research, but it is not necessarily a decisive edge.

Two further considerations must be mentioned. Just as the benefits of science are public and typically widespread, so does science have the potential to bring about significant and widespread negative consequences. Scientists at work developing synthetic diseases might have the best possible intentions, and their work might indeed be of great possible benefit. It is also of great potential harm. As with any other significant harms, the state has an obligation to regulate these potentially harmful activities to ensure the safety of its citizens. If a private group wishes to build a large building, the state regulates the construction to ensure the building is safe; similarly, science must be regulated, not just, as the next section will discuss, as regards how it works, but as regards what it is working towards, where this threatens well-being.

Second, in many cases the benefits of science are widespread and unavoidable even for those who might not wish to partake in the benefits, or who might, for one reason or another believe that the benefits were not true benefits at all. This point was made in the previous chapter—the anarchist who does not want the benefits of the law nonetheless continually receives these benefits whether he likes it or not. Similarly, if anyone had a moral objection to the computer chip, it would be virtually impossible to avoid benefiting from it nonetheless. A more realistic problem involves animal research, to which some object on moral grounds. While many steps can be taken by animal rights activists to minimize the ways in which they benefit from what they view as immoral science, it is unlikely that they receive no benefits from such research. In the event that embryonic stem cell research becomes common, and provides the benefits its proponents promise, it will become increasingly impossible for opponents of such research to avoid receiving its benefits.

## THE METHOD OF SCIENCE

It is in the discussion of the public nature of scientific method that we arrive at some of the most disputed, but also some of the most dubious claims regarding the immunity of science from political interference. Again, many scientists seem to think of science as something like sex, practiced behind closed doors, and thus owed a high and presumptive degree of privacy. But while there are aspects of science that are off-limits to political concerns, as I shall specify shortly, science is intrinsically not something that can be practiced behind closed doors in isolation from the public world with which the state is concerned.

This is most obviously true when human subjects are involved. Just as it makes no sense to suggest that scientific inquiry is immune from ethical considerations when the inquiry threatens the well-being, or autonomy, or privacy of those being studied, so it makes little sense to suggest that such studies are immune from the concerns of the state. The state exists precisely to protect justice and peace for its subjects in public contexts. Because the context of scientific experimentation is deeply public, if some experimental procedure is unfair, or threatening, or invasive, to a person, this is not relatively private unfairness or threat or invasion—it is not like bullying in a family, or a fight within a social club. Rather, such violations of justice are not only interpersonal but are carried out in the public context of the world of science.

This is of considerable importance in the area of embryonic research, especially when we compare this to the problem of abortion. Some believe that abortion is the morally wrong killing of a child, yet also believe that it should not be prohibited by the state (Cuomo, 1984). It is not clear that this is a completely coherent position, but one might argue in a limited way that the woman's womb is, like her house, a private domain regarding which she is entitled to a space for making her own decisions without interference. So abortion, though usually gravely immoral, should nonetheless be legal.

This argument is not the same as the perhaps more familiar antiperfectionist arguments that abstract from moral considerations, or hold that the state has no business taking controversial moral considerations into account. But it is similar to the common rationale for abortion in the United States and elsewhere in its emphasis on privacy. What is important about all research involving human embryos is that it is, by the account of science given earlier, deeply public. Science labs are public places, not to the extent that government buildings are, perhaps, but in the sense that their purpose is to render transparent the workings of nature to all, especially, but not only, those also within the scientific community, a public body.

For this reason, too, no scientific result from a genuine lab is destined to remain only in that lab: scientists want results that can and will be reproduced by other scientists around the globe. This desire is part of what it means to be engaged in science at all. A woman who opts for an abortion may hope that nobody knows, and may even hope that no one else ever undergoes the same procedure. But this is impossible for the scientist. The scientist acts in a public space, in a public manner, for public reasons, and with public aspirations.

There can thus be no political defense of destructive embryonic research that does not directly come to grips with claims and arguments about the humanity and personhood of the early embryo. Further, if, as I argued in Chapter 5, the human embryo is a human being, and hence a human person, then it is straightforwardly the case that the state is not only permitted, but obligated to protect the embryo from any threat to its life or well-being in the context of any form of scientific inquiry. The right to privacy is meaningless in this context.

Moreover, the force of this argument extends beyond questions of federal funding for embryonic research, or research carried out in federal facilities and so on to all privately funded and carried out embryonic research. While the distinction between "privately" and "publicly" funded research is not unimportant—it is very important where considerations of benefit are at stake—it is completely irrelevant in this context. It is inappropriate for the state to fund obscene or worthless art, but it might nonetheless be legally acceptable for some persons to produce such art on their own dime and for their own, or likeminded individuals' consumption. But this would not be parallel to the situation under consideration.

More parallel would be an artist whose work involved child abuse, or even animal abuse. Because the purpose of the state is to protect all persons in its midst, and to make possible both small-scale communities, and the more general community of good will that should exist amongst persons living together, all matters involving serious harms, and especially killing, are public in the relevant sense—they are matters of state concern. If we imagine a performance artist whose work involves actual pedophilia, or an artist who intends to kill someone, perhaps himself, as part of a performance, it is clear that these artists' activities are likewise public in the relevant sense.

Science that involves destruction of human embryos is thus public in important ways. So the case that scientific inquiry, insofar as it bears negatively on human well-being, is rightly subject to state regulation, control, and prohibition seems very strong.

Where confusion would appear to enter the discussion is in an elision between scientific method and the activities of scientists, on the one hand, and the content of scientific discovery, on the other. Again, the parallel with medicine and religion may be helpful. The state may play a role, positively and negatively, in the support and regulation of medicine, and it may play a role, positively and negatively, in the support and (minimal, but sometimes justified) regulation of religion. What the state has no competence over is what particular medical therapies and strategies are adequate or beneficial, or what particular claims of religious revelation or authority are genuine.

Similarly, the state has no competence over the truth claims made by scientists, or judgments of scientific adequacy. Of course, state-sponsored scientists may make such judgments, and the state may sponsor panels and other investigatory bodies. But the competence of the state as such does not extend to the truth or falsity of such bodies' findings. We saw earlier that it is a temptation of overly paternalistic or even totalitarian states to think that their competence does extend so far.

This sort of error is an error of principle; while the state might legitimately block the distribution of some instance of scientific knowledge—how to build an atomic weapon, for example—or even forbid some or all persons from working on some particular project, the state may never adjudicate the truth or falsity of scientific claims. But it is common to move from a discussion of *this* lack of competence to the broader claim that the state has no competence with respect to the regulation of the *activities* of science, or the *fruits* of scientific research and technological development. This move is fallacious. To say that stem cell research ought not to be pursued, or that research into lethal viruses should cease, is to say nothing about the truth or falsity of any claims made in consequence of such research. On the other hand, to stipulate that research about global warming must be false on the basis of considerations of national interest—the interest in the claim being false—would be an overstepping of boundaries.

A final point on the publicity of scientific method: Because scientific knowledge is of such significance, and because scientific method, including the publicity of method, is of such instrumental importance in the gaining of scientific knowledge, the state has an interest in promoting the publicity and transparency of scientific method. While under some circumstances it is important for a scientist to remain provisionally secretive about her work, and while there are legitimate concerns among scientists about the theft of their work, science depends upon a division of labor and sharing of information that deep secrecy makes impossible. The state should, therefore, take an interest in ensuring that the conditions under which scientists can feel comfortable in sharing information and knowledge and experimental results exist.

## THE EXPRESSIVE POWER OF SCIENCE AND THE STATE

I argued in Chapter 8 that a society expresses itself through its science, and the science of a society shapes the nature of the society that is expressed. This expressive power is magnified or diminished to the extent that the state takes a positive or negative interest in it. One reason that the value of participatory democracy has come to be more and more widely recognized is that the members of a society have an interest in this expression and identity shaping, and recognize the importance of the state in guiding such expression and identity shaping in directions consonant with the desires and values of its people (Gutmann and Thompson, 1996).

Where the regime in power can unilaterally decide, without significant input from the state's citizens, that its foreign policy will be structured according to a doctrine of preventative force, or nuclear threats, or that its domestic policy will hereafter be shaped by the imposition of religious law, or the neglect of the poor, or even by the pursuit of victory in the Olympics at any cost, including the genetic enhancement of its athletes' bodies, then the state is expressing itself, and shaping itself, in certain definite ways, but with little or no input from its members.

Such expression and self-creation is often a side effect of something chosen for some other reason—the state's governors may believe the ruthless foreign policy essential to the survival of the state. But to choose to make nuclear deterrence, and a willingness to eliminate millions of innocent persons, the cornerstone of a state's foreign policy constitutes the state in a certain way, and expresses that self-constitution. Citizens of a putatively free and democratic state should particularly object to the suggestion that such decisions may be made with no reference to the values of the people.[3]

In consequence, it is often an obligation of the state to ascertain what the thoughts, values, and desires of its citizens are in relation to both general plans for the promotion of science, and specific projects. So, on the one hand, a state might have resources enough either to provide more science funding, and to promote in various other ways the cause of science, or to engage in some other form of social works, such as a program of job creation for the poor, or the provision of better medical care to the uninsured, or even a greater emphasis on national sports. To some extent, such decisions will be matters of discretion—that is, under some circumstances, it will be morally permissible to spend the money, resources, and time one way, or another. In such circumstances, it should be a matter of public debate and deliberation: What sort of a society does the society in question wish to be? How does it wish to express itself, and be constituted by its decisions (Kitcher, 2001)?

On the matter of funding for particular projects, several points should be made. First, where a project is unambiguously immoral, it is simply wrong, regardless of the desires of the people, for the state to support it. If there had been unequivocal support in society for the sort of research done at Tuskeegee, this would hardly have justified it. But if the state approves such researches despite the general populace's lack of approval, then it wrongs not just the subjects of the experiments, but its other citizens as well.

Second, it is because the benefits of science and scientific technology are potentially so widespread, and because its method is so public, that science is so expressive of a culture, society, or state. So concerns that a form of science might wrongly express a culture will typically be related to concerns over the public nature of the benefits or methods of the science in question. The remainder of this chapter considers one particular area of science in which there is precisely such a convergence of concerns, the prospect of widespread government-sponsored research using human embryos.

## HUMAN EMBRYONIC RESEARCH AND THE EXPRESSIVE POWER OF THE STATE

Suppose that the United States were to support in a significant way destructive research on human embryos.[4] A considerable number of citizens of this country would be appalled at what they would consider the immoral destruction of human persons, and in this their concern would be importantly other related. But their concern would also properly be self-related in several ways.

First, they would worry that at some future time, possibly not too far into the future, the benefits of such research would be, practically speaking, unavoidable. Ordinary health care treatments and therapies, and possibly a host of other technologies might in time grow to be enormously, and complexly, tied to the research originally done on human embryos. While it might, to a point, be possible through a concerted effort to wall oneself off from these benefits, it would become increasingly difficult through time to do so.

What sort of a concern is this? It is not best understood as a concern about moral cooperation, for the deadly deeds will have already been done. But even if one has not cooperated in the wrongdoing that led to the received benefits, a person of good will could not help but feel that the widespread use of these benefits falsely expressed her moral views and her moral self. Similarly, persons of good will might, in some cases at least, recognize that certain sorts of benefits they presently receive were a consequence of historical mistreatment of black slaves. Even if no direct question of cooperation can arise here, such persons can still feel that the situation fails to express who they think they are morally.

Second, such persons will see embryonic research going on publicly, and increasingly commonly. It is true that they are not themselves involved in the research, but they will feel, as do the many persons now opposed to abortion, both that their culture tragically fails to express their moral ideals, and that because it is *their* culture, this makes it particularly hard to live with. Such feelings must have been common among people of good will who witnessed the segregation of blacks in the South prior to the civil rights movement. This expressive concern is only heightened and intensified, in the research case, as in the segregated South, by the publicity of the offensive actions.

We might compare these sorts of expressive concerns with others that people feel deeply about. Some object strenuously to any mention of God or religion in any public place or situation. I mean here not objections to premises derived from religious traditions being used in public deliberations, but to the more symbolic use of religious language as in the Pledge of Allegiance, or the oaths taken in court. By the public invocation of God, such citizens argue, the state expresses a certain type of ethos, or public character, specifically a theistic or even Christian ethos. This expressed character is viewed as so alien to these citizens that they feel themselves coerced or unfairly dominated.

To a point, this is a helpful analogy for the problem I am pointing to in science and the form of expressive power that science has, an expressive power that can be only magnified by the state. But there is a great disanalogy between the case of religious-symbolism objectors and embryonic-research objectors. While in both situations citizens believe that something deeply alien to who and what they are morally is being expressed socially, in the embryonic research case what is being expressed is, by the lights of objectors, murderous. This, I shall argue shortly, raises significant concerns for certain forms of research.

## DISPUTED CLAIMS AND EXPRESSIVE POWER

Considerations of the expressive power of science, and of the way in which the state can magnify or restrict that expressive power, are of particular importance because of the fact of widespread and sometimes radical moral disagreement. Consider again the case of religious expression. The use of theistic language in various political and social contexts is indeed intended to express the nation's self-understood relationship to the divine, a relationship of gratitude, humility, and reverence. But such expressions do not express the feelings, values, beliefs, etc., of all members of the country.

Some argue that the proper response to this is one of state neutrality, to be achieved by a complete elimination of all such symbolic references. However, the elimination of all public religious expression would express a different self-image of the state, and now one at odds with a large percentage of the country's theists (George, 2001, p. 6). The proposed state of affairs in which there are no public expressions of religious belief and reverence is not a neutral state of affairs, but one expressing something else, something likely to be offensive to believers, as the recent scuffles over the Ten Commandments monument in Alabama, or the contents of the Pledge of Allegiance, indicate.

In the case of religious symbols and language, what is primarily at issue is itself expression. In most cases in which it is the expressive power of science that is at issue, however, expression is only secondarily at issue. Proponents of some particular course of scientific inquiry typically have first-order benefits they hope to obtain—knowledge, technologies, and so on. Opponents typically wish to avoid first-order harms: the killing of unborn humans, or of animals, or the unjust appropriation of resources. It is because one views these courses of action as right or wrong that one also views them as expressive, and rejoices or worries at their further self-constituting features.

The view that I defended earlier in discussing the public benefits and method of science emphasized precisely these first-order benefits and harms: that some technology promises great benefits is a good reason to pursue it; that some scientific research would involve killing humans is a sufficient reason to avoid it. Especially where some form of inquiry violates a moral principle that it falls to the state to enforce, expressive concerns are irrelevant: the state may regulate lethal forms of inquiry without concern for how people feel about it.

However, I have already indicated one instance in which expressive concerns can tip the balance in favor of or against research, namely in cases in which it would be permissible but not obligatory for the state to promote, and perhaps fund some research. In some such cases, the fact that such research would or would not well express the considered views of society will constitute good reason for the state to promote or refuse to promote, fund, or refuse to fund. So the expressive potential of science is relevant here.

Such expressive potential is also relevant in a relatively (and fortunately) rare sort of case, in which the leaders, or a significant enough proportion of those leaders, and a majority, or a significant enough proportion, of the citizens, of a participatory democracy believe that some course of action is permissible, and wish very much to pursue that course of action, but in which a significant number of citizens, though not a majority, believe that the recommended course of action is deeply immoral, and thus object, beyond their stated first-order objections, that the course of action would violate their deepest moral sense of themselves. In such cases, it might be reasonable, and perhaps obligatory, for a state to refrain from promoting or funding some form of inquiry out of respect for those citizens, even though this might result in a significant loss of benefits.

In the case of religious expression, there seems to be a considerable amount of favor shown towards some such principle. The courts seem frequently to privilege the expressive concerns of atheists over theists, despite the fact that an atheist's deepest moral sense of himself does not, in the present situation, seem genuinely threatened. No atheist is called upon to say the Pledge of Allegiance, and atheists may take alternate forms of oaths that ordinarily refer to God. Nor do atheists seem significantly burdened by having to listen to the religious expressions of others. Nevertheless, a fair amount of concern for atheists has been shown in recent years, as in the Ninth Circuit Court of Appeals ruling on the constitutionality of the Pledge of Allegiance (*Michael A. Newdow v. US Congress et al.,* June 26, 2002).

Consider, by contrast, the expressive concerns of a significant minority in a state that practiced human sacrifice, or used rape as a weapon in war. These examples are imperfect because everyone who reads this will share abhorrence at such actions. But the point is to get such readers to recognize what a radical violation of their sense of their moral selves would be required to live in such a society, in which their deepest moral convictions on these matters were not shared. Similarly, citizens of good will in a state that supported slavery would feel that their deepest moral selves were being violated, and would feel compelled to question the legitimacy of their state. They are certainly incapable of doing nothing: those citizens who objected to the slavery practiced or permitted by their state could not simply object privately, but were morally obliged to contemplate even the strongest possible measures of response, such as armed rebellion.

To take a different example, Christians living in an Islamic state need not feel entirely morally alienated from their countries, if they are privately accorded religious liberty, even if a vast amount of public speech expresses Islam, and even though public Christian expression is somewhat restricted. The moral conscience of Christians need not be affronted by living in such a state, though of course they would have good reasons for desiring a freer society. More problematically, Christians governed entirely by Islamic law (*sharia*) would have strong moral grounds for disapproval, and might feel significantly alienated from the state in the way in which some Germans must morally have felt alienated from a Nazi state that persecuted Jews.[5] But both non-Christians and non-theists can live with a certain amount of religious and even Christian expression in their country, despite their objections: their deepest moral sense of themselves is not compromised by living in such a state.

By contrast, citizens who recognize the destruction of embryonic human life as murderous cannot live in a state that itself promotes such research without a radical violation of their moral sense of themselves. For believing Christians, Good Samaritan duties, reverence for human life, and a sense of the state as subject, ultimately, to God's law, are all too central to their moral sense of themselves for such state-sponsored murder to be anything but a serious attack on those moral selves, in addition to its wrongfulness as murderous. Citizens who felt this way, for example, would be morally justified in taking up arms to prevent this, if there were some hope, which there is not, that this endeavor would be successful. This can be recognized even by those who disagree with the claim about embryonic life: such persons can recognize the extraordinary gravity of the situation for one who believed it was taking of human life.

Political philosophers, politicians, and activists have all, in respect to the abortion debate, and increasingly in respect to the debate over embryonic life, asked what should be done about radical moral disagreement in a way that has presupposed that there was nothing that proponents of abortion or embryo research had to offer to opponents. Rather, because the premises of opponents of such procedures have been deemed "controversial" or "religious" or "such as a reasonable person could disagree with," philosophers, politicians, and activists have written exclusively as if all compromise needed to come from those opponents, and none from those in favor of such procedures.[6]

But no such compromise is possible on the issue of embryonic research. Publicly funded destructive embryonic research, much more than privately permitted abortion, is too great a burden—a moral burden—to ask objecting citizens to shoulder. States should not ask citizens to bear this burden, and should enact no legislation that would require them to bear it.

Could supporters of such research make the same sorts of arguments? No. True, supporters are being asked to give up something, namely, the potential benefits that might emerge from such research. So they are asked to bear a burden as part of the cost of maintaining the good will and moral integrity of citizens with whom they disagree. Proponents of the research are quick to capitalize on this, and frequently accuse opponents of "condemning" to death those who might otherwise be benefited, and of "holding hostage" the lives of the many for the sake of their moral or religious scruples. But this is entirely wrong.

First, opponents of the research stand to benefit from it every bit as much as proponents. The diseases for which embryonic research promises therapies are diseases that strike pro-lifers and their families, as well as the proponents of embryonic research. It is not at all as if opponents are offering to place all the burdens of a ban on such research on a different party's shoulders, while they reap the (moral) benefits of the ban. Rather, they offer to bear the burdens equally with others. Indeed, some of those who object *themselves* suffer from conditions that could possibly be treated by therapies developed from embryonic research.

Second, the benefits promised are deeply asymmetric with the harms being avoided. Ron Reagan, the son of the late former president, and others, have held out the idea that President Reagan's Alzheimer's disease could have been alleviated or even cured had embryonic stem cell research been permitted. No one can doubt that this would have been a good thing, but it must be kept in mind that President Reagan, at any rate, lived a full and long life before becoming sick. His illness and death were tragic in the sense that the illnesses and deaths of anyone can be called tragic, but he was deprived of relatively little by the absence of a cure that does not exist for any other person. Much more tragic, seemingly, are the deaths of millions of children to diseases that can be cured or prevented, and that are cured and prevented for those in wealthier nations. But stem cell research is not needed to provide immediate benefits to many of these young human beings. The asymmetry, then, is this: on one option, we could, without violating the consciences of our fellow citizens, save many children; on the other option we could, by violating the consciences of our fellow citizens, prolong the life of those who have lived full and reasonably long lives. Which choice is more reasonable?

It is true that many who suffer from diseases that could be possibly be treated from stem cell–based therapies are young people whose lives will be cut short by their conditions. But even here, the burdens are asymmetric, even if we abstract from the lives of the embryos themselves. No one's ability to live at home in their state and no one's moral sense of themselves are threatened by disease. Given the choice, it would be more reasonable to accept physical suffering than to accept the continued existence of great moral evil. I do not doubt that many citizens of good will in Nazi Germany would willingly have accepted a disease of the body rather than live in a state so deeply stricken with a disease of the soul. So even in the case of the burdens that the young would bear in the absence of a cure, there is a great asymmetry between the burdens of those asked to allow what they believe to be state-sponsored murder, and the burdens of those with serious illness. This asymmetry exists independently of the additional asymmetry between asking that embryos be killed in order that other human persons not suffer diseases encountered in the ordinary, though often tragic, course of life.

Finally, there is an asymmetry with respect to the notion of the burden's being imposed. For while the state would literally impose a burden upon those who morally object to embryonic research, no one imposes, in reality, a burden upon those who will get sick in the ordinary, albeit unfortunate natural course of events. Disease is inevitable, and unless it has been deliberately communicated to someone, it is not reasonable to speak of the burdens of disease as having been imposed upon someone. This is true even when human agents do bear some responsibility for the fact that someone is ill: it stretches the sense of the term to speak of smokers having their cancer imposed on them, whether by tobacco companies, or even by themselves, by virtue of their choice to smoke.

In consequence, proponents of destructive human embryonic research cannot utilize the same sorts of arguments in defense of such research that opponents can. The burdens they are asked to shoulder are not unfair, they are not moral burdens, and they do not threaten an agent's ability to view her state as legitimate. The fact that science is expressive and self-constituting of a society, and that the state can magnify or diminish that expressive power, grounds an argument against the state's involvement in embryonic research, and particularly against any form of funding of that research.

Two qualifications must be added. First, this argument applies primarily to state funding and promotion of this research. It does not, itself, apply to private funding and pursuit of such research. But this is a more limited qualification than might at first appear. Objectively, the arguments presented in Chapter 5, and earlier in this chapter, against embryonic research indicate that it is unreasonable for such research to be permitted *at all*. Further, these arguments are directly available to legislators: they do not need to be filtered through any liberal principle or strategy before they are rendered acceptable reasons for public action.

The argument that I have just given, therefore, does not begin from a premise that radical moral disagreement is a first-order consideration in discussion of these issues. Radical moral disagreement is not a principled first step in a discussion of embryonic research. Rather, the argument has accepted the assumption that in *fact* many people, and perhaps those in power, will not, for whatever reasons, recognize the soundness of the arguments against such research. The nature of the disagreement over such research then provides a premise in a second-order argument about how it would be reasonable for the state to proceed, not given the immorality of such research in first-order terms, but given the nature of the first-order concerns that those opposed to the research have, and the relationship these concerns would put such agents in to a state that funded and promoted such research. The argument thus abstracts from the truth or falsity of these first-order concerns only at this meta-level, and not at the primary level of moral and political analysis.

This explains the argument's relative weakness in the face of privately funded embryonic research: although such research is still public in the relevant ways, and although permitting such research does magnify that publicity and threaten the moral identity of many citizens of the state, it does not do this to the extent that public funding of such research would. So while it would be entirely reasonable, and indeed obligatory, for the state to ban entirely all research that was destructive to human embryos, the argument for such a ban on privately funded research seems to me to require the relevant first-order premises that assert the important truths about the nature and value of the human embryo. This is the argument's second qualification.

Two final points may be made. First, if we abstract from the particular interpretation of the term placed upon it by Rawls, the considerations urged here could be understood broadly in terms of the political demand for reciprocity. Here is a representative passage from Rawls:

> [T]he idea of political legitimacy based on the criterion of reciprocity says: Our exercise of political power is proper only when we sincerely believe that the reasons we would offer for our political actions . . . are sufficient, and we also reasonably think that other citizens might also reasonably accept those reasons. . . . To make more explicit the role of the criterion of reciprocity as expressed in public reason, note that its role is to specify the nature of the political relation in a constitutional democratic regime as one of civic friendship. (Rawls, 1999, p. 137)

To summarize, we might say that (a) a significant number of citizens may not reasonably accept destructive embryonic research, and (b) the funding of such research by the state would fail as regards the criterion of reciprocity and would thus destroy the bonds and the possibility of civic friendship.

Second, it might seem that the arguments put forth would justify a revision of governmental policy regarding the treatment of animals, despite the moral conclusions drawn in Chapter 6. In the current state of the animal liberation movement, I do not think this is so, for the following reasons. First, the number of animal rights activists seems considerably smaller than the number of supporters of embryo rights. Second, the ideological bonds that tie together those who believe in and practice animal rights are typically disparate and lack unity. Embryo rights activists almost unanimously believe that embryos should be accorded rights because they are human persons. But the supporters of animal rights range widely from rights theorists to utilitarians, to deep environmentalists, to those who believe that domination of animals is linked to gender domination. Third, it is not clear that there is a definite class of animals that all animal rights activists believe deserve protection. So the arguments of this chapter do not require that the state view animal research as it should view embryonic research.

This concludes my discussion of the politics of scientific inquiry. I have shown that the state should in most cases permit the free pursuit of scientific knowledge, should also, in many cases actively promote this pursuit, and should sometimes provide funding for those engaged in the pursuit, or those distributing its results. Further, the state may sometimes regulate and forbid certain forms of scientific inquiry, among them, research that destroys human embryos. However, the state never has authority over the truth value of science. Scientific inquiry does not, however, exhaust the forms of inquiry with which the state might concern itself. Before turning, in Chapter 11, to a discussion of the internal ethics of inquiry, I wish to expand the ethics of inquiry beyond scientific research, and to address the relationship between the state and two more forms of inquiry, inquiry in the humanities and journalism.

# 10 Humanistic and Journalistic Inquiry and the State

The two previous chapters focused on governmental concerns with scientific inquiry, broadly understood. Scientific research, including biomedical and technological research, are public forms of inquiry, and this publicity has consequences for politics.

But scientific research is not the only form of inquiry with which the state is potentially concerned, for the state funds public universities within which inquiry in the humanities is pursued, and both federal and state governments provide grants to scholars in the humanities. And questions concerning the relationship between the state and the profession of journalism are of continuing concern. Such questions are made more interesting by the ways in which humanistic and journalistic inquiries and investigations resemble, or fail to resemble, scientific research.

In Chapter 3, for example, I made the claim that the ethics of journalism is in many ways structurally similar to the ethics of science. Unlike police investigators, journalists do not have an authority that permits them to use certain techniques, such as coercion, or invasive searches, in pursuit of the truth. However, journalists do, like scientists, serve the common good in important ways. So one might think that the relationship between the state and journalism would be quite similar to the relationship between the state and science.

The humanities, on the other hand, would appear to be significantly different from the sciences in ways that might lead us to think that humanistic inquiry should be divorced from the concerns of the state. Addressing the humanities first, and then journalism, I argue for precisely the opposite of these two conclusions.

I look first at the dissimilarities between humanistic inquiry and scientific inquiry; I then argue that, despite these differences, state support of humanistic inquiry is justifiable. I then look at the ways in which journalism is similar to science. But I argue, despite these similarities, for a more hands-off policy when it comes to the state and journalism.[1]

## THE STATE AND THE HUMANITIES

Humanistic inquiry in many fields—in philosophy, political theory, literary studies, or culture studies, for example—resolves itself less frequently into consensus than does inquiry in the sciences. So there is less justification for speaking of a public body of knowledge of intrinsic benefit to society than there is in science. The instrumental benefits of the humanities are also typically less significant, judged from a particular perspective at least, than those of science. The number of socially useful inventions by philosophers and literary theorists is small; some would say the number of socially useful philosophers and literary theorists is even smaller.

Both these asymmetries, which track the first of the three ways in which I claimed that science was especially public, are related to further asymmetries connected to the other two ways in which science is public. One reason that inquiry in the humanities tends less towards agreed truth is that such inquiry does not have the very public experimental method of science. The humanities might therefore seem to be less expressive and constitutive of a culture than the sciences, although I shall provide reasons to question this claim.

One response to these perceived asymmetries has been the attempt to make the humanities "more scientific." Various attempts have been made to make philosophy more like science, such as logical positivism, naturalized epistemology, and American pragmatism. Similarly, attempts have been made to either eliminate humanistic inquiry, or limit it to those forms that might, at any rate, result in some distinct instrumental advantage. Philosophy and English departments are sometimes encouraged to focus especially on rhetoric or technical writing. Another response asserts that the state should simply not be involved in the funding of humanistic inquiry.

The question, then, is whether a defense of the humanities and its support by the state can be made that does not seek to assimilate humanistic inquiry to scientific inquiry. Such support might include funding public universities, issuing grants for research, and organizing cooperative ventures such as seminars.

The key for arguing for an affirmative answer is not to address each humanistic discipline one by one—a defense of philosophy, a defense of literary studies, and so forth—but to look at the humanities as a body. We will thereby see that the humanities constitute an important form of inquiry into human nature, and the human condition, and that these forms of humanistic inquiry are "liberal arts"—they constitute important forms of human freedom that should be encouraged.

It is important, first, to note the limitations of scientific inquiry. Science can show that this or that form of technology is possible, but it cannot show whether it is moral. A scientist can say many important things about the properties of ink and paper, but science tells us nothing about the nature or value of literature, nor does it have anything to say on particular works of literature. Scientific technique has been of importance in tracking political numbers and statistics, but it can say nothing about what forms of government and what sorts of political choices are reasonable. The natural sciences provide valuable tools for dating artifacts, but they cannot identify what historical events and persons are important for historical study, nor can they identify in what that importance consists. In short, science says nothing about the good, the right, the beautiful, the reasonable, the important, the valuable—nothing about any of these concepts of supreme importance to human beings.

These notions are important because of our lives are governed not just by what is true descriptively of us, and independent of our own action, but by what is true normatively, and by what we do, and fail to do, in response to normative concerns. Who and what we are is a function of who and what we should be. To say, as Aristotle does in the opening sentence of his *Metaphysics,* that all men desire by nature to know, should not be understood primarily as a kind of statistical claim about curiosity, but as a claim about what is good and right for us, translated into a claim about our nature. Because knowledge is good and right for us, the desire to know is natural.

The humanities in general are governed by these sorts of normative concerns. Of course, technique, description, analysis, even the use of the sciences, natural and social, can come into play in discovering, articulating, and synthesizing an understanding of the normative. So it should not be surprising to find large parts of humanistic inquiry that resemble scientific inquiry in one respect or another. Moreover, parts of the humanities, like the philosophical subfield of metaphysics, or history, are theoretical in a sense that contrasts with the practical. But the ultimate aim of metaphysics includes an understanding of our role in the cosmos, and the ultimate aim of history includes an understanding of what is humanly important in the past, and normatively relevant to the present, all understandings that are themselves partly normative, or normatively guided. So at root, the concerns of the humanities are normative and unscientific. But they are of central importance for our understanding of ourselves, and of the sort of world we should inhabit morally.

Because of this connection to the normative, humanistic inquiry is bound to be different as regards its conclusions than is science. Some believe that there is not the same consensus in the humanities as in science because the humanities are entirely matters of subjective "opinion." But even if, as I believe, there are truths in the humanities, it should be expected that they would be more difficult to obtain: they are not truths independent from us to be gained by detached assessment of a free-standing world, but truths involving us, and to the assessment of which we will bring desires, fears, hopes, and prejudices. The normative is not empirical, and so does not admit of interpersonal sensory checking and testing, and is, in some cases especially, deeply abstract. The normative is often filtered differently through different cultures in a way that facts about digestion are not.

One consequence of these differences is that not only the answers, but the methods of humanistic inquiry will be subject to disagreement, a type of disagreement that itself then creates further disagreements over results. Some of these disagreements can be resolved, and some are the result of culpable bias and error. But the persistence of much disagreement is something we should expect.

Still, consider how a culture determines itself when it decides that these normative questions are of no importance, even while praising and honoring the sciences. As a culture, it determines itself, ultimately, as a slave to nature in its entirely descriptive sense, a point made in a related context by C. S. Lewis in *The Abolition of Man:*

> At the moment, then, of Man's victory over Nature, we find the whole human race subjected to some individual men, and those individuals subjected to that in themselves which is purely "natural"—to their irrational impulses. Nature, untrammeled by values, rules the Conditioners and, through them, all humanity. Man's conquest of Nature turns out, in the moment of its consummation, to be Nature's conquest of Man. (Lewis, 1962, p. 47)

Such a culture asserts that the normative as such is of no importance to it—this goes beyond a rejection of any particular finding of the humanities, and threatens a radical curtailment of human freedom. Consider the consequences, for example, were moral inquiry not to provide a check to the scientific drive to remake human nature in the ways described in Chapter 7. The humanities are liberal in the sense that humanistic inquiry has as its aim the liberation of man from the sheerly descriptive constraints of nature.

Part of the original meaning of "liberal" in liberal arts was that the practitioners of such arts were free in a very straightforward sense: they were not slaves, nor were they lower-class workers striving merely to make a living. The humanities, the liberal arts, and culture all require leisure (Pieper, 1998). One of the most striking phenomena of travel to the poorest parts of the world is often the lack of leisured activity in contexts in which hard labor has made rest the only thing possible at the end of the day.

A democratic society, committed to the common good, has reason to avoid the radical separation of humanistic inquiry from ordinary labor approved of by Aristotle. All citizens are benefited from being introduced to the humanities and given at least an initial appreciation of the nature and importance of humanistic inquiry. Some who are so introduced will go on themselves to labor in the humanities, others to have only a dim recollection of "that philosophy class I took." But many will find their ability to appreciate art, their wonder at important questions, their critical reflection on ethical and political issues, and their respect for what is human, all to be enhanced. The humanities are thus a significant part of the common good.

This is certainly not to deny that the humanities contain their share of posers, and that at least some of what passes for humanistic inquiry is something else altogether, such as a thinly veiled attempt to promote a political agenda. My point here is merely to defend the claim that the humanities and humanistic inquiry are as such reasonable aspects of the common good that it is the state's mandate to promote. Moreover, such inquiry can be promoted relatively cheaply, especially relative to the possible rewards. There can thus be a legitimate role for the state in funding such inquiry in conjunction with a funding of the institutional context within which the fruits of such inquiry are publicized and passed on, and the methods of such inquiry made available to citizens.

This last point requires further articulation: it is, strictly speaking, neither research alone, nor teaching alone, of the humanities that the state is justified in funding, but both together. It is not research alone, for this will then lack the broad connection to the common good necessary for state funding. But it is not teaching alone either. Teaching without research grows quickly stagnant; to assume that there is a complete body of material in the humanities such as the Great Books that should serve henceforth as the body of humanistic material to be transmitted is self-defeating, for inquiry needs to be made into those books, to determine what they say. It is also short-sighted, in its assumption that nothing new about the human condition remains to be learned.

Further, it is in large part the art of inquiry itself that must be passed on to students: as much as, and sometimes more than, the wisdom of any particular text, it is the wisdom involved in how to approach a text, problem, or issue critically and reflectively that must be taught. This can be done only if the teachers themselves are inquirers. The university is sometimes thought of primarily as a repository of knowledge and teaching, rather than of inquiry and discovery (Newman, 1966, p. xxxvii). But this is to defeat a primary purpose of the university as a genuine home of inquiry.

In concluding this discussion, it is worth pointing out that the argument I have made for the importance of humanistic inquiry has worked by presenting a particular model of that inquiry, and what it is all about. Humanistic inquiry is shaped by broadly normative considerations, and is inquiry into the human condition and human nature, and the human place and role in the cosmos. To carry out such inquiry is itself an activity of tremendous human significance, and critical to the common good. Hence, the funding of this activity of the state is justifiable.

Insofar, however, as we can imagine a culture in which this understanding of the humanities is instantiated, and in which the state appropriately funds higher education, then we are in a position to rethink some of the earlier asymmetries between humanistic and scientific inquiry. For example, it would appear that a society that recognizes the importance of, and funds, for a large part of the population, humanistic inquiry does indeed thereby express and constitute itself as a society of a particular sort. Moreover, in such a society, there would be convergence in the humanities on at least one issue of crucial humanistic importance, namely, the importance of the humanities. And a crucial methodological disagreement would have been broadly resolved, namely, the disagreement over what, teleologically, the humanities were aiming at, and hence, over what a method, or the methods, of humanistic inquiry meant to achieve. In the sciences, method-ological unity, to the extent that it exists, is in large part a consequence of a shared understanding of the purpose of science—the empirically grounded understanding of the truth about the natural world. In the humanities today, by contrast, disagreement over whether there is a truth, and hence over whether the humanities are a form of inquiry, creates a meta-level of disagreement that does not exist to the same degree in science. But in the society that I have envisaged, *that* disagreement, at least, does not exist. So while there will, inevitably, be much first-order disagreement within the humanities, there will at least be harmony on the second-order method-ological commitment to the humanities as a form of inquiry into the truth about the human condition.


## JOURNALISTIC INQUIRY

In Chapter 8, I argued that science is best understood as a profession. Science was understood as a practice whose internal goods were of such social importance that institutional structures had arisen around the practice in order that those benefits might be more easily achieved, promoted, and dis-tributed. Journalism, too, should be considered a profession. This suggests that it should be supported by the state in the same way science is. What, then, are the goods that are internal to the practice of journalism, and how are they of such importance to the common good? I shall argue that jour-nalism serves the social good in three critical ways. But I shall then argue that despite this similarity with science, the state's relationship, both as to promotion and as to regulation, should be somewhat different from its nor-mative relationship to science.

Journalism plays (or ought to play) three beneficial roles for a flourish-ing community. First, journalism plays an important role in making avail-able the information necessary for individual choices and a correlative role, analogous and complementary to the role played by law, in solving coor-dination difficulties created by the numerous individual choices made in society. By making a variety of kinds of information available, it allows coordination among the choices made by individuals. While this role can be played by journalism even in tyrannical societies, still, such a coordina-tive function must be performed by journalism in a successful community, and it must be performed in a way quite different from its role in a totali-tarian or dictatorial state.

Second, journalism is essential to the public conversation by which a community assesses its needs, and deliberates about the appropriate means for satisfying those needs. Journalists provide a public space within which this necessary conversation can take place, and often contribute to that con-versation. Thus, journalism contributes to the possibility of a community's self-governance.

Third, journalism plays a role in society similar, but even more focused in some ways, to the expressive and constitutive role played by science, as discussed in Chapter 8. Journalism helps to form society as a "we," as agents bound by a sense of solidarity.

I have argued that science should be considered public in three ways: in its benefits, its method, and its expressive power. Journalism too could be considered public in three analogous ways, each corresponding to the types of benefits journalism provides. The information it provides that is necessary for individual choice and social coordination is like the knowledge benefits provided by science. Its role in fostering public deliberation is analogous to the public method of science. And, as mentioned, journalism's role in fostering social solidarity is also similar to the expressive and constitutive nature of science. However, in my taxonomy of the ways in which science is public, only the first, its provision of knowledge, was discussed in terms of its public benefit. Science's other two modes of publicity were considered independently of whether they should also be thought of as public benefits. With journalism, the case is somewhat different; the point of journalism is to be beneficial in each of these three ways. In what follows, I briefly discuss each type of benefit; I then argue that the nature of these benefits justifies a much more limited degree of state involvement in the profession of journalism than in science.

## Journalism and Individual Choice

At its most fundamental level, journalism is about inquiry, and the public articulation of the fruits of inquiry. But what sorts of inquiry, and of what benefit are its results? Unlike some branches of science, journalism is not concerned with systematic knowledge for its own sake. Rather, it is primarily concerned with seeking out and publicizing information of an instrumentally beneficial character. The instrumental benefits also differ from those of science. Journalism, unlike science, is concerned in large part with the provision of information that makes possible the sorts of decisions human agents need to make on a daily basis; and, by providing a common framework for such decisions for most agents in a society, journalism aids in the coordinating of the multitude of individual decisions by agents so as not to have social chaos.

This second function is analogous to one role of the law. Not every determination of the law is a matter of strict justice. Often, there are a variety of ways in which citizens could act, but it is necessary to determine one way, or a limited set of ways, in which they must or may act so as to prevent chaos, confusion, or gross inefficiency. Similarly, the institution of promising can coordinate two agents' actions in such a way as to prevent missed meetings, neglected work, or unnecessary duplication.

The importance of accurate and relevant information is of central importance both to individual choices and to the social coordination of multiple agents, all of whom must make individual choices. Errors of gaps in communication of the law, or the content of promises can negate the benefits of both institutions. But the need for accurate and relevant information to be used for individual choice and social coordination goes beyond what either the law or promises can provide. Journalism exists in large part to satisfy these needs.

To give a simple example: Several thousand people wish to attend a baseball game. But when and where is it to be held? Requiring all who wish to attend to call the box office for information, or simply relying on all ten thousand, or more, to show up eventually, is far from efficient. For a newspaper accurately to provide such information allows each of these thousands of citizens to decide whether they will go, and to arrange for going in an efficient manner. It further allows all these citizens to make their choices in a way that will not result in complete chaos.

The example might seem trivial, but the ability to make such everyday decisions, even outside the realm of the explicitly political, is a major benefit of modern life. And newspapers provide the citizenry of a state with the bulk of the information by which they govern their daily lives, including their daily political lives.[2] The very layout of most newspapers indicates an awareness of this purpose. "Community" sections, "Living" sections, "Religion" sections, and even classified advertisements provide information of clear importance to individual decisions; but because it is this set of information that provides the parameters for such decisions, the result is social coordination on a fairly wide scale.

This dual purpose of providing information for private choice and social coordination lies behind a number of roles played by the press that are often described as the press's "watchdog" function. Consider, for example, the difference between the press discovering that a certain form of medication is dangerous, and the government discovering the same thing. Even where the pharmaceutical company is criminally liable, only the government has the capacity for removing the food and punishing those responsible. But the press can make available information that may be used by doctors and patients to make effective and informed decisions. This is even more clear in those cases in which what the press reports is not something illegal. Although the government may take no action, information about a company's business practices, for example, may make possible new forms of behavior on the part of the citizenry: avoidance, protest, or political action.

The press plays a watchdog role in such cases. Yet the term is used most frequently to refer to the role the press plays in monitoring the actions of the state. The press reports on campaign finances, on who voted for what, on possible abuses of power and corruption of officials. The Watergate reporting by Carl Bernstein and Bob Woodward is perhaps the most famous instance of watchdog reporting with significant public consequences. But in a host of other ways, journalistic inquiry is aimed at providing information about governmental workings that makes possible reasonable decisions of the part of the citizenry.

Such decisions are often taken individually by citizens. But across a broad range of contexts, citizens also must deliberate and make decisions together. This is the second way in which the profession of journalism provides important public benefits.

## Journalism and Public Deliberation

Charles Taylor, in an essay titled "Liberal Politics and the Public Sphere," points to a modern transformation, documented by Jürgen Habermas, of the "opinions of mankind" into "public opinion." The older model of a commonly shared opinion of mankind was "seen as (1) unreflective, (2) unmediated by discussion and critique, and (3) passively inculcated in each successive generation. Public opinion, by contrast, is meant (1) to be the product of reflection, (2) to emerge from discussion, and (3) to reflect an actively produced consensus" (Taylor, 1995, p. 261; cf. Habermas, 1989). Central to the development of the notion of public opinion was the possibility of a common space in which the sort of public conversation necessary for a reflective opinion on public matters could develop. This common space was made possible by the developing eighteenth-century print media, in the form of books, pamphlets, and newspapers. At the heart of this common space, in turn, was a form of impersonal communication of ideas and arguments. As Michael Werner puts it, "The meaning of public utterance . . . is established by the very fact that [an] exchange can be read and participated in by any number of unknown and *in principle unknowable* others" (Warner, 1990, p. 40).

These developments make possible a central element of a flourishing civil society, briefly indicated in Chapter 9: the autonomous participation of citizens in deliberation about the common good, or, more simply, its "self-rule." We can see the importance of the development of a "common space" for self-rule in several ways. First, there can be no genuine self-rule if there is no common deliberation. Consider an organization in which five different interest groups independently work out an account of their needs, and then submit the account to a governing body, which determines which needs will be met and sets about meeting them. Absent some common communication and deliberation among the five groups, there is a strong sense in which the final decision cannot be said to be shared among all five, even if it is a decision in favor of an allotment that would have been agreed upon by all.

The level at which such common communication and deliberation takes place may vary: it may, for instance, be engaged in over the question of who should have the authority to determine the allotment, once the groups had individually and independently deliberated. This would be a rather thin notion of common deliberation. On the other hand, an arrangement by which no decision was reached until consensus was arrived at might be in practice unworkable. So a middle position suggests itself. Common deliberation is necessary both to determine who will bear the necessary authority in final deliberation and to provide guidance for that final determination.

In regard to these dual needs, the journalistic profession can benefit society in a unique way, both as a forum for common communication and deliberation and as a shaper of that communication and deliberation.[3] But the discussion of the common space also indicated the importance of a form of impersonal communication; and this can be seen to be important for a society's self-rule, and as part of the journalist's mandate.

Consider again the proposals put forth by each of the five interest groups. To the extent that the contents of these proposals turn on considerations that are relevant only to each of the interest groups individually, they may have no purchase for the other groups in a determination of priorities, allotments, and so on. It is only to the extent that proposals are made in terms of concerns that may be given consideration by the various members of the group that deliberation, rather than mere negotiation, is possible. Not all the concerns of an interest group are so frameable; but there still will be a set of concerns jointly shared by reference to which non-shared concerns may be seen to be of importance. So even when advocating personal interests, a group must be able to place such interests in a wider context of shared concerns, and the language of such shared concerns will be increasingly impersonal.

This impetus towards the impersonal raises questions in the ethics of journalism that will be important in later discussion of the state's relationship to journalism; for it might be thought that the considerations raised generate a mandate to the press to be maximally "neutral" and "objective," where the latter term is understood as requiring detachment from all particular concerns and interests. Objections to such a view are numerous, ranging from those who see the press as permissibly engaged in advocacy of certain positions to those who see the quest for objectivity or neutrality as self-deceiving. However, I suggest a model of the press that is both potentially partisan and objective in ways not appreciated by the objections.

That the press will be partisan in some respect is a function of the fact that any particular institution is itself a participant in the public life of its community. In the political realm, for example, editors, editorialists, and reporters are all participants in political life and discussion as well as the sustainers of that discussion, and they are participants together, not just as separable individuals. So a newspaper might well decide, as a corporate body, to engage in the political process on one side or another of an issue. This happens whenever a paper endorses a political candidate, and, perhaps more importantly, when a paper endeavors to shape public opinion on some matter of significant importance.

It is the manner in which such persuasion is engaged in that is crucial; for when a newspaper takes a stand on a public issue, it effects a separation between itself as a social and deliberating agent, and itself as an enabler of social deliberation and agency. So, to block dissenting voices from engaging in the discussion, to engage in purely rhetorical propaganda, or systematically to impugn, in a personal way, the motives and intentions of dissenters, is to violate the nature of the press as a common space for public impersonal deliberation, and its obligation, in the words of Davis Merritt, to be a "fair-minded participant" in the democratic process (Merritt, 1994, p. 23).

Correspondingly, we find two forms of objectivity at work when the press makes this separation. First, as with all participants in the discussion, the press must be objective not by maximal detachment, but by maintaining a commitment to getting at the truth of the matter under discussion. Here the necessary conditions for social agency impose obligations on the press as a sustainer of that agency. This explains the crucial function of the print media in fostering discussion—and in particular political discussion—by its straightforward investigation and reporting. Just as no individual's deliberation can be carried out without systematic attention to the best possible information, neither can a group's common deliberation. So the suppression or misrepresentation of truths in service of a particular agenda constitutes several sorts of failing: first, the basic sort committed by all who argue from untruths or half-truths to a favored position; second, and third, the failing peculiar to the press of insufficiently providing truth for the necessary framework of sound individual decisions, and for an effective common space for interpersonal deliberation and communication.

The first form of objectivity in the press, then, is its commitment to getting the truth, and presenting all relevant truths straightforwardly. The second form of objectivity takes us back to the impersonal mode of discourse appropriate to the public sphere, for the press plays a moderating role in the transmission of the discussion, its own contributions to that discussion included. It thus has an obligation to shape and direct the discussion as possible toward this impersonal form. An instructional aspect of the press's nature cannot be ignored here: the press must cultivate citizens who appreciate and participate in an appropriate form of public discourse, discourse whose aim is, in Taylor's words, a "common understanding," arrived at through reflective and critical discourse. This brings us to the third of the public benefits played by the press.

## Journalism and Social Solidarity

Journalism can help form a people's social sense as "one" or as "we." Taylor has pointed to the importance of such a social sense in discussing the value of patriotism and the necessity of freedom for self-rule: "We could say that republican solidarity underpins freedom, because it provides the motivation for self-imposed discipline" (Taylor, 1995, p. 193). In the absence of such a sense of solidarity, the motivation for engaging in the work of mutual deliberation and self-rule would tend to wane. Even the ability to conceive of oneself as a part of one's state might be compromised. One's basic ethical obligations toward others around one, obligations that are bedrock to the existence of society, might go unmet for lack of adequate motivation. So it is crucial to a society's existence that its members view themselves as in some sense one people.

Now this sense might be developed and sustained only at a very abstract level. There might, for example, be a mutual commitment to a constitution or a political regime. The press can play a crucial role in sustaining such a mutual commitment. But it has become increasingly clear, in a way that has introduced new difficulties, that the press has the power to foster, or destroy, ties on a more personal level. The speed and quality with which images are distributed throughout the world now, whether by newspapers, TV, or the Internet, has made it possible to be immediately apprised of the worst tragedies and finest successes of fellow citizens at the most distant removes from ourselves.

In turn, this seems often to have fostered a sense of connection and kinship with those at a distance, allowing all to share in the triumphs and tragedies of a few. One need only think of the response to the events of September 11, 2001, and the role played by the press in making such responses possible.

The press's power in these matters raises some of the questions of journalistic ethics discussed earlier in this book; questions about privacy, relevance, and taste have become more urgent as photographers record the grief of, and probe for information from, those most deeply involved in some form of horrible event. In Chapters 2 and 3, I addressed some of these issues by assessing the importance of privacy as an instrumental value, and looking at some of the boundaries separating privacy-respecting investigations of persons and failures to respect personal privacy, especially when the investigations concerned public figures and matters of public record and importance. But the question remains as to the boundaries of the private and public when reporters investigate personal tragedy. Further progress can be made by asking what purpose is served by reporting on such tragedies in the first place.

A major purpose of such reports should be to foster a sense of nearness across distance among citizens of a state (and perhaps even the world), and to facilitate the developing sense of the citizenry as "one people." But if this is so, then it gives us a foundation for further argument to the effect that there are limits on the extent to which the press should go in intruding upon the private lives of suffering citizens.

First, we may note the alienation often felt by those whose grief is probed too closely by the media, or who are shown in too vulnerable a way. Consider, for example, photographs of a drowned child, taken and published over the objections of the child's family. On the model of journalism I have been presenting, we can see why some attention should be paid to this story. First, as many defenders of the press point out, it is important to promulgate information about the dangers involved in, e.g., swimming pools, and the steps necessary to take to prevent further accidents. Reporting on such events is a public service.

Second, because such reporting draws us closer to those involved in the tragedy, and potentially in need, donations and offers of help may be made. This is made possible by the role the press plays in bringing us the story.

But calling it a "story" begins to indicate the danger here. The purpose of showing a family in pain is certainly not some form of *Schadenfreude* that we might experience. And yet, the more graphically the suffering is depicted, the more there is a tendency to objectify those involved, to indulge in a shiver at the horror they have experienced, and to treat the display as a peculiar form of aesthetic experience. This, in effect, must have exactly the opposite consequence of bringing the citizenry together in solidarity. It is akin to the freak show at the circus, not the social virtue of solidarity. The Society of Professional Journalists, which I criticized in Chapter 4 for its views on deception, here gets things right: "Avoid pandering to lurid curiosity" (SPJ, 1996, p. 2).

## THE STATE AND JOURNALISM

We have seen that journalism provides three crucial public benefits: the information necessary for individual choice and the coordination of such choices; the information and context necessary for social deliberation; and the information necessary for developing the virtue of social solidarity, and a sense of connectedness to others. Such benefits are of critical importance to society; moreover, they are, as discussed above, public in ways analogous to the public nature of science. Should the state, then, relate towards the journalistic profession in the way that arguably it should to the profession of science, providing funding and grants, overseeing projects, and also denying funding and sometimes legitimacy on the basis of political considerations? It should not.

This can be seen by recognizing the way that the state can threaten each of the three types of goods promoted by journalism if it intrudes too much into the practice of journalism. Consider first the good of providing information necessary for personal decisions and social coordination. This function could be governed by the state: the state could, by direct operation of the media, or by a combination of threats and inducements, determine what information was provided to citizens through the media. In effect, this would mean that the state was the arbiter of judgments of relevance of information, and hence, of opportunity, for information determines the context of choice. Totalitarian governments exercise precisely this option, but even in more democratic governments a state-owned and -controlled press is possible.

In the United States, by contrast, the press enjoys a wide autonomy in deciding what should count as relevant and necessary for the decisions of ordinary agents. This autonomy can be abused, and sometimes is, whether as a result of ideology or financial considerations. But in principle, a press free from governmental interference in such judgments seems closer to the decisions of the people, more responsible to what they take to be their needs, and potentially less manipulative. By contrast, to give government the power to determine what information is relevant to individual choice creates opportunities for oppression, subtle or not. Governmental control over information risks creation of a system of coordination notable for its monotonous sameness.

Such considerations are only magnified when the object of the press's scrutiny is government itself. The watchdog function of the press would be seriously jeopardized by the state's control of the press. Who would expect that a government would be inclined to freely part with information that could potentially be damaging, or used for criticism of the state?

The press must be independent of the state in the sense of ownership and direct control. But a government too inclined to censor the press could accomplish much of the damage that state ownership could. A fairly robust notion of freedom of the press as regards reporting emerges: content-based restrictions on what the press publishes should be rare, and permissible only in cases of extreme emergency.

What about the ethical guidelines I have discussed already on matters such as privacy and truth telling? Should the state be charged with the job of restricting the work of the press when it violates the privacy of others? I believe, contrary to some commentators, that the general manner in which the courts have decided to approach privacy issues where the right of a free press is concerned is fundamentally correct. Rodney Smolla writes that there are two strains to American privacy law in these regards: "The first involves claims of 'intrusion.' The second involves claims of 'revelation.'"

> [The former] all in one way or another seek to impose liability for invasive *conduct* of some kind, divorced from any information that might have been gathered and subsequently disseminated as a result of the invasion. When used against the media, these are commonly described as "news-gathering torts," in the sense that they focus on actions antecedent to any publication or broadcast of material. "Revelation" privacy claims may similarly involve tort of criminal law actions broader than the common-law tort of "publication of private facts," although that tort is probably the legal doctrine most famously associated with the revelation strain of privacy. (Smolla, 2003, p. 89)

Smolla points out that the law, and the courts, have been much more favorably inclined to accept a defense based upon freedom of speech and press when charges are brought on the basis of revelation than on the basis of intrusion. Where information has been *obtained* in a way that violates the right to privacy, for example, through surreptitious surveillance, or breaking and entering, the courts are likely to side with the plaintiff. But where the objection to publication has to do with *what* was published, the courts routinely side with the press.

I believe this approach to be fundamentally sound for legal purposes, though not for ethical purposes. As I argued in Chapter 3, the press has no authority, in a way analogous to the authority of public officials, that entitles it to an immunity against ordinary laws protecting individuals against intrusions on privacy. But in most cases, for the courts to rule against the press on grounds of *what* was published would involve the state in precisely the sort of control over the press deleterious to the free provision of information to citizens. Smolla quotes a crucial passage from the Supreme Court's ruling in *Miami Herald Publishing Co. v. Tornillo* that makes precisely this point:

> A newspaper is more than a passive receptacle or conduit for news, comment, and advertising. The choice of material to go into a newspaper, and the decisions made as to limitations on the size and content of the paper, and treatment of public issues and public officials—whether fair or unfair—constitute the exercise of editorial control and judgment. It has yet to be demonstrated how governmental regulation of this crucial process can be exercised consistent with First Amendment guarantees of a free press as they have evolved to this time. (Smolla, 2003, p. 92)

However, while legally this division is sound, ethically there is more to be said. The distinctions raised in this chapter, and in Chapters 3 and 4, have wider application than should be legally enforced. For example, not all lies are legally actionable. Yet all lies are immoral, and should be avoided by journalists in pursuit of the truth. Further, there are many truths about persons that should reasonably be considered private, even when obtained by entirely legal means. Photographs of grieving families should not be splashed over newspaper front pages, nor should such families be hounded, nor should their neighbors be encouraged to reveal personal and private facts about them. Even within the lives of public figures, as argued in Chapter 3, a division should ethically be made between the private and the public, a distinction that journalists should respect even when the law does not.

Similar considerations can be raised in relation to the other two benefits provided by journalism. Earlier, in discussing the role the press plays in providing a public space for the common deliberation of citizens, and the resolution of public opinion, I discussed the press's obligation to objectivity: objectivity in the sense of providing the truth, and in the sense of providing an impersonal framework of debate that was common, and not narrowly prejudiced towards one side, even though that might be the side supported in argument by journalists, individually or corporately. By this means, the press makes it possible for genuine debate to happen, genuine both for being rational, rather than merely rhetorical, and for being truly multisided and non-exclusionary.

The press's objectivity can, however, be jeopardized. Indeed, government interference is not necessary for effective threats to journalistic objectivity and integrity on these matters. As the press has become more politically powerful and socially homogeneous, it has also become more adept at excluding voices, denigrating opposing views, and occasionally skewing its reporting in favor of one side's facts over another. On the other hand, overwhelming corporate interests, a gross consumerism, and a market mentality can contribute to a press concerned only with the lowest common denominator. Such a press is pandering, unchallenging, and oriented above all to financial gain; it can play no helpful role in the deliberative life of the state.

But similar threats loom when the press is controlled, or even financially supported, by the state. Those in power have a clear interest in structuring deliberation in one way rather than another, and in suppressing, or minimizing the voices of dissent. A free press is no guarantee of objectivity, but it makes it more likely than a government press.

Finally, similar considerations govern the state's relationship to the press over the issue of social solidarity. It is true that the state has a legitimate interest in a patriotic citizenry, and a love of country. But such notions do not admit of only one interpretation; citizens can be patriotic in varying ways, and to varying degrees. For the state to make creation of social solidarity its business would, however, again risk a dangerous homogeneity and exclusiveness. In addition, it would by definition involve a top-down, rather than a bottom-up approach. This would infringe upon citizen autonomy in determining the nature of the society and societies to which they wished to belong. A free and diverse press is thus more likely to serve this function adequately than a press controlled or paid for by the government.

The upshot is that although the journalistic profession, like the profession of science, serves the public good in crucial ways, the state should be more distant from journalism than from science. This should not be surprising, however, in light of some further comparisons. The one domain of science that I deemed absolutely free from state interference was the domain of truth: the state has no say over what is scientifically determined to be true or not. But the state did have a say over the proper treatment of other persons, thus legitimating some kinds of interference. It also had a reason to support science financially, to the extent that modern science could not be carried out without some form of financial assistance. But this created various obligations on the part of the state to verify that public money was being spent legitimately for the common good, and not in a way that violated the deepest moral sense of citizens. Finally, because of the power of science, the state could justifiably oversee projects that threatened the well-being of society, such as research into dangerous weapons systems or diseases.

With journalism too, we see that the state should not interfere in the truth claims of journalists. But unlike most science, journalism is often concerned with truth claims that bear on the state itself—claims about its policies and their effectiveness, about officials and their behavior, and so on. While the state can fund a great deal of science in such a way that does not seriously threaten the objectivity of scientists, state funding of journalism almost inevitably threatens journalistic objectivity. But if the state takes a hands-off attitude to journalism in this way, it thereby also frees up journalists from the kinds of state scrutiny that come with the provision of financial and other assistance. Finally, while the press can be powerful, and can make and unmake governments, the power of the press is typically predicated on the misdeeds of those they investigate. Research into nuclear weaponry is inherently dangerous; investigation into the integrity of government officials is dangerous, for the most part, only when that integrity is questionable.

So a concern that is at root very similar—for the truth—in both science and journalism, generates different kinds of conclusions about the extent to which state involvement, support, and regulation of the profession is called for. The politics of inquiry, across science, the humanities, and journalism, is oriented to the pursuit of the common good, but achieves that good in diverse ways.

# 11 The Vocation, Practice, and Progress of Inquiry

Previous chapters of this book have been concerned with a person-centered ethics of inquiry. Person-centered considerations are well known in the ethics of biomedical and scientific research. Nor are they foreign to the ethics of journalistic or military investigation. But Chapter 10 began with a discussion of a form of inquiry for which person-centered ethical considerations seem less salient, namely, inquiry in the humanities. Yet humanistic inquiry seems no more immune from ethics than scientific inquiry.

This raises the possibility of a different ethics of inquiry, not person centered, but focused on truth, the good, or end of inquiry. Such an ethics could be considered "internal" to inquiry, since it emerges from consideration of inquiry's nature. These final two chapters are concerned with the internal ethics of inquiry.

For reasons that I will make clear, this ethics especially governs agents who have made a significant commitment to inquiry, possibly a vocational commitment. The next section articulates the nature of such a commitment, and why, and under what circumstances, a life of inquiry could be a reasonable one. Given, however, that the internal ethics of inquiry is to be understood as starting from this point, then the internal ethics of inquiry should be primarily concerned with the virtues that a morally responsible inquirer, considered as an inquirer, ought to have; for a vocational commitment, if honored in action through time, shapes in deep and abiding ways the character of the agent who makes, and successfully keeps the commitment. Correlatively, the nature of the vocational commitment is better understood through understanding the types of differences in character that commitment ought to make. To use an analogy: a marital commitment shapes in deep and abiding ways the character of a spouse, but a spouse's understanding of the nature of the commitment will in turn be shaped by recognition of the types of virtues demanded by the commitment, and even more by the acquisition of those virtues.

In consequence, any ethics of an activity that can reasonably be seen as vocationally directed will be to a great extent a virtue ethics. This is not to deny the existence of moral norms and rules, even moral absolutes: adultery is a violation of a categorical norm within a marriage. But a virtue approach can provide a more robust understanding of the point and purpose of the commitment, and of the moral demands associated with that commitment, than a rules-based approach: understanding the commitment to marriage as intrinsically demanding a special kind of fidelity can thus aid in appreciation of the norm against adultery.

The long-term goal of the discussion of vocational commitments, and the role that inquiry can play as the nub of such a commitment, is the investigation, in Chapter 12, of the virtues of inquiry. More preliminary spadework will be necessary, however. I argue in this chapter that the MacIntyrean concept of a practice can again be of aid, this time in understanding the relationship of virtues to inquiry. I also utilize MacIntyre's understanding of the nature of progress in inquiry to show that the virtues of inquiry are truly internal to inquiry, and not externally imposed burdens. Finally, I address the communal and cooperative nature of inquiry, a topic initially discussed in Chapter 8, on the nature of scientific inquiry.

## INQUIRY AS A POSSIBLE VOCATIONAL COMMITMENT

Much of the person-centered ethics of inquiry applies to any agents who happen to be involved in inquiry of some sort. Whatever form of inquiry one is engaged in, one cannot kill, lie, or use manipulative means to obtain information. But some of the norms investigated had more actual application to those who were involved not just in occasional or one-off inquiry, but in systematic, long-term inquiry: the inquiry characteristic of those who are scientists, academics, and so on. For these types of agents, norms governing inquiry have more play in their lives, because their lives are, to important extents, deeply structured by the activity of inquiry and its purpose.

If lives can be so structured by this activity, and its purpose, then a significant part of an internal ethics of inquiry should have special application to those whose lives are so structured. In particular, the internal ethics of inquiry should say something about the conditions under which the commitment to structure one's life that way is made, about what it means for a life to be so structured, and about the subsequent consequences for the individual's responsibilities.

This requires first saying something about the nature of a vocation, and a vocational commitment (see Finnis, 1980, pp. 113–39; Tollefsen, 2004; cf. Rawls, 1971, p. 433). I am using the notion of vocation here in a broadly secular way. From the perspective of natural reason, and the norms of practical reasonableness, the importance of such a commitment is clear. As I have stressed more than once, human beings are faced with a multiplicity of goods among which to choose. This creates a problem for practical reason: how to choose reasonably among the multiplicity, given that maximization is recognized as an inadequate strategy.

Among the demands of reason in responding to this problem for choice is a demand that agents not pursue goods in a way that is purely serial, or randomly oriented towards different goods at different times. Adequate pursuit of any good can be achieved only by focus and commitment: to become an adequate carpenter, doctor, or musician, one must devote a part of one's life to that good or activity so as to be able, through time, to achieve the excellences necessary for achievement in that domain.

Further, because of limits of time, ability, and the inevitability of conflict, it is unreasonable for an agent to make too many such commitments, or to make such commitments with no thought to how they may be jointly pursued. An agent who seeks to become excellent at the violin is in most cases not also going to be able to achieve excellence at surgery. In any event, an agent who plays in a major symphony and who also is a surgeon in a busy medical practice, is unlikely to have a soundly structured life. Harmony of commitments is necessary, and this, in turn, requires hierarchy: some commitments must be such as themselves to play a structuring role in ordering other commitments in their appropriate places.

Some activities are more capable of playing such a structuring role than others, and some are more worthy of being allowed to play such a role than others. Some activities are pursued primarily for the sake of instrumentalities such as money; these are ill suited to play a major structuring role in an agent's life. In other cases, the relationship between activity and basic good is so immediate, and the demands so significant, that the activity must play a structuring role, or the agent will fail at it. Marriage and the religious life, for example, cannot be pursued half-time, or in a way subordinate to other pursuits, except at the expense of success itself.

Having entered into such an activity, and made the necessary commitments, an agent is bound to shape her character in such a way that that activity and its good or goods will be evident in understanding most of the major, and many minor, events of her life narrative. That the agent is married, for example, will play some role in explaining why such a job was accepted, why certain decisions were made about where to live, how to act, what not to do, and so on. In other words, a particular vocational commitment sets some of the standards by which moral judgments are rightly made for the agent in question. But even within the framework set by such overarching commitments, other quite extensive commitments must be made that will also play a significant shaping role in the arc of an agent's life. So a married agent who pursues a career in, say, medicine, will lead a life shaped powerfully by the medical profession; so powerfully, indeed, that at times a difficult negotiation is necessary between the demands of work and the demands of marriage.

This is an especially pressing difficulty in the case of a profession like medicine, because this seems capable on its own of giving a fairly full vocational structure to an agent's life: that I am a doctor, or that I wish to become a doctor, are thoughts that can shape my life through time, and dominate decisions at a time. Doctoring is both important and tremendously difficult to do well; it is, therefore, not surprising that for some agents the medical vocation has a certain primacy. Recognizing that marriage and children, for example, would be incompatible, or greatly strained, by a life tending to the health of distressed patients in the third world, an agent might choose not to marry, so as to maintain a higher level of commitment to her vocational activity.

For such an agent, the structure of the demands of practical reason will take on a hue borrowed in considerable measure from the good or goods at which the activity in question aims. Someone who has made a vocational commitment to medicine cannot drive by an accident, or turn off her beeper because she is at a fine dinner with friends; nor can she agree to perform useless but desired surgery upon a wealthy patient. Her sense of the demands made by her vocational commitment shapes her particular sense of what virtue and duty demand, and thus, ultimately, shapes her character.

This is true, to continue with the medical case, even in those cases in which medicine is subordinated to some further commitment, as when the agent is married, or is in a religious order. Medicine is too significant a practice—indeed, it is a profession—for it to play a minor role in shaping an agent's responsibilities, and thereby her character. The examples given above, of driving by an accident, and so on, are still special responsibilities to a married doctor. So, while the vocational ethics of a profession will be somewhat more stringent for an agent with no other vocational commitment, much can be done working out a vocational ethic without attending to whether the agent also has some other more supervisory vocation such as marriage.

So far, the discussion has concerned what a life shaped by a vocational commitment looks like, in very broad terms, and what the consequences of that commitment are, morally speaking. To reiterate: the commitment structures other subordinate commitments and activities; and the commitment determines the content of a number of obligations and virtues that flow from the commitment's particular nature. How should agents go about making vocational commitments? It is tempting to think that it is sufficient for an agent to make such a commitment that she want or desire the form of life in question: surely if an agent wants to be a doctor, and is willing to do the work, then it is perfectly acceptable for her to make the commitment to become a doctor.

Such a view is in error: the desire to pursue, in a substantive way, a life commitment, though important, is insufficient to make such a commitment reasonable, and in many cases, a commitment guided only by such desires will be disastrous. Someone who wishes to become a doctor is not thereby entitled to become one: prospective doctors must pass numerous tests to ensure that they are by nature suitable candidates for the medical profession. They must be bright enough, potentially skilled enough, and have at least minimal moral dispositions to care for it to be prudent for medical schools and practices to offer them opportunity to serve in the profession.

An agent considering whether or not to embark on a professional route should consider for herself whether she is gifted in the right ways for this to be an appropriate commitment. Indeed, because no profession has a flawless way of eliminating inappropriate candidates, agents considering a vocational commitment have a strong obligation to scrutinize whether they really should be pursuing their goals themselves. While medical schools typically can weed out candidates for the profession who are insufficiently intelligent (medically intelligent—a fine candidate for philosophy might be a terrible candidate for medicine), they seem less able to determine whether a candidate lacks the character traits and virtues that would make medicine a reasonable life commitment.

All this has a clear bearing on inquiry. As I will elaborate shortly, inquiry should be considered a practice; indeed, as we saw in Chapter 8, some forms of inquiry become sufficiently embedded in institutional structures, due to their social importance, that they become professions, with the scientific profession as a paradigm. But it is a practice commitment to which can, and sometimes should, play a vocationally structuring role in an agent's life. There are several reasons for this. First, inquiry is extremely difficult. It requires skills that are not to be obtained all at once, and inquiry into a worthwhile subject matter will not be quick. Rather, inquiry will be pursued more successfully if pursued over a longer and more sustained period of time than not. Inquiry that is pursued briefly, sporadically, without sustained attention, or with constant interruption is typically a failure.

In addition to skills, inquiry demands a range of virtues that flow from the particular nature of the good sought—truth—and the nature of that good's pursuit. Like medicine, the character traits that inquiry demands are pervasive through an agent's life. Susan Haack remarks that she would find it odd to hear of someone that he was a good man but intellectually dishonest; but likewise it would be problematic to say of an agent that he was a brilliant scientist, but otherwise dishonest (Haack, 1998, p. 15). The commitment to truth required by a vocational commitment to inquiry should be seen globally across an agent's character, and not merely in some isolated domain. I will return to this point in the next chapter.

Three final points may be made. First, inquiry can play the kind of overarching structuring role characteristic of the objects of major vocational commitments. Agents can see their lives as dedicated to inquiry, and other activities as subordinated to the life of inquiry. Agents who are committed to inquiry make certain sacrifices with respect to other goods, for example, spending less time exercising or learning how to play the piano. Second, particular obligations can flow from the vocational commitment to inquiry. Consider the obligation that committed inquirers might have to reasons opposed to what they take to be the truth. Such reasons support belief that not-p, even though the inquirer believes overall that p is more likely to be true. It seems plausible that vocationally committed inquirers have a special obligation to defeated considerations—an obligation to give them further consideration, demonstrate the ways in which they are epistemically inadequate, and so on (Tollefsen, 2003b). Similarly, some have suggested that a heightened skepticism might also be a particular obligation of a professional inquirer (Zagzebski, 1996, p. 224). Such considerations suggest that, like medicine, inquiry can form the focal point of an agent's vocational commitment.

Finally, a vocational commitment to inquiry, even if not undertaken in conjunction with a commitment to marriage or religious life, cannot be an all-encompassing commitment. The good of knowledge simply cannot have a bearing on all upright choices one makes throughout a life—many other duties will intervene, other goods must be pursued, and so on. Indeed, Germain Grisez has argued that only one good, the good of religion, can play such an all-encompassing structuring role (Grisez, 2001). Nothing I say here should be understood to deny that unique role for the good of religion in an upright agent's life, nor to imply that the demands of inquiry can enter into every single choice a vocationally committed inquirer makes. Nothing so extensive is necessary to sustain my argument.

In the case of both medicine and inquiry, the commitment to a life of this type of activity is, in reality, a commitment to the good of that activity. In the case of medicine, this is health; in the case in inquiry, the good is truth. The choice of inquiry as a vocational commitment is, first and foremost, a commitment to the good of truth as a good that will play an overarching structuring role in one's life.

So the agent considering a vocational commitment to truth and inquiry must assess herself—her capacities, her personality, or incipient virtues and potential skills—in light of this good and its requirements: does a commitment to this good, as opposed to some other(s) make sense given her natural talents, dispositions, desires, and incipient virtues? Plato, in the *Republic*, makes a similar suggestion in discussing the character traits that should be sought after for potential philosophers. No one, says Socrates, can follow such a way of life unless he is "by nature good at remembering, quick to learn, high-minded, graceful, and a friend and relative of truth, justice, courage and moderation" (487a). Socrates argues that the Guardians of the Republic should make these assessments, but it is more reasonable, following the discussion of autonomy earlier in this book, to hold that agents considering a life of inquiry should ask themselves whether, in addition to the desire to pursue the truth through systematic inquiry, they also have these traits and virtues. But Plato's list is helpful: agents who have poor memory skills, who are not quick to learn, who do not care deeply for the truth, or who are unwilling to work hard for it, even if they are willing to work hard for something else, should not make such a commitment.

This is a decision of *moral* significance; those who take vocational commitments lightly, or who make serious mistakes in making such commitments, significantly reduce their own possibilities for a fulfilling life; and frequently are unjust to others insofar as their bad decisions have negative consequences for others, including the waste of others' time that necessarily will occur in a form of activity as social as inquiry is.

So a morally reasonable agent will have an adequate sense of the importance of making a serious and well-informed commitment, and will take into account the factors that make this a reasonable commitment to make. Such an agent will be disposed to give similar consideration to the particular areas of inquiry in which she intends to involve herself. Not every possible subject is equally worthy of consideration. An agent should have some idea of why her field of study and inquiry is important. Moreover, it would seem inappropriate to think of one's inquiry-related projects as *merely* a serial set of projects, even if each were individually important, unrelated to one another, and to be pursued *seriatim,* one as soon as the previous was completed. It would be more desirable for an agent to see her life of inquiry itself as hanging together as a whole, and this would most likely be possible in view of similarities and relationships between projects pursed, and perhaps because of some systemic relationship between the variety of projects pursued and some larger problem or domain of knowledge on which the agent wished to make progress. This latter sort of consideration is one that could only be dimly conceived early in an inquirer's career; more reasonably, it would be a kind of regulative ideal for the agent: to see her work in inquiry as overall coherent, as unified and unifying in her life; even errors should be seen as related to the overall task. And, as we shall see, the overarching body of knowledge to which an agent should see herself as contributing will be a body of knowledge not possessed alone, or entirely, by the agent herself, but by the agent in her particular community of inquiry.

One might object that not every agent who pursues a life of inquiry does so from a desire for truth in itself; some desire riches and fame; others desire the truth as a means to technological accomplishment. With regard to the first, the desire for riches or fame, this issue will arise repeatedly in the next chapter, in the discussions of moderation and justice. I would here only suggest that while such desires can be reasonable, insofar as one needs money, and insofar as it is just that one be rewarded for what one has accomplished, to make these one's ultimate ends, and to make inquiry merely instrumental to these ends, is both to demean the value of truth, and to risk positively damaging it, insofar as one's desires for money or fame could lead one to suppress truth when that was to one's advantage. Even though it need not be one's only end, for the genuinely vocational inquirer, truth must remain an end in itself, something viewed as valuable just because truth is basic to human well-being. Rightly to order one's life to inquiry does require that one commit to the pursuit of truth as intrinsically valuable.

With regard to the second point, agents who pursue a course, or even a life of investigation into some domain primarily for instrumental reasons— they desire to build bridges, or to heal bodies—should not be considered vocationally committed *inquirers*. Truth is important to such agents, as the benefits they seek would not be promoted by error. But truth is not the primary end of their activities. Their vocation is thus not that of the inquirer, nor should one expect there to be complete overlap between the virtues of inquiry and the virtues of whatever good is the true object of their vocational commitment. For similar reasons, police detectives and journalists are probably not vocational inquirers. The internal ethics of inquiry, consequently, has a lesser hold over such agents.

Having said something about the circumstances under which an agent reasonably commits herself to a life of inquiry, my ultimate goal is to say something more substantive about the ethics of inquiry for those already engaged in inquiry. This requires that more be said about the nature of inquiry itself, for it is the nature of the activity that shapes the ethical demands the activity makes on agents. My starting point will be a focus on two aspects of inquiry. The first is its nature as a practice. This will involve as well a discussion of the communal and historical nature of inquiry. These aspects are critical to an understanding of the role that the virtues play in an inquirer's activities.

The second focus, which is also MacIntyrean in inspiration, will be on what constitutes successful progress for inquiry. In other words, when is it reasonable to assess a course of inquiry in some subject area as moving forward? This focus is crucial, because I claimed in Chapter 1 that the internal ethics of any activity is such that violation of that ethics is damaging to the activity itself. Unlike the case of the external ethics of inquiry, in which adherence to moral norms might result in some limitations on what could be accomplished, in the internal ethics, ethical behavior and success are mutually joined.

## PRACTICES, VIRTUES, AND GOODS[1]

Recall MacIntyre's definition of a practice:

> . . . any coherent and complex form of socially established cooperative human activity through which goods internal to that form of activity are realized in the course of trying to achieve those standards of excellence which are appropriate to, and partially definitive of, that form of activity, with the result that human powers to achieve excellence, and human conceptions of the ends and goods involved, are systematically extended. (MacIntyre, 1984, p. 187)

In Chapter 8, I articulated an understanding of practices, using examples such as the game of basketball. Here, my initial discussion will focus on the role that practices play in leading to virtues; I will also discuss the relationship between practices, communities, and history, or tradition. In Chapter 12, having argued that inquiry should be considered a practice, or a family of related practices, and having discussed the nature of progressive inquiry, I will discuss the specific virtues of inquiry.

According to MacIntyre, practices are the contexts in which virtues initially emerge. Thus, in *After Virtue,* MacIntyre shows how, in a shared activity in which several agents pursue some common good, the virtues of justice, courage, and honesty are required. If agents are afraid to take certain risks in promotion of the good, and in extending their understanding of the good, then the practice in question will grow stagnant, the good will not be progressively pursued in more successful ways. So courage is necessary in the activities of a practice.

Similarly, if agents are dishonest or unjust to one another, then they introduce differences in the relationships between agents that are not intrinsically related to the pursuit of the goods of the practice. The relationship between teachers and students, for example, must be rationally ordered with reference to the goods mutually pursued, and the roles teachers and students play in that pursuit respectively. When arbitrary distinctions are made because of, for example, the attractiveness of one student over another, the intelligible order of the practice, and hence its orientation to its good, diminishes.

There is a necessary relationship between a practice and a community. A community is not a mere aggregate of individuals, even if they are related by mutually accepted rules, such as the law. Rather, a community exists when a number of individuals are engaged together in the pursuit of a good that cannot be understood merely as itself an aggregate of the goods of the various individuals. Individuals in a genuine community do not see their good as fully intelligible apart from the good of those others with whom they work in pursuit of the good. And so it is for those engaged in a practice: genuine excellence at basketball is something that can be understood, appreciated, and achieved only from a standpoint that sees the good of basketball as a common good. When basketball players begin to think only in terms of their own individual satisfaction or excellence, they cease to pursue the particular excellences of the practice of basketball and cease to be members of a genuine community of ballplayers.

I will argue that any systematic form of inquiry should be understood as a practice, and thus as an activity pursued most properly in a community. But it is worthwhile here to draw another parallel between a characteristically MacIntyrean theme, and the natural law approach followed throughout this book. MacIntyre's account of the virtues and the context in which they are possible depends upon two further concepts, the narrative unity of a life, and tradition. The former of these will bring us back to the notion of a vocational commitment; the second will illustrate an historical and cultural feature of the circumstances in which particular forms of commitment are possible.

A practice alone is insufficient to ground a full conception of virtue because agents typically inhabit multiple practices—those of their occupation, of family, of religion, and so on. Agents must harmonize their pursuit of the various practices of which they are a part. Moreover, agents must do this not just now, but through time, so that order is introduced into their lives viewed as extended in time. Thus, the life of a well-integrated agent has the unity of a narrative, not by nature or accident, but because the agent has acted so as to bring that unity into her life.

But any agent asking herself how she shall introduce such unity, which practices she shall privilege, and how she shall pursue those practices must stand in a particular relationship to her own past, the past of her practices, and the past of her community. She must, that is, have a respect for her tradition, for it is in tradition that the resources for asking and answering questions about the good and its pursuit may be found. Agents cannot, on MacIntyre's account, radically distance themselves from their historically particular circumstances when asking questions about how they should live; even a radical rejection of tradition must emerge from an engagement with the tradition-based claims being rejected. Thus tradition is the final concept necessary for a full understanding of virtue for MacIntyre.

Some of the MacIntyrean scheme of practices, communities, narrative forms of life, and tradition is straightforwardly compatible with the basic goods approach of this book. We have seen this in the overlapping need for ordered commitments in an agent's life. Similarly, the concept of a community, and its importance for genuine flourishing overlaps both accounts. What might seem at variance, over the two accounts is the MacIntyrean emphasis on practices, by contrast with my account of basic goods, and the MacIntyrean emphasis on tradition, with its somewhat unsettling hint of relativism.

Without claiming that the following account is entirely true to MacIntyre's intentions, I argue that both practices and tradition can and should play a role in the basic goods–based natural law account of this book; for the basic goods can be pursued in a potentially infinite variety of ways, and with regard to at least some of those ways, they can be pursued in ever deeper ways. But just as no individual can successfully pursue any good to a significant degree of depth if he does not focus, not just on a good, but on a particular path to the good, so successions of agents through time cannot explore the depths of excellence in the pursuit of goods if they do not capitalize on the pursuits of those who have gone before them. This requires that, in some areas of pursuit of the basic goods, the particular mode of pursuit become progressively more specified as being of this rather than that aspect of the good, as being in this rather than that mode of pursuit, of using these rather than those resources, techniques, and skills, and so on. But this, in fact, is simply to say that the pursuit of the basic goods across generations, if it is to be progressive, must specify itself into a series of practices, in which the wisdoms, techniques, and foci of past generations are made more determinate in a variety of ways.

Practices, then, are the result of such a historically determining and specifying pursuit of some basic good or goods; the practices of writing sonnets, painting portraits, farming, doctoring, or lawyering, are all consolidations of past advances in the pursuit of goods, consolidations that have increased the potential depth to which the goods may be pursued, but, through the development of conventions, techniques, and skills, narrowed the breadth of ways within which the goods may be pursued, consistent with membership in the practice. This does not mean that agents involved in a practice are rigorously bound to the conventions and rules established already; practices are in decline when agents see rote conformity as their only available mode of life in a practice. But a practice does specify the mode of pursuit of a good in a way that can only develop across a more or less significant amount of time. None of the practices just mentioned could have sprung up whole all at once.

By the same token, agents will be unable to participate in the practices, even with a view to radical innovation, without a strong sense of the past of the practice. MacIntyre writes that a tradition is a continuing argument through time, and in a sense, so is a practice: a continuing argument over how to shape in a number of particular ways the pursuit of some facet of the basic goods. Agents with little sense of why the practice they inhabit is as it is will tend to see its particularities as arbitrary; agents who reject altogether the contingent starting point of a practice at a time will miss out on the accumulated resources of the practice's ancestors.

## INQUIRY AS A PRACTICE

Is inquiry a practice? Strictly speaking, we should, no doubt, be speaking of the practice of inquiry in this or that domain of knowledge, just as we would speak of the practice of writing love sonnets, or the practice of portrait paintings. Yet we may also speak of the practice of writing poetry and the practice of painting with a good deal of sense. It is in this sense that I speak of a practice of inquiry.

Inquiry meets all the criteria of a practice that MacIntyre lists in his famous definition, particularly when it is considered at some further degree of specification, such as "philosophical inquiry," "historical inquiry," "scientific inquiry," and so on (and these too could be further specified). In each case, there is a socially established and cooperative form of human activity. It is true that there are individual inquirers, and there are those such as Socrates, of whom it is difficult to see how he is engaged in an *already* socially established activity. But Socrates' very social form of inquiry did in fact quickly lead his students to develop and systematize a form of activity etiologically related to his, and the new practice of philosophy also possessed a very social existence in the Platonic and Aristotelian schools. And while some may inquire individually, with little reference to a broader community, this would seem to occur only at the outset of the existence of a particular form of inquiry, or in a way that is both parasitic on the social activity and in some violation of the norms of inquiry. Henry Cavendish, for example, was a scientific loner; but his ability to accomplish what he did was dependent upon the fruits of others' past intellectual labors, and his refusal to publish seemed then, as it seems now, a violation of the ethos of science. Robert Merton quotes Aldous Huxley's articulation of this: "'Our admiration of his genius is tempered by a certain disapproval; we feel that such a man is selfish and anti-social'"(Merton, 1973a, p. 274).

Other salient aspects of the definition of a practice also have bearing on the practice of inquiry. For example, forms of inquiry are identified and individuated by their coherent and ordered domain-specific truth goals: this form of scientific inquiry wishes to understand the truth concerning this set of problems; that form of philosophical inquiry wishes to understand the truth concerning that set of problems, and so on. So forms of inquiry themselves take on a coherent shape in consequence of this ordering: the activities of the members of the practice, their techniques and tools, their aims, their desires, are all ordered towards the same end. Further, that shape will inevitably be of a significant degree of complexity, if the inquiry is not to be brief, trivial, or unsuccessful. At least two forms of division of labor will develop: the various tasks necessary to progress in the inquiry will need to be divided up amongst various participants, and those working on this, rather than that, aspect of a problem will divide to varying degrees over the way in which, in particular, they will approach the problem (see Kitcher, 2001, pp. 106–16).

Finally, since inquiry is to be understood in terms of its truth relatedness, and specific forms of inquiry in terms of their specific truth goals, inquiry generally, and all particular forms of inquiry, have an internal good, and specific forms of excellence that are partly constitutive of the achievement of that good. The nature of these excellences—the virtues of inquiry—will be the focus of the next chapter, but we can also see that MacIntyre's final point holds of inquiry too. As the virtues of inquiry are more deeply understood, and more deeply manifested, the understanding of the nature of inquiry and its good is likewise extended, with a consequent deepening of the achievement of excellence in inquiry.

This raises a crucial issue concerning the nature of inquiry, and its status as a practice. It is essential to anything that can be a practice, and to anything that already is a practice, that progress be possible, for practices are just the medium of specification of the pursuit of basic goods through time, across generations, by which participation in those goods is to be deepened, albeit in an increasingly narrow sort of way. It is for this reason that MacIntyre spends a good deal of *Whose Justice, Which Rationality* discussing the nature of progress in the particular form of inquiry of most interest to him, namely, moral inquiry. In the next section, I highlight MacIntyre's account of progress in moral inquiry, an account that itself derives from Platonic, Aristotelian, and Thomistic reflection on the nature of inquiry; but what MacIntyre argues regarding moral inquiry, I will suggest is true more broadly of inquiry as such. This suggestion will set the stage for a more extensive investigation into the nature of the virtues of inquiry.

## PLATO, ARISTOTLE, AND AQUINAS ON
## PROGRESS IN MORAL INQUIRY

A core concern of *Whose Justice, Which Rationality* involves the nature of moral inquiry, and what the standards for such inquiry, and the defense of its achievements, would have to be like. In MacIntyre's narrative, a series of advances are made by Plato, Aristotle and Aquinas in understanding what progress in inquiry involves. There is a tradition of inquiry about inquiry here, and understanding this tradition is necessary for understanding the role moral norms and virtues play in assessing activity within this tradition.

MacIntyre credits Plato for the recognition of four features of progressively successful inquiry:

- Later stages "presuppose the findings of the earlier," and thus "afford us a point of view from which it would be possible to identify and to characterize the findings of earlier stages in a way which that would not have been possible at those stages" (MacIntyre, 1988, pp. 79–80).
- Where there has been earlier unresolvable disagreement, later stages must "provide an explanation both of why the disagreement occurred and of why it was then and with those resources unresolvable" (MacIntyre, 1988, p. 80).
- Later stages must provide "a successively more adequate conception of the good of the inquiry" (MacIntyre, 1988, p. 80).[2]
- This concept of the good of inquiry is a conception of "what it would be to have completed the inquiry." MacIntyre characterizes this as a conception of the *arche* of inquiry, the *arche* being what we are aiming at, and what, if we had it, would provide unity of explanation to everything achieved within the inquiry (MacIntyre, 1988, p. 80).

The discussion of Aristotle highlights two further features:

- The first concerns the sort of progress associated with correction of error: "It is in practice one of Aristotle's criteria for a successful correction of a false view that we are able to explain why we might expect such a view to be generated if our overall standpoint is correct" (MacIntyre, 1988, p. 118).
- Success requires a confrontation between "alternative and rival opinions, especially of those most cogently argued, by each other, so that we may arrive at a conclusion as to which of these best survives the strongest objections which can be advanced on the basis of the others" (MacIntyre, 1988, p. 118). This requirement has its roots in Socratic dialectic and Plato's use of that dialectic.

MacIntyre's discussion of Aquinas makes clear how much of Aquinas's conception of inquiry makes use of and elaborates on the previous considerations.

For example, Aquinas systematizes the use of dialectical confrontation with rivals in his use of the *Quaestio*. But Aquinas further recognizes the extent to which it is impossible to characterize rival views in a neutral manner; thus the characterization of a rival account as a failure from one's own perspective must be supplemented by a new stage of inquiry:

- Having characterized the contentions of a rival view in one's own terms and addressed it as such, it is then necessary that one approach the rival view from its own perspective, entering into that perspective empathetically, and asking "whether the alternative and rival tradition may not be able to provide resources to characterize and to explain the failings and defects of [the first] tradition more adequately than they [the proponents of the first tradition] using the resources of that tradition, have been able to do" (MacIntyre, 1988, p. 167).

We have here a series of standards by which inquiry may be judged successful or unsuccessful. Again, it is crucial that any effort, at this point, to introduce moral standards by which inquiry may be judged be such that an intelligible connection may be seen between the criteria for successful inquiry and the criteria for morally upright inquiry; for in the absence of such an intelligible connection, moral standards will simply be imposed externally in the activity of inquiry. If there is a genuine internal ethics of inquiry, however, such as I will develop in the next chapter, then the internally immoral pursuit of inquiry will constitute a failure of inquiry as such. It will thus be one project of the next chapter to show how successful progress in inquiry requires the virtues.

MacIntyre, in the various passages quoted and discussed, has primarily been addressing the nature of *moral* inquiry. Can the account be extended to inquiry as such? It seems so, for theoretical inquiry is a practice, perhaps even more than moral inquiry is; it is systematic, cooperative, and historical. And it is, for many, life shaping and architectonic, requiring commitment and a will rightly oriented towards its end. All forms of inquiry seem characterized by the need for authority for initiation into the practice, for openness to and participation in constructive criticism, and to the possibility of error rooted in moral failure.

In consequence, the same conditions that MacIntyre applies to progressive moral inquiry also characterize progressive theoretical enquiry. Such inquiry builds upon the past, for example. Later stages of inquiry explain earlier errors and disagreements, and reveal an increasingly clear conception of the goal of inquiry, and of what it would mean to complete the inquiry. All inquiry proceeds through dialectical exchange with rival views, but this dialectic can be thwarted by an insufficiently sympathetic understanding of those rival views. From all these similarities, it seems, we can conclude that all systematic inquiry requires, for its success, the virtues. It is, therefore, to the virtues of inquiry that I now turn.

# 12  The Virtues of Inquiry

[W]e . . . need to become self-conscious about the moral requirements
of inquiry itself.

—MacIntyre (1995, p. 351)

It is now time to turn to a positive account of the virtues of inquiry. The
virtues in question will be character traits that are internally related to the
particular good of the practice of inquiry. This does not necessarily mean
that the relevant virtues will have different names from the more generally
familiar virtues, such as the cardinal virtues. Rather, what will often be the
case is that virtues that are typically important in a wide variety of domains
will become specified in particular ways in accordance with the nature of
the practice. An obvious case of this is the virtue of intellectual courage. So I
will, in many cases, articulate a particularly inquiry-based account of virtues
such as moderation or justice, known initially from other contexts.

Because the cardinal virtues are the most general and widely applicable
virtues, it is natural to look at their relationship to inquiry. I will argue that
there is an inquiry-specific account to be given of justice, courage, temper-
ateness, and prudence. Beyond this list of virtues, three others stand out as
important to inquiry. First, because inquiry is intrinsically truth related, the
most specifically truth-related virtue, honesty, has a special application to
inquiry. Second, Aquinas draws our attention to a virtue he calls studiousness; this too should be considered a virtue of inquiry. Finally, as I argued
in the previous chapter, inquiry is a viable candidate for a vocational commitment. This means that the demands of inquiry on an agent's character
extend across his entire person, both at a time, and through time. We should
thus investigate the virtue of integrity in the context of inquiry. In all, seven
virtues require an accounting.

## HONESTY

Genuine inquiry begins and ends with truth. It begins with truth for one is
no real inquirer if one does not have a concern for the truth. It ends with

truth for this is what inquiry aims at, without which inquiry cannot be considered wholly successful. And a vocational commitment to inquiry and its goods is above all a commitment to truth and the knowledge of truth.

This has a number of consequences for considering the way in which an inquirer's character is shaped. First, for the vocationally committed inquirer, truth is an architectonically shaping good, just as, for the doctor, health is. Thus truth enters into the explanation of much, perhaps all, that she does: her decisions about what job to take, about what projects to pursue and what not to pursue, her sense of what is important for her to attend to on a day-to-day basis—all these will be shaped by the overall commitment to truth

Such a commitment would not begin, or not be maintained, unless the agent's will had become oriented towards the truth in a particular way: the vocationally committed agent must have a love of truth, perhaps even a passion for truth. Philosophers from Plato to Peirce draw attention to this requirement. Inquiry as a way of life begins, and is sustained, by this love. As Plato argues, such a love has as its corollary a hatred of all that is false (*Republic*, 485c).

Related to this will be the way in which truth shapes up for the inquirer as an absolutely unweighable good (MacIntyre, 1998). Truth is not to be bartered or sold for some other benefit as if something else were of more worth; for the truth-loving agent such a price on truth is inconceivable. To give the truth a price, such that the truth could be abandoned for that price, would be as well to put a price on one's own integrity, to will that the ordered structure of one's character could be abandoned for the sake of the relevant price.

Correlative to the commitment to truth that the honest inquirer has is the joy of the inquirer who has found the truth. It is not the joy of one whose reputation is now to be made, or who expects rewards and fame. Rather, because the activity of the inquirer is oriented above all, at least insofar as she is an inquirer, towards the truth, the accomplishment of this end is a recurring source of joy, the satisfaction of the will. At the same time, however, the honest inquirer will not see the quest for truth as simply a quest to attain a single specified goal, but as an ongoing pursuit to know the truth more deeply.

All these characteristics go some of distance towards sketching the nature of a vocationally committed inquirer who possesses the virtue of honesty. Honesty is, from one point of view, *the* virtue of inquiry precisely because its starting and ending points are the same as inquiry's: truth. An honest inquirer is characterized above all by a love for truth, and by the consequences of this love in her character. As Peirce says, "A scientific man must be single-minded and sincere with himself. Otherwise, his love of truth will melt away, at once. He can, therefore, hardly be otherwise than an honest, fair-minded man" (Peirce, 1955, p. 41).

The honest inquirer does not, therefore, shade, ignore, or cover up the truth. Such actions would involve a rejection of truth as the unweighable and ultimate end of inquiry, and would, moreover, undermine inquiry from within. The honest inquirer is committed to considering all the relevant evidence, not just the evidence that suits her wishes, and to uncovering more evidence irrespective of what the evidence might show.

Susan Haack has distinguished two ways in which inquiry might fail in respect of the commitment to truth, and thus as regards the virtue of honesty. She characterizes both as "pseudo-inquiry": sham reasoning, and fake reasoning. Of sham reasoning, Haack writes that its characteristic feature is "the 'inquirer's' prior and unbudgeable commitment to the proposition for which he tries to make his case" (Haack, 1998, p. 9). And of fake reasoning, she writes that this is "making a case for some proposition advocating which you believe will advance yourself" (Haack, 1998, p. 9).

Many abuses of intellectual honesty in inquiry are well described as instances of sham reasoning—perhaps because they have already accepted some proposition through social faith, believing it largely as a way of getting on with others, perhaps because they cannot bear to be wrong about what they pre-reflectively think, and perhaps again for more exalted theoretical reasons, such as a commitment to an overarching worldview, agents will inquire with a view to making a pre-ordained case. As Haack points out, this cannot really be considered inquiry at all.

Haack points to recent "advocacy" research as an instance of sham reasoning. Such research has done considerable damage in the humanities, and the social sciences, as academics have pursued research agendas that only thinly cover political agendas (see Searle, 1999). Topics, questions, and evidence are considered untouchable if they threaten political convictions, whether on the left or the right. One might object that this is true also of religious faith. However, while faith involves reasonable belief for reasons that go beyond the available epistemic reasons, reasonable faith does not go *against* the evidence, nor does it deny evidence, nor do reasonable believers wish to continue to believe if their belief is false. Truth, and the desire for truth, are central to reasonable, as opposed to blind, faith: those who believe with a reasonable faith believe they have an authoritative, personal guarantee of the *truth* of their beliefs. But no such guarantees are or can be claimed for mere political positions. An agent whose inquiry is guided by the unshakeable conviction of correctness, and whose conviction thereby leads to ignoring evidence, or denying the possibility of certain directions of research has an unreasonable faith that is not consistent with the virtue of honesty.

Haack's fake reasoner is one who does not have a love of truth as central to his character. The fake reasoner—the one who argues for a position to advance himself, and not because he believes in the truth of the asserted view—is deeply dishonest. By entering into the activities and subpractices constitutive of inquiry, such as assertion, argument, criticism, and so on, and of the transmission of the fruits of inquiry, by writing and publishing, the fake reasoner leads his interlocutors to believe that he is engaged in these activities with a view to achieving their purpose: knowledge of the truth. But this is no part of what he really desires, no part of what he is really doing. Fake reasoning is thus a form of lie.

In Chapter 5, I argued that lying is intrinsically and absolutely wrong in all circumstances. Lying necessarily creates a disharmony in the character of the liar between internal and external, a disharmony contrary to the good of integrity. I also suggested that the ethics of lying and dishonesty, while in one sense external to the ethics of inquiry, would also turn out to be internal to that ethic. Recall the analogy: whether capital punishment is morally right or wrong, it might be additionally or independently wrong for a physician to be an executioner, for this would be in conflict with her ethos as a physician, her dedication to healing. Something similar is true of the ethics of lying: while it is wrong always and everywhere for any agent to lie, it is especially egregious for an inquirer to lie. Even a white lie is of greater significance, because of its tension with the inquirer's architectonic commitment to truth. As Plato, again, says of those with a philosophic temperament, "They must be without falsehood—they must refuse to accept what is false, hate it, and have a love for the truth" (*Republic,* 485c).

This discussion of honesty and lying raises two related issues. The first is that honesty and truth telling might seem not really to be best described as parts of the ethics of inquiry. One who lies has already made an assessment as to what he believes to be the truth; scientists who lie, by making up data, for example, are either not inquiring, or have already inquired and are subsequently falsifying their results. Similarly, the philosopher or historian who knows Plato's views on some matter, or who knows the true history of some matter of controversial social importance, but who, whether in court, or in a popular piece of writing, or on television, doctors his true views so as better to promote a favored cause, does not lie as a part of inquiry. And while the plagiarist is dishonest, the inquiry concerning which he is dishonest is over and done with. His offense does not seem to be internal to the ethics of inquiry as such.

But this is to take too narrow a view. Inquiry is both a social and a continuing activity, spread out across many agents and multiple times. There is a division of labor in all inquiry, even in philosophy, and all inquirers rely upon the work of those who have preceded them for their appropriate starting points. Agents who lie about what they know commit an offense *against* inquiry so conceived, even if not an offense within inquiry: they make it increasingly difficult, perhaps impossible, for other agents to rely on their work, to know the truth about some area in which they might need to depend upon the work of others. Dishonesty is neither merely keeping something for oneself, nor an innocent subordination of truth to some other set of values. It cuts deep into the social fabric that binds all inquirers, present and past, into a single community.[1]

The second point is that much of the ethics of inquiry is overdetermined by its virtues, for the verdict against any form of dishonesty as being a violation against inquiry will be supplemented in the discussion of justice; the social nature of the violation of truth makes such dishonesty, as we shall see, a matter of injustice in inquiry.[2] Plagiarism, too, can be addressed under both headings: it is an unjust taking from another, and, as a species of dishonesty, it is a violation of the commitment to truth. It is an offense against inquiry, so considered, just insofar as it creates obstacles to the work of others—for example, by preventing someone from discovering what else of interest the plagiarist's source might have had to say, and by violating the spirit with which a community of inquiry is constituted.

Bernard Williams has written, in *Truth and Truthfulness,* of the virtues of accuracy and sincerity (Williams, 2002). He considers these to be the most important truth-related virtues. Accuracy, however, is an aspect of honesty, rather than an independent virtue, and sincerity involves both honesty and intellectual integrity, which I shall address in due course. Still, Williams's point is essentially correct, and in a way that brings out the communicative function of honesty. The honest agent does not simply refrain from lying, nor does she remain silent with her understanding. She transmits the truth. This can be done only if she is meticulous as to what she is transmitting, being neither careless, nor obscure, but clear and efficient; i.e., accurate. This is a case in which a virtue demands a set of skills: an honest inquirer who cannot write clearly, who cannot communicate her ideas, arguments, or theories, cannot adequately put her virtues into action, and is thus only imperfectly virtuous.

A final point to be made about honesty, which could be reiterated with respect to all the virtues, is that it does not stand, as a virtue, in independence of moral norms or rules. The content of the character of an honest inquirer cannot be fully determined except by acknowledging the role that moral absolutes have played in shaping it. So, the honest inquirer, as motivated by love of truth, will never violate the absolute moral norm discussed in Chapter 4: never lie. This norm, like the virtue of honesty, which, in relation to truth, it shapes, is the cornerstone of the commitment made by an honest inquirer to the good of inquiry.

## COURAGE

Reflection on some of the threats that can lead us away from the virtue of honesty highlights the importance of courage. Courage, according to Aquinas, is a virtue not of the concupiscible, but of the irascible appetite (1981, I-II, Q. 60, a. 4). It is concerned with fending off challenges to an agent's commitment to action. Among those challenges, the greatest is fear of death, and in some extreme cases inquiry has been accompanied by the threat of death: Socrates and Solzhenitsyn both pursued moral inquiries (and Solzhenitsyn later pursued historical inquiries) in face of a threat of death. Scientists who inquire into the nature or cure of infectious diseases have, at times, pursued their researches despite threats to their health. But even short of the fear of death, agents can face challenges towards which the spirited combativeness of courage is appropriate.

Since courage combats fear, it is worthwhile, in considering intellectual courage, or the courage of the inquirer, to consider some of the various types of threat, and their corresponding fears, that are peculiar to inquirers, beyond the threat of death. Among the forms of fear to which inquirers are especially subject are:

- Fear of the truth.
- Fear of the consequences of the truth.
- Fear of society's response to the truth.
- Fear of failure in the attainment of the truth.

## Fear of the Truth

Much that we believe is believed unreflectively. Yet in many cases, our personal investment in such unreflective belief is very great. Most agents consider their identity to be a function in part of the web of beliefs they possess, unsurprisingly, since core beliefs in that web concern the nature of the human person, and the nature of the cosmos. Many of those beliefs—beliefs about the gods, about morality, about the nature of the world and cosmos, about our social role and how others in our social world think about us—translate into action. In consequence, inquiry that threatens various of the these unreflective beliefs thereby threatens to undermine in significant ways our self-conception, and our general modes of action. The Copernican revolution and the Darwinian paradigm shift both ruptured a great part of ordinary agents' conception of themselves and their world. This was, and is, greatly feared, even by those who pursued their cosmological or biological inquiries rigorously (Kitcher, 2001).

Of course, some of these fears may have been unjustified: the Galilean hypothesis no longer seems incompatible with the Christian worldview, and many believe the Darwinian view can likewise be shown compatible (John Paul II, 1996). St. Augustine held that Christians should not fear the truths of science, holding that these, and the truths of faith, could not conflict. Moreover, there have on the other side been courageous investigators into the truth of Christianity or some denomination thereof, investigators such as John Henry Newman, or the many atheists who have become converts (Newman, 1968). But few can genuinely know the full effect of their inquiries on their self-conception and world conception ahead of time, and there are sometimes reasons to think the effect will be quite great. This is an obvious cause of fear that intellectual courage combats.

Nor does the truth threaten only non-reflectively held beliefs. Because the investment of an agent in beliefs that she takes to be well-grounded, and into the truth of which she has already inquired, is so great, it can take a special degree of courage for a scientist, a philosopher, a theologian, or a police detective, to acknowledge the possibility of error and re-investigate, and to give new evidence a fair hearing.

One possible response to such uncomfortable truths as these is that perhaps we should not, therefore, put such a premium on truth. If the truth would make us uncomfortable, threaten our worldview, self-identity, or self-respect, then perhaps we should not pursue the truth or value it so highly. Such a response is possible with regard to all the fears that inquiry might induce. But a worldview based on false beliefs, and a self-conception founded on ignorance or error, are not themselves real goods to protect. It is rather our feelings of discomfort and unease that we are trying to prevent, thus subordinating the value of a basic good to the value of a mere subrational aversion. Such acquiescence in one's subrational feelings over the real benefits promised by an intelligible good is unreasonable, and incompatible with a will to ideal human fulfillment.

There are, however, instances in which the pursuit of some inquiry would not be appropriate because it threatened genuine goods; some research into the conditions necessary for production of certain kinds of weapons, for example. But the good in question in the examples above is only the good of avoiding discomfort from replacing false with true beliefs, and even if the discomfort is great and threatening, this should not distract an agent from the demands of intellectual courage.

## FEAR OF THE CONSEQUENCES OF TRUTH

Related to the worry that Darwinism might undermine an agent's self-conception and sense of privilege in the universe is a worry sometimes put forth by non-religious defenders of religion. The worry is that religion is such a significant part of our ordinary motivation for morality that if religion were to crumble, then so would the social fabric of society. On this sort of account, the consequences of inquiry, and of the truth, might be such that inquiry should be suppressed. Or again, perhaps a biological or sociological investigation could show that our ethical concepts were the result, not of reasoned reflection, but of some biological imperative; this might undermine our moral intuitions and motivations. Accordingly, someone might argue against such an investigation from fear of such consequences.

This argument is different from that in Chapter 9 about the social goods and evils that particular discoveries might bring about. It might well be the case that research into some horrific weapons system could have such ill possible consequences that it should not be conducted. But failure to carry out the research is not acquiescence in ignorance or falsity. It is true, when we "relinquish" the possibilities for knowledge in some area, that we are willing to remain ignorant about that domain of knowledge; but we remain entirely self-aware concerning our ignorance of the matter (Joy, 2000). By contrast, when it is suggested that we should not inquire to closely into the truth of some theory because of the social consequences of the truth, the benefits that we wish not to give up are themselves predicated, not just on our ignorance, but on our suppressing our awareness that we are in ignorance. Yet it is not clear that such a view can even be coherently held: we would need the thought that we should maintain religious beliefs for their social consequences, yet we would also need to be aware that those beliefs would be shown false if we inquired too closely. But the view that there are some areas of inquiry, whose consequences could be disastrous, that should be left alone, can stand the burden of self-scrutiny, and regularly does, when we decide on any one of a number of matters not to pursue some avenue or other of inquiry.

## Fear of Society's Response

Society can see itself threatened, as to both its self-conception and its stability, by various sorts of inquiries. Moreover, society can exert a variety of pressures, threats, and negative inducements to inquirers to either abandon some line of inquiry, or to pursue it in a biased and non-objective way.

Concern for the threat posed by society to the inquirer is found, again, in the *Republic*, which in many ways deserves to be considered the founding text in the ethics of inquiry. In a passage in which Socrates refers to both the threats and the promises made by society, he says,

> When many of them are sitting together in assemblies, courts, theaters, army camps, or in some other public gathering of the crowd, they object very loudly and excessively to some of the things that are said or done and approve others in the same way, shouting and clapping, so that the very rocks and surroundings echo the din of their praise and blame and double it. . . . [And] don't you know that they punish anyone who isn't persuaded, with disenfranchisement, fines, or death? . . . No, indeed, it would be very foolish even to try to oppose them, for there isn't now, hasn't been in the past, nor ever will be in the future anyone with a character so unusual that he has been educated to virtue in spite of the contrary education he received from the mob (492c-e).

Two institutionalized forms of pressure deserve special notice. First, both the state and its laws, and, second, the academy, can bring such threats to bear on inquirers in an especially pressing way. There are well-known examples of states explicitly threatening inquiry by forbidding forms and conclusions contrary to the ruling party's ideology, as in the former Soviet Union under Stalin. Again, this is to be distinguished from a state's legitimately forbidding immoral or dangerous forms of research, or legitimately refusing to fund even legitimate research whose relation to the common good was insufficiently apparent.

The case of academia is even more problematic. As universities, both public and private, have become increasingly homogeneous, politically and ideologically, and as advocacy research, political correctness, and a liberal orthodoxy have become dominant, it has become increasingly difficult to argue or inquire honestly, and without a predetermined agenda, in various areas, particularly those touching upon the most important cultural and moral issues of the day. Thus, open argument and debate about issues such as abortion, marriage, and the legitimacy of war have become increasingly rare, and scholars arguing for the less "acceptable" position on these issues have come to feel increasingly threatened in the university environment. The pressures exerted range from threats of social ostracism, to denial of tenure or promotion; these are circumstances calling for intellectual courage.

At the same time, it should be said that, as important as intellectual courage is, it is also a virtue the value of which is widely acknowledged, and the mantle of which is frequently claimed. It is, moreover, relatively easy to mistake simple opposition to one's claims for something more sinister: an attempt to thwart inquiry, or silence its results. It is tempting to simulate the virtue of courage by inquiring into, and proclaiming the truths of, so-called "subversive" or "transgressive" viewpoints, not because one views them as legitimate areas of inquiry, or as domains of significant truth, but precisely to flout one's lack of concern for the mores or morals of the day. In the end, true intellectual courage cannot be dissociated from intellectual honesty and its love of truth; there is a deep unity of the virtues of inquiry.

## Fear of Failure

The most realistic fear in inquiry is of failure. Inquiry is difficult, and inquiry into the most important matters especially so. This is important: the love of truth that drives inquiry is not simply a desire to gain as many truths as possible; it is a desire for important truth, systematic in nature. In consequence, it can be a form of intellectual cowardice to pursue only simple, or disjointed, or manifestly apparent truths, rather than to pursue the complex, systematic, and perplexing. Similarly, an over-reliance on the work and authority of others can be indicative, not of an appropriate intellectual humility, but of fear of failure in the event that one should think for oneself. Intellectual risk is a necessary element in intellectual success; thus, the virtue of courage, in the context of inquiry, requires that one resist more the one side of James's dichotomy: fear of error versus love of the truth (James, 1951).

## MODERATION

Moderation occurs twice in my catalogue of inquiry's virtues. In the first case, moderation signifies the control of non-epistemic appetites that can conflict with the life of inquiry. In the second case, moderation enters in as the virtue Aquinas called "studiousness," a virtue concerned with the appropriate structuring of the desire for truth. Conceptually, this virtue seems different enough, however, from our ordinary conception of moderation, to justify separate treatment.

Plato argues that moderation of non-epistemic desires is necessary for inquiry—indeed, he argues that such moderation is a consequence of the passionate desire for truth characteristic of the philosopher:

> [W]e surely know that, when someone's desires incline strongly for one thing, they are thereby weakened for others, just like a stream that has been partly diverted into another channel . . . Then, when someone's desires flow towards learning and everything of that sort, he'd be concerned, I suppose, with the pleasures of the soul itself by itself, and he'd abandon those pleasures that come through the body . . . Then surely such a person is moderate and not at all a money lover. (*Republic*, 486d)

Plato's argument is often viewed with skepticism. For one thing, the empirical evidence seems to be against it: Bernard Williams and Susan Haack have both pointed to James Watson's account of how the desire for fame "and the uncomplicated desire to do down Linus Pauling" led to the discovery of the structure of DNA (Williams, 2002, p. 142; Haack, 1998, p. 9; Watson, 1968). We can even find scientists admonishing each other that they *must* desire goods such as fame and possess "a burning desire for reputation" (Cajal, 1999, p. 29).

These writers, while either acknowledging, or extolling, the role of non-epistemic desires in inquiry, are nevertheless at pains to point out that what the inquirer must want a reputation *for* is to have found the truth. Watson did not desire to be famous for having appeared to discover the truth about DNA, but for having in fact discovered it. And so Williams calls it a "Platonic misunderstanding" to think that the desire for fame will "corrupt or undermine the search for truth" (Williams, 2002, p. 142).

I do not think, however, that it is a *complete* misunderstanding. While Williams is correct to say that non-epistemic desires—for reputation, money, or power—need not inevitably corrupt inquiry, it is true that they can: academic fraud exists, and frequently occurs from a desire to be known as the discoverer of some truth, or to reap the rewards for some discovery. Such desires can lie behind the forms of pseudo-inquiry diagnosed by Haack: it may be precisely because an agent desires above all an academic reputation that she grows unconcerned for the truth, particularly in the humanities.

Such desires can further undercut inquiry, not by leading to deliberately deceptive or fraudulent work, but by leading to sloppy, careless, or self-deceptive work. The desire to be famous for having discovered the truth can lead one to think one has discovered it, despite the holes in one's theory and problems with one's evidence. Did the self-described "discoverers" of cold fusion really intend to deceive the scientific community, or did they allow themselves to be led by their desires—for money, fame, reputation—into seeing what was not really there to be seen (Resnick, 1998, pp. 11–12)? One's desires can lead one to pursue avenues of inquiry not because of their importance, but because they are in fashion, when a sober assessment would indicate that they were unworthy of attention. In consequence, a moderate inquirer should at least maintain an appropriate level of critical scrutiny of his non-epistemic desires to ensure that they do not impair the truth-aptness or significance of his work.

Indirect consequences are also possible. Consider the inquirer whose desires for drink, food, society, or other pleasures are allowed to grow and to dominate his life. Such an agent can come undone as an inquirer: his competing desires will not corrupt his work, but will prevent it from taking place at all. Alcoholism is an extreme case, but even drinking enough to induce a hangover on a day when one plans to work on one's research constitutes a failure of moderation that impedes inquiry. And any inquirer must be able to deny himself the opportunities for various pleasures that present themselves on a daily basis: the invitation to skip work to go to the movies or to play golf, the pleasures of socializing, the prospect of enjoying the sights, sounds, and smells of the local coffee house, and so on.

It is therefore no misunderstanding, Platonic or otherwise, to suggest that moderation plays a crucial role in the life of a committed inquirer. The vocational inquirer must have a sense of where all her other desires, especially her subrational desires, stand in relation to her vocational commitment in importance and in function, and she must have successfully structured her character around this conception.

There is more to Plato's concern, however, than simply a worry that desires will corrupt inquiry. There is, additionally, the suggestion picked up on by Williams that there is something unseemly, something despicable even ("To despise them for seeking fame is itself to suffer from a Platonic misunderstanding . . ."), in some of these desires, the suggestion that one's love of truth is brought into question by the presence of these desires.

Plato's suspicion seems to rest on two further assumptions, neither of which is essentially related to the worry that non-epistemic desires will corrupt inquiry. The first is the assumption that, as one's desire flows more strongly for some one end or good, then other desires will flow more weakly. The second is that insofar as one understands the value of one's epistemic desires—the desires for truth, knowledge, and wisdom—one will see the objects of other desires in a new, negative light, and as somehow unworthy of one called to the pursuit of truth.

It is worth reconstructing these suggestions in terms, not of Platonic psychology, but of the moral psychology and theory of value articulated earlier in this book. For Plato, the soul is tripartite, made of reason, spirit, and the desires. But both the spirited part of the soul, and the reasoning part of the soul have their own desires, and in the case of reason's desires, these are for what is most truly real. Moreover, the reasoning part of the soul is, for Plato, most truly constitutive of what one is. In consequence, both assumptions make good sense: an agent who has recognized both the worth of the objects of reason's desires, and the relation of reason to her true self, will come to look upon non-epistemic desires as insignificant, or trivial, and will have less of her self to give to them. These desires will then, to use Plato's image, "dry up" as the stream of reason's desire grows.

On the view I have articulated, the human person is a unity of body and soul; so Plato's dualism cannot be relied upon to defend a quasi-ascetic account of the life of inquiry. However, subrational desires are not for intelligible goods, and thus do not orient an agent genuinely to human fulfillment. Moreover, pleasure is not itself a basic good; it does not give anyone intrinsic reasons for its pursuit. Goods such as fame, money, and power are mere instrumentalities, and also give the clear-headed agent no intrinsic reason for action. Finally, none of these reasons can play a satisfyingly architectonic role in an individual's life.

This last point requires further articulation: subrational desires, such as desires for food, sex, and other pleasures, do not in themselves promise an agent anything of depth, breadth, or substance. Insofar as a particular desire is satisfied, the desire ceases to exist and the agent once again requires a new motivation for action; typically, in an agent who has given himself over to the satisfaction of subrational desires, this will be the pursuit of the satisfaction of a new desire. But the serial satisfaction of desires is, taken as a life plan, radically unsatisfactory: it has no wholeness to it, being composed only of a series of discrete incidents. It offers no opportunities for excellence, no opportunities for growth, and, by the nature of desires themselves, no opportunities for mutual pursuit among multiple agents. So the pursuit of subrational desires and sense pleasures does not offer the possibility for structuring a life in a humanly fulfilling way.

In the case of the desire for instrumentalities such as fame, power, and money, Aristotle's well-known arguments indicate how such goods are deficient from the standpoint of an agent seeking to structure her life in a fulfilling manner. Fame and power both depend, for example, on other people, not just for their continued existence, but for the very content of the activities that sustain them: what brings fame today might not bring it tomorrow. Money's inability to constitute, or purchase, a life worth living is also apparent on very little reflection.

By contrast, the life of inquiry is aimed at a genuinely basic human good, knowledge of truth. It is capable of providing a significant degree of structure to an inquiring agent's life—the pursuit of knowledge is vocational in a strong sense. Further, the good pursued by the life of inquiry is not simply a set of truths, but of truths that hang together systematically. The sort of systematic truths pursued in such inquiries have both breadth and depth: knowledge of new truths opens up new avenues for investigation that promise to build upon the old, and agents can work together in pursuit of a more perfect body of knowledge. Finally, the objects of knowledge—at least some kinds of knowledge—have a significance that makes them special relative to the objects of other possible pursuits. Knowledge of the nature of the human person, of nature, and of the divine are substantive and significant in a way that sensible pleasures are not.

In consequence, from the standpoint of an agent committed to the pursuit of knowledge over a lifetime, and of matters both substantive and systematic, the appeal of goods such as sense pleasures and instrumentalities such as power, fame, and money really should begin to wane. It will seem inappropriate, for example, for the agent to value knowledge and fame equally, or to see both as jointly constitutive of the goodness of her life. Watson thus could be expected, if he truly loved knowledge, to be willing to sacrifice fame for the sake of knowledge, if it turned out that the two were not, in his particular case, compatible. Were it the case, for example, that the discovery of the structure of DNA would not, for some set of reasons, bring fame to Watson in his lifetime, he would think it unfortunate, but he should also think it beneath his dignity to cease his pursuit of the structure of DNA to do something else more conducive to fame and reputation.

A moderate asceticism, then, is appropriate in a variety of ways: agents given too much to the satisfaction of their desires will run the risk of being, if not positively fraudulent inquirers, nonetheless unreliable and inattentive. And agents genuinely committed to a lifetime of inquiry should, normatively, give less attention to various other desires and concerns, which will seem to some extent or other trivial by comparison with the good of her vocation.

It is *only* a moderate asceticism, however. For sensible pleasures can be integrated into the pursuit of intelligible goods. This is most obvious in the case of pleasures associated with food, drink, and sex. The pleasures of the table are integrated into the pursuit of life and health, and can be integrated into the pursuit of sociability, aesthetic pleasure, and rest. The pleasures of sex can be integrated into marriage. And some of these pleasures can be integrated, albeit somewhat indirectly, into inquiry itself. It is no accident that the pleasures of food and drink play a fairly significant role in inquiry considered as social: those who inquire together, argue together, read, write, and dispute together, typically find it pleasurable also to eat together, to relax with wine and lighter conversation together. Even Plato, who might be expected to argue a more strongly ascetic line, portrays Socrates, in the *Symposium*, as one who freely integrates the pleasures of eating, drinking, and joking into philosophical discussion and dialectic, albeit without gluttony, drunkenness, or buffoonery. A wise soul may be dry, but it should not be parched.

## STUDIOUSNESS

I have discussed the moderation of non-epistemic desires—desires such as those for food, drink, and sex. But there is also a desire for knowledge, which,

Aquinas argues, must be moderated for the sake of virtuous study. Aquinas calls this virtue studiousness, and contrasts it with the vice of curiosity.

There is an aspect of Aquinas's discussion of studiousness and curiosity that seems initially puzzling, however, and will result in some reordering on my part of his account. This peculiarity emerges from his claim that the desire that studiousness moderates is twofold: "As regards knowledge, man has contrary inclinations. For on the part of the soul, he is inclined to desire knowledge of things, and so it behooves him to exercise a praiseworthy restraint on this desire, lest he seek it immoderately: whereas on the part of his bodily nature, man is inclined to avoid the trouble of seeking knowledge" (Aquinas, 1981, II-II, Q.166, a.2, ad. 3). Aquinas goes on to say something puzzling to modern ears: that the moderation of the desire to know is more essential to the virtue of studiousness than is the keenness of interest that overcomes the inclination to avoid the trouble of seeking knowledge. This is puzzling because for us, studiousness has come to mean precisely the virtue of having sufficient discipline to overcome the tendency to rest, and because, where intellectual labor is concerned, that tendency can seem particularly prominent. A. E. Housman's called the love of truth "the faintest passion," and this, to us, seems correct (Frankfurt, 1992).

However, it is possible to explain why this is especially so today, in a way that differs from the past. Sustained inquiry is a consequence of leisure; cultures in which the daily imperative is to produce enough food to survive are not well known for their intellectual achievements. It is only with a degree of freedom from such imperatives that philosophy, the arts, and the sciences become possible. Accordingly, when a space of leisure opens up, and men no longer are entirely exhausted by the demands of their bodily needs, then the desire for knowledge really can assert itself as in some way naturally stronger.

We live today, however, in a world in which our leisure is dominated by consumer goods and by the promise of pleasures of the body, and in which our various forms of entertainment and even knowledge make increasingly scant intellectual demands. The lives of children are dominated by television and video games, the lives of adults by the pursuit of money and sex. The lives of university students, somewhere between childhood and adulthood, seem dominated by alcohol, sex, and football; indeed, Murray Sperber has argued that these interests are actively encouraged by university administrations to distract students from their instructors' lack of interest in them (Sperber, 2001). This is not the leisure of an intellectual culture. For, in addition to raising the sorts of problems mentioned in the discussion of moderation, the modern world of leisure creates a further difficulty: when the intellect is insufficiently exercised, when its rigorous formation is not attended to in childhood, and when a capacity for sustained attention is not created and fostered, the act of the intellect becomes increasingly and distressingly, taxing. Intellectual laziness and inertia are thus conditions internal to leisure in the modern world, in a way in which they were not when leisure seemed desirable precisely because of the opportunities it offered for the life of the mind.

For us, then, Aquinas's claim about the moderation of the desire for knowledge being the essential part of studiousness seems truly puzzling: for us, the disciplining of the mind through, and for the sake of, study, and the overcoming of intellectual sloth is the great task of the day. Accordingly, this is how I conceive of this fourth virtue of inquiry: studiousness is, above all, a kind of discipline in the soul, to resist laziness and pursue the truth despite our deep inclination to stasis, sloth, and the like. Indications of this virtue are to be seen in the practical disciplines that the inquirer subjects herself to, such as a fixed schedule and degree of organization, a refusal to fool herself into thinking she is accomplishing something simply by being in her study, a resolution to avoid daydreams, a willingness to accept and adhere to deadlines, and so on.

Ramon y Cajal, in *Advice for a Young Investigator,* writes:

> In Spain, where laziness is a religion rather than a vice, there is little appreciation for how the monumental work of German chemists, naturalists, and physicians is accomplished—especially when it would appear that the time required to execute the plan and assemble a bibliography might involve decades! Yet these books have been written in a year or two, quietly and without feverish haste. The secret lies in the method of work; in taking advantage of as much time as possible for the activity; in not retiring for the day until at least two or three hours are dedicated to the task; in wisely constructing a dike in front of the intellectual dispersion and waste of time required by social activity; and finally, in avoiding as much as possible the malicious gossip of the café and other entertainment—which squanders our nervous energy (sometimes even causing disgust) and draws us away from our main task with childish conceits and futile pursuits. (Cajal, 1999, pp. 37–38)

Cajal's advice in some cases overlaps with a concern for ordinary moderation, but in general he seems to have diagnosed the necessary response to a culture that treats laziness like "a religion rather than a vice." The virtue of studiousness is necessary, and practical steps must be taken for that virtue to take root.

The most interesting part of Aquinas's discussion of studiousness is his discussion of the vice of curiosity. The rest of this section will rather closely follow that discussion, with some commentary. St. Thomas's discussion is divided into two parts: the first concerns curiosity regarding intellective knowledge, the second, curiosity regarding sense knowledge. Concerning the first, he initially notes that knowledge is in itself good, though it may be evil accidentally, as when it leads to pride, or when one uses the knowledge for some evil purpose. But moderation concerns primarily the *desire* for knowledge, so that desire is disordered if an agent seeks knowledge to take pride in it, or to bring about some other evil.

Could there be, in addition to these accidentally evil forms of knowledge, some form of knowledge that is *in itself* illicit? The possibility of such "forbidden" knowledge occurs occasionally in fiction, and in some understandings of religious restrictions on knowledge, such as the proscription against eating the fruit of the tree of knowledge in the Garden. But Aquinas asserts the contrary: all knowledge is in itself good; it is forbidden only in consequence of something that is accidental to it considered as knowledge—its leading to harm, its association with other vices, and so on.

In discussing those "who study to know the truth in that they may take pride in their knowledge," Aquinas first quotes Corinthians viii.1, "Knowledge puffeth up," and then Augustine, on those who "imagine they are doing something great" in knowing the world, rather than knowing immaterial and divine things. Not only is the pride itself a vice, but the desire is disordered: right-willed inquiry is in important ways not oriented to the self.

Aquinas then discusses briefly four ways in which the desire for learning or knowledge can be inordinate: when a man is withdrawn from an obligatory study to something less profitable; when a man studies in order to learn from one from whom it is unlawful to be taught; when a man desires to know the truth about creatures without referring his knowledge to God; and when a man studies to know the truth above the capacity of his own intelligence. In each case, the desire for knowledge must be restrained and reordered if the agent is to have the appropriate virtue.

Is the right ordering of intellectual desire an aspect of the internal ethics of inquiry, as I have defined it? Do the disorders of desire diagnosed by Aquinas hamper the progress of inquiry? Or is their wrongness external to the search for truth? In three of these cases, the disorders are clearly internal. Consider first the inquirer whose desire for knowledge leads him to abandon what is otherwise obligatory. The obligation might be itself non-inquiry related, as when a man ignores his family to pursue his studies. In such a case, the moral issue is probably best described as part of the external ethics of inquiry. But in other cases, inquiring agents must discipline their desire for knowledge in order that they may continue to pursue some line of investigation that has become obligatory for them rather than allow themselves to digress in pursuit of some avenue of inquiry that seems, at the moment, new and interesting.

How does an agent come to have an obligation to some particular pursuit of knowledge? Given the account of inquiry as vocational, this should be easy to see. Any vocational commitment requires specification in a number of ways, and also requires that the specifications be adhered to with a will that overflows from the overall vocational commitment. A husband's commitment to his wife to live with her until death generates a number of specifying commitments: to take a job, to do various things domestically, to attend to her needs in particular ways, to avoid flirting with a colleague. If the mode of satisfying these subordinate commitments were to shift regularly, there would be an overall failure in the husband's ability satisfactorily to honor his vocational commitment.

Similarly, an agent who makes a commitment to inquiry must specify that commitment by choosing avenues of inquiry and particular projects that further the goods of that commitment. Because the consequences of abandoning such specifications and projects regularly would be so negative for the agent's ability to honor her overall commitment, specified commitments to projects and avenues of inquiry create at least presumptive obligations for inquirers, which are violated when the force of desire for some other kind of knowledge leads an agent to abandon the initial commitments.

Aquinas's third example, of the agent who fails to refer his knowledge to the divine, might seem not to be an internal failure of the ethics of inquiry. One might think, if one was a believer, that the ethical failure here was one of respect for God; or one might think, if one was not a believer, that there was no failure whatsoever. However, it is clear that if there is a creator God, then reference to Him, and his work, is necessary for a *full* understanding of the nature and working of the created world. Moreover, it may well be the case that this further understanding itself generates epistemic advantages. The fundamental intelligibility of nature, for example, seems strongly guaranteed in a theistic world; and it is arguable that a theistic worldview served to promote the advance of science in the modern world (Jaki, 1980). Accordingly, it is critical for any serious inquirer to wonder, and investigate, whether such claims are, in fact, true. So even if one is not a committed religious believer, one has an obligation to ask at least how one's work and conclusions fit into a broader understanding of the cosmos, and the meaning of things.

Aquinas's fourth example, the agent who desires and studies above his intellectual capacity, is a failure internal to inquiry and often is an ethical failure: agents who commit substantial parts of their lives to inquiry must give thought to their capacities and abilities, and refrain from pursuing something for which they have little aptitude, however attractive it might otherwise be.

So three out of four sorts of failure are failures in the internal ethics of inquiry. The difficulty is Aquinas's third case of inordinate desire: the case of the agent who studies in order to learn from one from whom it is unlawful to learn. Aquinas's example is of one who seeks to learn the future from demons. Secular examples are also available. Gregory Reichberg, in his discussion of studiousness, suggests that it might be wrong to learn from Nazi scientists (Reichberg, 1999). But it appears that the Nazis' failures are best explained in terms of the distinctions of the first half of this book: they violated person-centered norms in a host of ways, the wrongness of which was not consequential upon the fact that they were engaged in *inquiry*. So how could learning from them be a failure in the *internal* ethics of inquiry?

This is an appropriate place, however, to rethink the strict wall between the external and the internal ethics of inquiry. Could one, for example, have all the internal virtues of inquiry, as discussed so far—honesty, courage, moderation, studiousness—and yet be in other respects highly immoral in one's inquiry? Could an internally virtuous inquirer also be willing to violate the rights of research subjects, experiment on them without their consent, or engage in unfair research? I want to argue that the answer to this cannot be unconditionally affirmative.

The reason for this is that the truly virtuous inquirer, who has made a vocational commitment to inquiry, has a love of truth. It is not a love of this truth or that, or this type of truth or that, but of truth as such. Plato makes a similar claim: the lover of wisdom, he writes, loves the whole of wisdom. And truth itself is a whole. There are many truths, but all, in the end, hang together in an ordered fashion. These truths, which together comprise the truth that is the overall object of the inquirer's passion, include practical truths, the truths of ethics. One cannot be a genuine lover of truth but be indifferent to the truths of ethics.

Thus the Nazi scientists' love of truth was, considered as such, deficient; they may have been lovers of truths, but they were not unconditional lovers of the truth. Indeed, we may see this in an assessment of how they stood in regard to some of the virtues of inquiry discussed so far. The Nazi scientists were not honest: their work was carried out for the sake of ideological ends, and was shaped accordingly. And they were, in all likelihood, intellectual cowards, afraid to acknowledge plain truths about the human persons they subjected to their brutal experiments. Their lack of the virtues of inquiry shows forth in much of their science, which was wasteful and inefficient by any reasonable scientific standards even apart from its obvious moral deficiencies (Cornwell, 2004).

The relationship is different going in the other direction. It seems that one *could* honor the external ethics of inquiry, yet fail to have the internal virtues of the vocational inquirer. This is indicated by the fact that not all who engage in inquiry, even over extended periods of time, are vocational inquirers; police investigators and journalists are unlikely to be inquirers on my account. Yet they must adhere to the external norms developed in the first several chapters.

This does not yet address the status of Aquinas's claim that it manifests the vice of curiosity to seek knowledge from one from whom it is impermissible to learn and whether such curiosity is a failure of the internal ethics of inquiry. I suggest the following, which I take to be partly convergent with Reichberg's solution. First, by "those from whom it is unlawful to learn," I will understand Aquinas to mean something like "those whose knowledge does not proceed from a morally virtuous disposition towards knowledge." This will cover Aquinas's example of demons, for the demons, although they sometimes have genuine knowledge, including knowledge of the future, do not value that knowledge in itself, but only insofar as it can be used for the ruin of souls. If falsity can do the job better than knowledge, demons will feel free to use falsity. Similarly, if my account of the Nazis is correct, they violated not just external norms of inquiry, but internal norms as well. They were not genuinely vocational inquirers, in the sense described in this and the previous chapter.

Second, we should distinguish between "seeking to learn from," and "obtaining knowledge from." We might obtain knowledge of many things from those who had gained their knowledge illicitly; we might even obtain knowledge from those who did not themselves really have knowledge. But Aquinas is warning against intellectual submission to those who are themselves not in possession of the virtues of inquiry. This is a legitimate warning. The professor who is careless of the truth, or an intellectual coward, or who is insufficiently dedicated to truth, or for whom the intellectual life is a cover for a political agenda, is a teacher to whom one should not submit oneself as a learner. One might learn a great deal; but one would risk moral corruption insofar as one was committed to genuine inquiry. Likewise, to learn from demons is incompatible with a will to genuine inquiry and truth, because the demons have no such commitments. Aquinas's norm, then, turns out to be part of the internal ethics of inquiry for learners.

It remains to say something concerning Aquinas's treatment of the vice of curiosity as regards sensitive knowledge. St. Thomas asks whether there is a vice of curiosity about sensitive knowledge, in addition to intellectual knowledge. He argues that there is, calling it concupiscence of the eyes, following Augustine. And, citing Bead, Aquinas lists the learning of magic arts, sightseeing, and the discovery and dispraise of our neighbor's faults, as instances of this sin. Aquinas argues that curiosity about sensible things is sinful when it detracts from some more useful consideration, and when it is directed to something harmful. Sightseeing in the strict sense—looking at the bizarre, the unusual, the freakish, simply out of curiosity—is the model of the former; prying for the sake of gossip is a model of the latter.

Both are vices to which inquirers are subject. The appeal of unusual sights and sounds, of the sight of the weird, bizarre, or even ugly, of pain, or death, has a hold over many of us that is not always easy to acknowledge. Giving in to this appeal can be demeaning, and can distract from legitimate studies (of course, one can always *call* the weird, bizarre, and ugly legitimate fields of study). And academics are as prone to trade in gossip and rumor as anyone—especially when the objects of their inquiries are their colleagues and rivals. What would the academic novel be, otherwise? So both of Aquinas's points are well taken within the framework of the internal ethics of inquiry.

## JUSTICE

To address justice in inquiry, it is necessary to recall its social nature. Consider first an agent's initiation into the life of inquiry. This is made possible only because, at a very general level, the agent has been taught her language, and the variety of ordinary linguistic and ratiocinative skills that make inquiry possible. At a more specific level, it is made possible only because the agent has been taught by experts in her field how to inquire: how to think about what constitutes a legitimate problem for inquiry, what methods are reasonable, what unreasonable, and what as yet insufficiently understood, what bodies of knowledge may, and what must be relied upon in her work, and so on. All this is made possible, in turn, by the vast body of accumulated knowledge and methodological sophistication that preceded her teachers, made their inquiries possible, and generally sustained a culture of inquiry in that particular area.

Agents in all the inquiring disciplines work together to some extent. In the humanities, the communication of theories, and the discussion and mutual criticism of views constitute the bare minimum of social necessities for successful inquiry. In the sciences, the degree of collaboration is much greater, as discussed in Chapter 9: the scientific method itself is social, requiring that scientists test and reconfirm, or falsify, the work of their peers. There is a division of labor such that inquirers may rely on the work of many others, even as they are retesting or scrutinizing the work of some, in advancing the course of inquiry.

This is quite summary. But it indicates the extent to which justice must play a role in responsible inquiry. There will be issues of both distributive and commutative justice, that is, justice regarding the distribution of goods, such as resources, and also what Finnis calls the "incidents of common enterprise," such as jobs, offices, and roles; and justice in matters of interpersonal treatment in regards to which there is no obvious issue of distribution. Outside the area of inquiry, commutative justice includes concern for wrongful harm and restitution, truth telling, and concern for the person of another, as well as contracts and other voluntary agreements. But, over both types, it will be helpful to remember Finnis's thumbnail sketch of the virtue of justice: "Justice, as a quality of character, is in its general sense always a practical willingness to favor and foster the common good of one's communities, and the theory of justice is, in all its parts, the theory of what in outline is required for that common good" (Finnis, 1980, p. 165). The account of justice in inquiry, then, must look to what a willingness to favor and foster the common good of the community of inquiry involves.

Some conclusions follow from the account above of initiation into inquiry. Central to that account is a condition characterized by MacIntyre as one of dependence: learners and inquirers are dependent upon their teachers for the skills and nurturing necessary for them to achieve an eventual state of independence (MacIntyre, 1999). Their teachers provide them with the whole range of skills, sensibilities, and dispositions that make it possible to inquire soundly. Thus agents must be willing, for the sake of initiation into the practice of inquiry, to subject themselves to authority within their discipline, and in particular to the authority of their teachers. All inquirers are thus in a condition, from the very beginning, of radical debt with respect to others from whom and with whom they have learned how to inquire, and what virtues and rules were necessary for that inquiry. How is that debt to be repaid? How is justice in inquiry to be served in this regard?

There is an obvious problem with respect to the debt we owe our teachers: some of those teachers are dead, and many more are beyond the possibility of adequate recompense in those respects in which they have benefited us. This is itself, however, a key premise in a Platonic argument,[3] the conclusion of which is that those who have been aided to success in inquiry by others incur an obligation to themselves take up the burden of teaching with respect to those only now beginning the practice of inquiry.

Obedience to authority and gratitude, then, are elements of a just inquirer's character, and shape her activities. But the core of justice in inquiry concerns one's relation to those with whom one inquires, either immediately, or insofar as they are part of the larger community of inquiry. Within this context, I incur obligations both to acknowledge the role others have played in my community of learning, and to keep up my part in the constitution of that community. Unacknowledged taking, especially where some in particular have played a crucial role in the prosecution of inquiry, is an injustice. This should not militate against the very ordinary way in which members of a community may, without repeated acknowledgment, continuously rely upon the division of labor mentioned above; but special contributions should be acknowledged, and the contribution of another should not be claimed as one's own. Failure of attribution and plagiarism are serious offenses against the internal ethics of inquiry.

Further, because of the reliance of others within the community of inquiry on me, I must be forthright and generous in sharing the fruits of my inquiry. This is a point touched upon in the discussion of honesty: dishonesty in inquiry is a failure not only of that virtue, but of justice, in at least two ways. First, in the community of inquiry, it really is true that a lie violates the structures of will and commitment on which the community is founded and exists; for the community of inquiry is founded on a commitment to truth, and this is ruptured when inquirers lie to one another, either by misrepresenting or concealing what they know, or by claiming to know what they do not.

Second, progress in inquiry is halted when inquirers, relying upon the work of others, either pursue avenues of research that depend upon what they take to be true but is not; or pursue avenues of research the truth of which is already known to someone; or fail to pursue avenues of research because they are convinced that the truth already is known to someone. In each of these ways what is due to an inquirer—the aid of open communication—is denied, and an injustice is done to her. Moreover, I must keep up my part in the community of learning by subjecting my conclusions, and the conclusions of others, to public scrutiny. Inquiry has its potential freeriders, and I must make a commitment to share, to criticize, and to accept criticism in a way that acknowledges the cooperative nature of my pursuit.

There is a tension, however, between what Robert Merton identified as the norm of "communalism" in science, and inquiry generally, and the actual practice of inquiry, involving as it does both competition and secrecy (Merton, 1973a). Do these acknowledged facts about inquiry as it is actually practiced vitiate the account of justice in inquiry given so far? Competition and secrecy are, in the actual world, inevitable and ineliminable; it would be a blow to the account if the prospect of even approximate justice in inquiry was impossible. In what follows, I argue that competition and secrecy within inquiry *are* compatible with justice. The account will not justify the whole of the contemporary practice of inquiry, but it will show that it is not inevitably corrupt in virtue of the presence of these properties.

Competition has been with us in one form or another since the beginning of the development of practices; MacIntyre's narrative in the early chapters of *Whose Justice? Which Rationality?* gives us a good idea of the tension between the competitive spirit, with its focus on victory and rewards, and the pursuit of the goods internal to any practice. Yet the benefits of competition for practice are undeniable. Consider the context of play. Even very skilled and social play with a ball and a hoop can be improved by the introduction of certain kinds of structural elements: a beginning and an end to the play, for example. But ad hoc or arbitrary endings are less satisfying than endings that correspond to some genuine completion—that one player or group has scored such and such an amount; alternatively, genuinely arbitrary endings, such as ceasing play after forty-five minutes can be rendered satisfying if a conclusion is built into the ending—whoever has the most points at the end wins.[4]

The introduction of endings brings with it the introduction of winning and losing. This, in turn, naturally marks the beginnings of competition: each participant in the form of play will desire to be the winner, will work harder, and will practice longer, to be the winner. One overall consequence of this is that the quality of the game will improve with the introduction of competition. Notice that this account of competition is so far independent of any role that the notion of reward plays. But reward might appropriately also be introduced, because competition gives us a reasonably good way of determining whether the condition appropriate to reward exists, namely merit.

Two aspects in the account converge here: reward is appropriate to merit; and competition, which tends to increase merit, also tends to identify it. So competition does not seem naturally unjust; rather, it seems initially conducive, whatever long-range problems it might also bring, with the demands of justice.

The ability of competition to play this dual role—increasing and identifying merit—is not limited to the context of play. Rather, the introduction of competition, whether through formal institutions or through informal social pressures, can play both roles across other practices—hence the competitive quality, in Greek life, of the practices most central to the culture: games, yes, but also politics, philosophy, and law. There are differences across each practice in terms of what can count as a "win" and what should count as appropriate merit and reward. But in general, the consequences are roughly the same: an increase in the quality of performance and product, and a mechanism by which rewards for performance and product may be distributed.

Why should such a story not also pertain to the context of inquiry? Indeed, in certain respects, inquiry provides its own natural end points towards which a competitive impulse will tend, since inquiry aims at truth. It is therefore natural for a competitive culture of inquiry to develop, with an attendant structure of rewards. Merton has drawn our attention to the peculiar nature of the rewards granted within the West's culture of inquiry: the primary form of reward allotted to the meritorious in inquiry centers around reputation, the eponymous naming of discoveries, and posthumous fame (Merton, 1973b).

The competitive impulse in inquiry, though it can become warped, and can generate failures in justice, and the other virtues, is thus not fundamentally incompatible with justice, nor with the other virtues discussed above. The account of moderation as incompatible with an overwhelming desire for fame or reputation is compatible with recognition that merit does deserve reward; with recognition that merit generally increases under the influence of competition; and with the self-conscious, albeit limited and disciplined, desire for victory and reward within the context of inquiry. Watson *may* have been immoderate in his desire for reputation, and he certainly was if, counterfactually, he would have abandoned his inquiries for some more prestigious line of investigation, but it was morally possible for him both to be a just and a moderate inquirer, and to desire reputation and reward for his discoveries.

What of secrecy? Secrecy seems *prima facie* to be even more opposed to the ethos of inquiry, with its communalism and openness. But a role for secrecy follows from the account given so far of competition, and just reward. In inquiry, competition is oriented around successful achievement of the ends of inquiry—the discovery of particular truths. In this, inquiry is analogous to team sports. However, with qualifications, a game, or even an argument presented in a law court, is such that the achievement of the end, and progress towards the end, is available for public inspection pretty much throughout. Cheating on the basketball court is witnessed by fans and referees; cheap shots in the law are rebuked by judges and ignored by juries. And, when the game or the trial is over, it is relatively apparent to most whether there has been a fair play of the game or a fair trial.

By contrast, in inquiry, progress, while public in various senses discussed in Chapter 9, is not always *apparent*; there are no referees during the process of investigation, and while there are institutional checks on the validity and accuracy of results, there are not naturally such checks on the fairness by which the results were obtained. It will not, therefore, be obvious to external observers when scientist A announces the results of his work that A has, in fact, stolen much of his data, or his hypotheses, or his procedures, from scientist B, as it is evident to observers that player A has obtained the ball by means of a cheap foul on player B. But if it is B's work that has generated the results, then it is B who deserves recognition and not A. In consequence, it will be to B's advantage, and reasonable *up to a point,* for B to prevent A from obtaining access to her data, hypotheses, etc., by keeping them secret.

There are other, more external, reasons that secrecy is involved in research and inquiry. Some data must be kept confidential to honor the privacy of research subjects; some work is related to trade secrets; and research might be kept secret for various prudential motives, such as safety concerns. Such concerns are not internal to the ethic of inquiry. But the concern for secrecy I have identified above is internally related, for it is a means by which fairness may be maintained between the various participants in the community of inquiry, some of whom will, under real-world conditions, violate the fair terms under which the community generally operates.

Both competition and secrecy are sometimes abused: scientists hoard their results, data, or methods for self-centered motives, and competition on occasion threatens the sprit of inquiry, and generates wrongful motives and actions. The institutional culture within which inquiry takes place sometimes actively contributes to such threats. Such qualifications aside, however, competition and secrecy are not incompatible with justice in inquiry.

## PRUDENCE AND INTEGRITY

Prudence and integrity represent, in a way, the beginning and the end of the virtues of inquiry. Prudence is the beginning of inquiry, for without the practical knowledge possessed by the prudent agent, inquiry would go astray from the beginning; and integrity is the end of virtuous inquiry, because intellectual integrity supervenes on the character of an agent possessed of all the virtues of inquiry.

Prudence is an intellectual virtue; it is not a habit of either the will or the passions, but is the virtue of the practical intellect insofar as the agent is disposed to deliberate well about means to ends. Aristotle and Aquinas contrast prudence to those virtues of the appetites, such as temperance and fortitude; without prudence, these virtues would be inadequately guided in action. Without these virtues guiding the appetites, however, the appropriate ends of the agent would not seem desirable, for the end appears to the agent in accordance with her character. This interrelationship is one source of Aristotle's and Aquinas's insistence on the unity of the virtues.

Aquinas writes that prudence is the complement of all the virtues (1981, II-II, Q. 166, a. 2, reply to objection 1); the discussion so far of the five moral virtues of inquiry bears this out. In the discussion of each, what was at stake was a consideration of how an agent with such a virtue would or would not approach inquiry. The honest inquirer will not lie, and will have an adequate sense of how open she must be about the truths she knows and is pursuing. The courageous inquirer will pursue those truths that are worth finding out despite the risks. The moderate agent will know what pleasures are a risk to inquiry, and the studious inquirer will know when disciplined activity is called for, and when it might be necessary to take a break. The just agent knows how best to acknowledge the role of others in her inquiries, whether those others are dead or alive, directly or indirectly responsible for her ability to inquire successfully. Prudence is responsible in each case for the appropriate determination of answers to such questions. So prudence determines the appropriate act of the virtuous inquirer in any context in which the other virtues have application.

Moreover, prudence enters into the life of inquiry in ordering the commitments and activities of such a life with the agent's life overall. This will involve ordering the life of inquiry in a way that is subordinated to more important or architectonic life commitments, and ordering subordinate commitments, decisions, and actions, within the life of inquiry as appropriate. Of the life of inquiry, the agent must ask: Is such a vocational commitment appropriate for me? If so, to what particular field of inquiry? What sorts of projects should I undertake with a view to pursuing such a field? How is the systematic pursuit of inquiry to be related to my marriage, or religious obligations? And so on.

Similarly, Aquinas's discussion of curiosity also incorporated moral questions for which a prudent determination was necessary. From whom would it be inappropriate to learn? What forms of knowledge are beyond my grasp? How is my field of knowledge to be ordered to higher things, such as knowledge and love of the divine? Prudence is the beginning of systematic lifelong inquiry, because it is required if an agent is to judge that inquiry is indeed a reasonable lifelong activity for her, if she is to judge concerning the various forms of inquiry available to her, and if she is to judge about how to "place" inquiry within the structure of her life overall.

So prudence has a twofold role, placing inquiry within an agent's life, and determining within inquiry what the demands of the various virtues are from context to context. This accords with the general definition of prudence as concerned with means rather than ends, for end is a relative term. Inquiry is an end for agents who have committed themselves to the pursuit of knowledge, and the agent must prudently deliberate in a variety of situations as to how best that end may be pursued. But relative to the end of a well-lived life, the pursuit of knowledge through inquiry is a means, and an agent must deliberate prudently as to whether it is an appropriate means for that agent in pursuing that end.

If prudence is the beginning of virtuous inquiry, then integrity is its end. Intellectual integrity supervenes in a virtuous inquirer on her various other virtues. This is one reason why intellectual integrity is frequently described in ways that make it seem identical to some other virtue, particularly intellectual courage or moderation.

Recall, from Chapter 2, the complexity of the human being. We are rational volitional, and passionate, and each of these aspects of the human being may come into conflict with others. But if we have made wise structuring choices, are of good character, and have educated our passions adequately, then we will be persons of integrity: in internal harmony across the various aspects of our person.

What, then, is intellectual integrity? There are some straightforward parallels between the account of ordinary moral integrity and the picture of the virtuous inquirer limned thus far. For example, the person of intellectual integrity has made a reasonable commitment to the life in inquiry, and has both integrated that commitment into more architectonic commitments, and integrated subordinate commitments into the framework provided by the commitment to inquiry. The virtuous inquirer has organized the projects and goals of his life of inquiry, and pursues them in a reasonable and orderly fashion—he is not blown hither and yon by the winds of intellectual fashion, or chance interests and curiosities.

The virtuous inquirer likewise does not let his desires get out of hand, so that they rule or even threaten his choices about what to inquire into, or his choices about how to inquire, or his subsequent judgments on the matters into which he is inquiring. And, having a passion for truth as such more than for the truth that pleases him in some other respect, his judgments as to the truth do not stand in an uneasy tension with his desires; rather, the truth works on his character, as the nature of his desires and wishes, insofar as they bear on the matters into which he inquires, themselves become shaped by what he recognizes as true.

While intellectual integrity is frequently mistaken for intellectual courage, it is a broader dispositional feature of the agent. The two virtues are related however: the inquirer who lacks intellectual courage allows the process of inquiry and resultant judgments to be shaped by her fears—fear of the truth, of society, of the consequences of the truth, and of failure. She avoids what she knows she should investigate, overlooks important evidence, or willfully believes, or claims to believe, what is false. These are all failures of courage, but in virtue of this, they are also failures of integrity.

Integrity, then, supervenes on the presence, in the agent, of all the virtues of inquiry; the agent whose inquiry is governed by this family of virtues is herself an internally unified person. In closing this discussion, however, it is worth noting two further types of harmony that flow naturally from the discussion of integrity, and the virtues of inquiry.

First, agents may stand in analogous relationships of harmony or disharmony to others; they may be friendly, of good will, or positively cooperative with others, or they may be surly, uncooperative, or downright hostile. Moreover, tensions in the social realm may have consequences for personal integrity and vice versa; consider again, the agent whose inquiry is misshapen for fear of what the crowd will think. Second, agents may stand in a harmonious or non-harmonious relationship to the divine. Some agents acknowledge and worship, others deny and scorn what they take to be the transcendent source of meaning. Both forms of harmony are also implicated in the discussion of the virtues of inquiry; for, on the one hand, the social nature of inquiry demands that the interpersonal harmony of justice be present within the community of inquirers. Moreover, recall from Chapter 9 the various ways in which inquiry, especially scientific inquiry, was to be considered public apart from its method: it is public in its benefits, and its expressive power. So the demand for social harmony extends, for inquirers, beyond their limited community of inquiry to the polis of which they are citizens.

On the other hand, consider again Aquinas's account of curiosity. It is part of the vice of curiosity that the curious agent neglects to frame his inquiries in the larger context of awareness of recognition of the role of the divine in knowledge—as, that is, an object of knowledge, and the source of all else that is knowable. The suggestion that knowledge of the divine is the end of all inquiry is impossible to follow through in this book, but it is relevant to the discussion of integrity: the forms of harmony that integrity requires naturally radiate out from the person of integrity to the social world around, and to the source of that world, the divine.

## CONCLUSION

This chapter and the previous one constitute the core of the internal ethics of inquiry: a virtue ethics that governs the activity of gathering and assessing evidence, and that flows from an inquirer's commitment to truth as the end of inquiry. In establishing this ethics, I have moved well beyond the person-centered requirements of biomedical and scientific research; yet, since medical and scientific researchers can and ought to have a commitment to truth as a central part of their life plan, the discussion of this chapter applies to such inquirers just as it applies to inquirers in philosophy, or history.

Neither the person-centered nor the truth-centered ethics of the first and second part of the book, respectively, can be considered complete. Many questions remain, and not every possible topic has been addressed. Some of these questions and topics will be obvious, especially within established fields of research and investigative ethics; it is incumbent on the goods-based approach to address remaining and disputed questions in these areas. But it is perhaps worthwhile to indicate three further areas where an expanded ethics of inquiry should proceed.

First, an obvious parallel to the ethics of inquiry is to be found in the literature on the ethics of belief. Indeed, some of W. K. Clifford's complaints about violations of the ethics of belief, in his famous essay of that name, involve failures to inquire (Clifford, 1979). At the same time, belief is an end of inquiry: we inquire in order to judge, and judgment brings about belief. What, then, is the relationship between the internal ethics of inquiry and the ethics of belief? In what ways are the two continuous, and in what ways discontinuous with one another?

Second, what is the appropriate institutional context for inquiry? Is, for example, and as I believe, the university the true institutional home for systematic inquiry into the most important things? Does inquiry suffer when the core values of its institutional home become transformed so as to place less emphasis on the internal goal of inquiry, truth? What if the understanding of the value of truth is instrumentalized, or denied altogether? What sorts of external rewards and inducements are conducive to inquiry, and what sort corrupt? Such questions are equally important for inquiry in the humanities and sciences (D. Bok, 1982, 2004; Merton, 1978b).

Third, what is the relationship between the life of virtuous inquiry, as described in this chapter, and the divine? Is inquiry, as I suggested earlier, into the nature and existence of the divine somehow morally obligatory? If so, what results does such an inquiry turn up, and how do the results of that inquiry bear, in turn, on future inquiry, and, especially, on the ethics of inquiry? And, in a question relating the concerns of the previous paragraph to the concerns of this one, how should we rethink questions about the institutional context of inquiry in light of answers to these questions concerning the divine? Can there be a religious institution that is also a genuine university and home of inquiry?

All such questions are, as I conceive it, of importance to a fully worked-out ethics of inquiry. Yet the work done in this book should at least make clear that the virtues of inquiry must play a role in the ethics of belief; that no institutional setting for inquiry can be successful if it fails to respect persons or cultivate the virtues of inquiry, and that our relationship to the divine is, in all likelihood, compromised by failures in the ethics of inquiry, and promoted by virtuous inquiry. An expanded ethics of inquiry must therefore build on the foundation established here, a foundation that conceives of respect for persons in terms of the goods constitutive of human flourishing, and the internal ethics of a practice in terms of its virtues.

# Notes

## NOTES TO CHAPTER 1

1. See Aquinas (1981, II-II, Q. 64, a.2). Aquinas's view is criticized in Boyle (1989) and Brugger (2004).
2. The paradigm statement of this form of liberalism is Rawls (1996). For a libertarian view, see Engelhardt (1996).
3. Strictly speaking, Aristotle holds that contemplation is the highest good. But I will typically speak of the value of knowledge in discussing this view, as few think that contemplation as Aristotle understood it—of the unmoved mover—is the highest, or dominant, good. If knowledge is viewed as the highest good, the claims of inquiry against morality emerge straightforwardly.
4. Philosophers in particular have been susceptible to the charms of this position. See Slade (1999) who attributes to the ancients the view that "the best kind of activity is not ruling but contemplative knowing," and that therefore philosophy is the "contemplative fulfillment and perfection of man" (p. 56).
5. This view was earliest, and, in my view, most successfully presented in the twentieth century, by Germain Grisez, Joseph Boyle, and John Finnis. See Grisez (1965), Grisez, Boyle, and Finnis (1987), and Finnis (1980). The Grisez–Boyle–Finnis approach has been followed especially by Robert P. George (1999). More recently, and in slightly differing ways, a goods-based view has been developed by Chappell (1997), Oderberg (2000), Murphy (2000), and Gomez-Lobo (2002).
6. Chappell (1997, pp. 14–15) helpfully names this the "Problem of Reconciliation."
7. Not all basic goods theorists acknowledge the agent neutrality of the goods; see Murphy (2001).
8. Kraut (1989) accepts a version of the Single End View; but to accommodate natural intuitions about the legitimacy of goods that do not seem instrumental to contemplation, he is forced to abandon Aristotle's eudaimonism, and hold that some goods are pursued for their own sake but not for the sake of happiness. A particularly stark statement of the SFE view's instrumentalism occurs in the *Eudemian Ethics* at 1249b16–19: "What choice and possession of the natural goods—whether bodily goods, money, friends, or other goods—will most of all produce contemplation of god, that choice or possession is best and this the finest standard." The translation is Richardson Lear's, p. 120, fn 60.
9. The second-tier status of the non-contemplative life cannot be avoided by the DFE view; even on Richardson Lear's version, which attributes significant value to the life of active virtue as an imitation of the best, i.e., contemplative, life, still, the life of practical reason is only an "approximation" of the best life.

10. In particular, an ethics of truth seeking has begun to be articulated, in various ways, by Haack (1998), Williams (2002), Frankfurt (2004), and Lynch (2004). Epistemologists pursuing "virtue epistemology" have also been important in this regard: see, e.g., Zagzebski (1996).

11. See Dellapenna (2006) for an account of the former; Hwang Woo-Suk is a Korean scientist who announced breakthrough discoveries in cloning and stem cell research. His claims turned out to be fraudulent.

## NOTES TO CHAPTER 2

1. See, for example, Michael Gazzaniga's personal statement in PCB (2002).

2. The Nuremberg Code, the Helsinki Declaration, and the *The Belmont Report: Ethical Principles and Guidelines for the Protection of Human Subjects of Research*, are reprinted in many texts, including Barnbaum and Byron (2000, pp. 28–43).

3. "Autonomy" comes from the Greek for "self rule." Some important recent sources of philosophic reflection on the idea include Faden and Beauchamp (1986), Raz (1986), and Dworkin (1988). I am working in this section with the notion of "personal autonomy" in Joseph Raz's (1986) sense, rather than (Kantian) "moral autonomy." My primary concern is with the value of personal autonomy, understood in a largely Razian way.

4. One agent can tempt another to a violation of harmony or friendship, however. The basic goods approach marks this difference between goods discussed in the text with the terms "substantive" and "reflexive"; reflexive goods require a choice as in part constitutive of their existence. See Grisez, Boyle, and Finnis (1987, p. 107).

5. My argument here owes much to that of George (1993, Chapter 7).

## NOTES TO CHAPTER 3

1. Not all accept the autonomy framework, however. See, for criticism, O'Neill (2003).

2. Not all; it is important that the options offered to patients for their consent be fair and involve no other wrongdoing.

3. See, for voices critical of the requirement of consent to sociological research, and a discussion of the role internal review boards (IRBs) should play in vetting such research, Shea (2000).

4. Miranda rights must be read to a suspect before he or she may be interrogated. These rights include the right to remain silent and refuse to answer questions, the right to an attorney, and the warning that anything said by the suspect may be used in a court of law. After each right is read the suspect must be asked, "Do you understand?" See Stuart (2004).

5. As Deni Elliott, director of the Ethics Institute at Dartmouth College, says, "The need for reporters to be honest, straightforward and clear extends even to the sleaziest of sources. What if it were known that reporters would deceive only the bad guys? If reporters always seem friendly, still sources would never know if reporters were being honest with *them*" (Elliott, 1991, p. 3).

6. The Society of Professional Journalists' "Code of Ethics" states that journalists should "avoid undercover or other surreptitious methods of gathering information except when traditional open methods will not yield information vital to the public" (SPJ, 1996). This is, however, an extremely broad exception, ruling out hardly anything.

7. Or the vice president's. See Safire (2000).

## NOTES TO CHAPTER 4

1. The view articulated here resembles that in Veatch (1987).
2. See the "Declaration of Helsinki," Part II: "In any medical study, every patient—including those in a control group, if any—should be assured of the best proven diagnostic and therapeutic method."
3. The American Sociological Association's updated "Code of Ethics" states that "informed consent is a basic ethical tenet of scientific research on human populations" (ASA, 2005, p. 12). The Code requires informed consent in a wide variety of circumstances, but still allows waivers to be obtained when there is only minimal risk to subjects and the research could not otherwise be carried out. Similarly, deception is now said to be typically wrong, although there are, again, a number of circumstances specified in which deception is still permissible. My arguments in this chapter are intended to question the claim that deceptive research is *ever* permissible.
4. Benjamin Constant's essay, which provoked Kant's famous response, made this point: "To tell the truth is thus a duty: but it is a duty only in respect to one who has a right to the truth. But no one has a right to a truth which injures others." Quoted by Kant in "On the Supposed Right to Lie from Altruistic Motives," in S. Bok (1989, p. 268).
5. Finnis's summary of Aquinas's position helpfully points in both directions—towards the agent's integrity, and towards the interpersonal communicative context in which integrity is ruptured: "It is a moral direction of reason, an implication of the good of reason itself [*bonum rationis*] as that good involves (we may say) the person's integrity or authenticity—harmony of inner with outer aspects of the person—precisely as that integrity or authenticity bears on and indeed makes possible interpersonal communication" (Finnis, 1998, p. 161).
6. "The Baltimore Affair" designates an incident in which Nobel Prize–winning David Baltimore published a paper, with several co-authors, subsequently suspected of containing fraudulent data. See the discussion in Resnick (1998, pp. 6–8); After accusations of plagiarism, Stephen Ambrose and Doris Kearns Goodwin both acknowledged errors in their citations in published work; Michael Bellisiles resigned from his position as Professor of History at Emory University after allegations that he had falsified evidence from probate records on the rate of gun ownership in early America.
7. In 1992, for example, ABC reporters for *Prime Time Live* concealed their identities to obtain jobs at Food Lion, a grocery chain, in order to expose Food Lion's unhygienic meat-packaging practices. Investigative journalism owes its existence to the work of Nellie Bly, who in the nineteenth century simulated indigence and mental illness to achieve entry into an asylum.
8. For example, the famous Joseph D. Pistone, who posed as Donnie Brasco in the mob: Pistone (1997). More recently, see William Queen, who went undercover with the California motorcycle gang the Mongols. He tells his story in Queen (2005).

## NOTES TO CHAPTER 5

1. Parts of the following chapter are derived from Tollefsen (2006b). The argument of this chapter is greatly expanded, and many objections addressed, in George and Tollefsen (2008).

2. Locke writes that a person "is a thinking, intelligent being, that has reason and reflection, and can consider itself as itself, the same thing, in different times and places" (Locke, 1975, II: xxvii, §9).
3. An early paradigm of this view: Tooley (1972).
4. For example, Moore and Persaud (1998): "Human development begins at fertilization, the process during which a male gamete or sperm . . . unites with a female gamete or oocyte . . . to form a single cell called a zygote. This highly specialized, totipotent cell marks the beginning of each of us as a unique individual" (p. 18). Similar views are held by Carlson (1999), Larsen (1997), and O'Rahilly and Muller (1994).
5. Not that either thinks that heaps are genuine entities. It should also be noted that Van Inwagen and Merricks disagree about the extension of the term "real entity," Merricks ultimately reserving it only to beings that are free self-movers, Van Inwagen more permissively holding that all organisms are composite but genuine entities. Finally, it should be pointed out that both think that simples are genuine entities. Such differences are not essential to the arguments of this section.
6. Some Catholics disagree, however, with the claim that embryo adoption is morally permissible. See the essays pro and con in Brakman and Weaver (2008).
7. At least one twin, however, of a pair of identical twins, must come to exist later than the one-cell stage. This does not mean, as I have shown, that the one-celled embryo was not a distinct individual human being.

## NOTES TO CHAPTER 6

1. However, even field studies can be interventionist and experimental, and there are often effects on animal behavior that can be attributed to human observation; see Farnsworth and Rosovsky (2003).
2. "Integrity" is here used in a sense only analogous to that in the phrase "personal integrity." But animals are complex, albeit not as complex as human beings, and that complexity can be well or poorly integrated into a unity.
3. Wilson (2002) considers the claim that cruelty to animals is wrong for reasons similar to the reason it is wrong to destroy a work of art; his discussion focuses on the notion of uniqueness of the work of art, a respect in which works of art differ from animals (pp.18–20).
4. Wilson (2002) also draws attention to the normative importance of the fact that cruelty involves the infliction of pain "for trivial reasons" (p. 22).
5. This example, of William Carroll's, was related to me by Ed Munn.
6. According to the AMA, "virtually every advance in medical science in the 20th century, from antibiotics and vaccines to antidepressant drugs and organ transplants, has been achieved either directly or indirectly through the use of animals in laboratory experiments" (American Medical Association, 1996, p. 77).
7. F. Barbara Orlans writes that "[h]istorically, a real problem existed in U.S. junior and senior high schools in the 1960s to early 1980s. Youths from age eleven to seventeen sought to impress judges of science-fair competitions by attempting highly invasive experiments on live animals. Often the students conducted these experiments in their homes, and supervision was absent or cursory. Extreme animal suffering occurred. Typical were high school student projects of attempted mammalian surgery, blinding, injection of lethal substances, and starving animals to death" (Orlans, 2003, pp. 288–89).

## NOTES TO CHAPTER 7

1. Nevertheless, there is far from complete compliance with this norm. See Amnesty International (2005).
2. Shue (1978) distinguishes between "interrogational torture" and "terroristic torture." Here, I am concerned only with the former. A focus on torture as an interrogational tool also characterizes most of the philosophical essays in a recent collection of essays on torture (Levinson, 2004).
3. This much quoted description is to be found in the August 1, 2002, memorandum from Jay Bybee, Office of Legal Counsel of the Department of Justice, to Alberto Gonzales, Counsel to the President, on "Standards of Interrogation." See also Isikoff, Klaidman, and Hirsh (2005).
4. After work on this chapter was completed, I participated in a seminar held at the University of Notre Dame on torture. There, Germain Grisez argued that there could not be an absolute norm against torture, since the infliction of severe pain without damage would be torture but, under some circumstances, not impermissible. I think there is something stipulative to the definition of torture; my stipulative definition has as a consequence that there is an absolute norm. But Grisez and I agree, I believe, on the morality of inflicting pain.
5. The broad sense of integrity here is in contrast to the more narrow sense of person integrity used in Chapters 2 and 4, in the discussion of lying. In the narrow sense, as pointed out, one is entirely responsible for one's own integrity and for any damage to it.
6. Some of the contributors to the Levinson collection, such as Dershowitz and Elshtain, distinguish between "torture lite" and more significant life and health threatening forms of torture. The former include, according to Mark Bowden, "sleep deprivation, exposure to heat or cold, the use of drugs to cause confusion, rough treatment . . . forcing a prisoner to stand for days at a time, or sit in uncomfortable positions, and playing on his fears for himself and his family. Although excruciating for the victim, these tactics generally leave no permanent mark and do no lasting physical harm" (Mark Bowden, "The Dark Art of Interrogation," *Atlantic Monthly,* October 2003, quoted in Elshtain, 2004, p. 85).
7. The agent who "remains innocent, chooses, that is, the 'absolutist' side . . . not only fails to do the right thing . . . , he may also fail to measure up to the duties of his office" (Walzer, in Levinson, 2004, p. 62).
8. GNR stands for genetics, nanotechnology and robotics, of which artificial intelligence is a branch. Also common is NBIC, which stands for the convergence of nano-bio-info-and cogno-sciences, i.e., nanoscience and technology, biotechnology and medicine, information technology, and cognitive and neuroscience (see Roco and Bainbridge, 2000).
9. See also the various statements and documents available at www.transhumanism.org.
10. "The Defense Advanced Research Projects Administration is providing tens of millions of dollars to MIT, Duke, and other universities through their 'Brain Machine Interfaces Program' aimed at permitting soldiers to communicate with equipment, and each other, at the speed of thought. A lot of research is focused on creating new materials that can coexist with neurons indefinitely, and can be made into nanoscale electrodes" (Hughes, 2004, p. 40).

## NOTES TO CHAPTER 8

1. Material in this section is drawn in part from Tollefsen (2002).

2. According to Barnbaum and Byron (2000), "A recent study reported that 98 percent of new drug studies that received funding from the drug's manufacturer were positive, compared to only 79 percent of studies that received no industry support" (p. 309). But for some competing considerations, see Cherry (2006).

## NOTES TO CHAPTER 9

1. For example, from the National Science Foundation: "The National Science Foundation (NSF) is an independent federal agency created by Congress in 1950 'to promote the progress of science; to advance the national health, prosperity, and welfare; to secure the national defense . . . ' With an annual budget of about $5.91 billion, we are the funding source for approximately 20 percent of all federally supported basic research conducted by America's colleges and universities. In many fields such as mathematics, computer science and the social sciences, NSF is the major source of federal backing" (NSF, 2007).
2. We see here an overlap with the concerns of Charles Fink, expressed in Chapter 6, concerning the expenditure of money on animal research that could be used for more immediate humanitarian concerns.
3. Of course, in any given state with this, or any of the other policies mentioned, the citizens of the state might support the policy in question. Then there is no expressive gap of the sort I am here discussing.
4. Similar concerns are raised when states support such research. So the argument below applies to the various projects states such as California and New Jersey have pursued.
5. That is, from the Nazi state that persecuted Jews in the years prior to the attempted genocide. One should have no allegiance whatsoever to a state one knows to be murdering Jews or others by the millions.
6. The discussion of abortion in Gutman and Thompson (1996) is a case in point.

## NOTES TO CHAPTER 10

1. Two kinds of inquiry I do not address in this chapter: military and police investigation, as it has already been discussed in earlier chapters, and inquiry in the social sciences, an adequate approach to which would incorporate elements of both the discussion of science and the discussion of the humanities.
2. For an early discussion of the role of the press in political coordination, see de Tocqueville (1988, pp. 517–20).
3. The role I describe here is similar to that ascribed to the press by defenders of "public journalism." My version is more similar to the "republican" than the "procedural" version of public journalism, however. See Glasser (1999).

## NOTES TO CHAPTER 11

1. Material in this and the following two sections is drawn from Tollefsen (2006a).
2. MacIntyre typically uses "enquiry." In this chapter and the next, I have changed quotations from MacIntyre from this to "inquiry" in order to maintain continuity with the rest of the work.

## NOTES TO CHAPTER 12

1. It is for this reason, I believe, that MacIntyre considers trust to be important in inquiry: "Any adequate answer [to the question about the moral requirements of inquiry] will have to specify both what the functions are of truthfulness, trust, and truth in the work of cooperative enquiry itself and what the relevance of the conception of truthfulness, trust, and truth required by such enquiry is to the moral life in general" (MacIntyre, 1995, p. 361).
2. Aquinas indicates this connection between truth and justice: " . . . truth is a part of justice, i.e., allied to it as a secondary to a principle virtue" (1981, II-II, Q. 109, a. 3. Reply).
3. From the *Republic,* on why the philosopher must return to the cave (520a-d).
4. My thinking on this matter has been aided by work with Ryan Walsh, Princeton '06.

# Bibliography

Allen, A. L. "Why Journalists Can't Protect Privacy." In *Journalism and the Debate over Privacy*, edited by C. LaMay, 69–88. Mahwah, NJ: Lawrence Erlbaum Associates, 2003.

Allen, C. "Spies Like Us: When Sociologists Deceive Their Subjects," *Lingua Franca* 7 (1997): 30–39.

American Medical Association (AMA). "Use of Animals in Biomedical Research: The Challenge and Response." In *Animal Rights: Opposing Viewpoints*, edited by A. Harnack. San Diego: Greenhaven Press, 1996.

American Psychological Association (APA). "Ethical Principles of Psychologists and Code of Conduct." 2002 http://www.apa.org/ethics/code2002.html

American Sociological Association (ASA). "Code of Ethics." 1999. http://www.asanet.org/members/ecoderev.html.

Amnesty International. "2005 UN Commission on Human Rights: The UN's Chief Guardian of Human Rights?" Executive Summary, 2005. http://www.web.amnesty.org/library/index/engior410012004.

Angell, M. "The Ethics of Clinical Research in the Third World." *The New England Journal of Medicine* 337 (1997): 847–49.

Angell, M. "Investigator's Responsibilities for Human Subjects in Developing Countries." *The New England Journal of Medicine* 342 (2000): 967–68.

Aquinas, St. Thomas. *The Summa Theologica of St. Thomas Aquinas*, 5 vols. Translated by the English Dominican Fathers. Westminster: Christian Classics, 1981.

Aristotle. *The Complete Works of Aristotle*, 2 vols. Edited by J. Barnes. Princeton, NJ: Princeton University Press, 1984.

Baker, L. R. *Persons and Bodies: A Constitution View*. Cambridge: Cambridge University Press, 2000.

Barber, B. *Consumed: How Markets Corrupt Children, Infantalize Adults, and Swallow Citizens Whole*. New York: Norton, 2007.

Baumrind, D. "Research Using Intentional Deception: Ethical Issues Revisited." *American Psychologist* 40 (1985): 165–74

Bezanson, R. P. "The Structural Attributes of Press Freedom: Private Ownership, Public Orientation, and Editorial Independence." In *Journalism and the Debate over Privacy*, edited by C. LaMay, 17–59. Mahwah, NJ: Lawrence Erlbaum Associates, 2003.

Boethius, A. M. S. "Contra Euthychen et Nestorium." In *Tractates and the Consolation of Philosophy*, translated by H. F. Stewart, E. K. Rand, and S. J. Testor. Cambridge, MA: Harvard University Press, 1918.

Bok, D. *Beyond the Ivory Tower: Social Responsibilities of the Modern University*. Cambridge, MA: Harvard University Press, 1982.

Bok, D. *Universities in the Marketplace: The Commercialization of Higher Education*. Princeton, NJ: Princeton University Press, 2004.

Bok, S. *Lying: Moral Choices in Public and Private Life.* New York: Vintage Books, 1989.

Boonin, D. *A Defense of Abortion.* Cambridge: Cambridge University Press, 2003.

Boyle, J. "Sanctity of Life and Suicide: Tensions and Developments Within Common Morality." In *Suicide and Euthanasia: Historical and Contemporary Themes,* edited by B. Brody, 111–50. Dordrecht, Netherlands: Kluwer, 1989.

Boyle, J. "The Absolute Prohibition of Lying and the Origins of the Casuistry of Mental Reservation: Augustinian Arguments and Thomistic Developments." *American Journal of Jurisprudence* 44 (1999): 43–65.

Boyle, J. "Limiting Access to Health Care: A Traditional Roman Catholic Analysis." In *Allocating Scarce Medical Resources: Roman Catholic Perspectives,* edited by H. T. Engelhardt and M. J. Cherry, 77–95. Washington, DC: Georgetown University Press, 2002.

Braine, D. *The Human Person.* Notre Dame: University of Notre Dame Press, 1992.

Brakman, S., and D. Weaver, eds. *Embryo Adoption and the Catholic Moral Tradition.* Dordrecht, Netherlands: Springer, 2008.

Brugger, E. C. "Aquinas and Capital Punishment: The Plausibility of the Traditional Argument." *Notre Dame Journal of Law, Ethics and Public Policy* 18 (2004): 257–372.

Bybee, J. "Memorandum from the Office of Legal Counsel of Department of Justice, to Alberto Gonzales, Counsel to the President, on 'Standards of Interrogation.'" August 1, 2002. http://www.washingtonpost.com/wp-srv/nation/documents/jojinterrogationmemo20020801.pdf.

Caplan, A. "Stem Cell Therapy Raises Ethical Issues: Should Human Embryos Be Used for Research Therapy?" November 5, 1998, MSNBC. http:// www.msnbc.com/news/212154.asp?cp1=1.

Carlson, B. *Human Embryology and Developmental Biology.* St. Louis, MO: Mosby, 1999.

Cassell, J., and A. Young. "Why We Should Not Seek Informed Consent for Participation in Health Services Research." *Journal of Medical Ethics* 28 (2002): 313–17.

*Catechism of the Catholic Church.* 2nd ed. New York: Doubleday, 2003.

Cajal, R. Y. *Advice to a Young Investigator.* Cambridge, MA: MIT Press, 1999.

Chappell, T. D. J. *Understanding Human Goods.* Edinburgh: Edinburgh University Press, 1997.

Chappell, T. D. J. "The Polymorphy of Practical Reason." In *Human Values: New Essays on Ethics and Natural Law,* edited by T. Chappell and D. S. Oderberg, 102–26. New York: Palgrave Macmillan, 2004.

Cherry, M. J. "Financial Conflicts of Interest and the Human Passion to Innovate." In *Research Ethics,* edited by A. S. Iltis, 147–64. New York: Routledge, 2006.

Christakis, N. A. "The Ethical Design of an AIDS Vaccine Trial in Africa." *Hastings Center Report* 18 (1988): 31–37.

Clark, E. *The Want Makers: The World of Advertising: How They Make You Buy.* New York: Viking, 1989.

Clarke, S. (1999) "Justifying Deception in Social Science Research." *Journal of Applied Philosophy* 16 (1999): 151–66.

Clifford, W. K. "The Ethics of Belief." 1879. http://www.ajburger.homestead.com/files/book.htm.

Coetzee, J. M. *The Lives of Animals.* Princeton, NJ: Princeton University Press, 2001.

Cornwell, J. *Hitler's Scientists: Science, War, and the Devil's Pact.* New York: Penguin Books, 2004.

Cuomo, M. "Religious Belief and Public Morality: A Catholic Governor's Perspective." *Notre Dame Journal of Law, Ethics and Public Policy* 1 (1984): 13–31.

Dellapenna, J. W. *Dispelling the Myths of Abortion*. Durham, NC: Carolina Academic Press, 2006.

Dershowitz, A. M. *Why Terrorism Works: Understanding the Threat, Responding to the Challenge*. New Haven, CT: Yale University Press, 2002.

Dershowitz, A. M. "Tortured Reasoning." In *Torture*, edited by S. Levinson, 266–67. Oxford: Oxford University Press, 2004.

De Tocqueville, A. *Democracy in America*. Translated by G. Lawrence. New York: Harper & Row, 1988.

Dewey, J. *Reconstruction in Philosophy*. Boston: Beacon Press, 1957.

Donagan, A. *The Theory of Morality*. Chicago: University of Chicago Press, 1977a.

Donagan, A. "Informed Consent in Therapy and Experimentation." *Journal of Medicine and Philosophy* 2 (1977b): 307–29.

Douglas, H. D. "The Moral Responsibilities of Scientists (Tensions Between Autonomy and Responsibility)." *American Philosophical Quarterly* 40 (2003): 59–68.

Elliott, C. *Better Than Well: American Medicine Meets the American Dream*. New York: W. W. Norton, 2003.

Elliott, D. "Thou Shalt Not Trick Thy Source." *FineLine: The Newsletter on Journalism* 3 (1991): 2–3.

Ellis, C. *Fisher Folk*. Louisville: University of Kentucky Press, 1986.

Elshtain, J. B. "Reflection on the Problem of 'Dirty Hands.'" In *Torture*, edited by S. Levinson, 77–89. Oxford: Oxford University Press, 2004.

Engelhardt, H. D. *The Foundations of Bioethics*. 2nd ed. New York: Oxford University Press, 1996.

Etzioni, A. *The Limits of Privacy*. New York: Basic Books, 2000.

Farnsworth, E. J., and J. Rosovsky. "The Ethics of Ecological Field Experimentation." In *The Animal Ethics Reader*, edited by S. J. Armstrong and R. G. Botzler. New York: Routledge, 2003.

Feldman, N. "Ugly Americans." *New Republic* 32 (2005, May 30): 23.

Fink, C. "Animal Experimentation and the Argument from Limited Resources." In *Research Ethics: Text and Readings*, edited by D. R. Barnbaum and M. Byron. Upper Saddle River, NJ: Prentice Hall, 2000.

Finnis, J. *Natural Law and Natural Rights*. Oxford: Clarendon Press, 1980.

Finnis, J. *Fundamentals of Ethics*. Washington, DC: Georgetown University Press, 1984.

Finnis, J. *Moral Absolutes: Tradition, Revision, and Truth*. Washington, DC: Catholic University of America Press, 1991.

Finnis, J. *Aquinas: Moral, Political, and Legal Theory*. Oxford: Oxford University Press, 1998.

Finnis, J., J. Boyle, and G. Grisez. *Nuclear Deterrence, Morality and Realism*. Oxford: Oxford University Press, 1987.

Ford, N. *When Did I Begin? Conception of the Human Individual in History, Philosophy and Science*. Cambridge: Cambridge University Press, 1988.

Frankfurt, H. "The Faintest Passion." *Proceedings and Addresses of the American Philosophical Association* 66 (1992): 5–16.

Frankfurt, H. *On Bullshit*. Princeton, NJ: Princeton University Press, 2004.

French, H. "AIDS Research in Africa: Juggling Risks and Hopes." *New York Times*, October 9, 1997, p. A1.

Fukuyama, F. *Our Posthuman Future: Consequences of the Biotechnology Revolution*. New York: Farrar, Straus and Giroux, 2002.

George, R. P. *Making Men Moral*. Oxford: Oxford University Press, 1993.

George, R. P. *In Defense of Natural Law*. Oxford: Oxford University Press, 1999.

George, R. P. *The Clash of Orthodoxies*. Wilmington, DE: ISI Books, 2001.

George, R. P., and C. Tollefsen. *Embryo: A Defense of Human Life*. New York: Doubleday, 2008.

Gertner, J. "Proceed with Caution." *New York Times Magazine,* June 6, 2004, p. 36.

Glasser, T. L. "The Idea of Public Journalism." In *The Idea of Public Journalism,* edited by T. L. Glaser, 3–18. New York: Guilford Press, 1999.

Glendon, M. A. "Transcript of the President's Council on Bioethics." April 25, 2002. http://www.bioethics.gov/transcripts/apr02/apr25session3.html.

Gomez-Lobo, A. *Morality and the Human Goods: An Introduction to Natural Law Ethics.* Washington, DC: Georgetown University Press, 2002.

Green, R. *The Human Embryo Research Debate.* Oxford: Oxford University Press, 2001.

Grisez, G. "The First Principle of Practical Reason: A Commentary on the *Summa Theologiae,* 1–2 Question 94, Article 2." *Natural Law Forum* 10, 1965: 168–201.

Grisez, G. "Against Consequentialism." *American Journal of Jurisprudence* 23 (1970): 21–72.

Grisez, G. *The Way of the Lord Jesus Christ: Living a Christian Life.* Vol. 2. Quincy, IL: Franciscan Press, 1993.

Grisez, G. *The Way of the Lord Jesus Christ: Difficult Moral Questions.* Vol. 3. Quincy, IL: Franciscan Press, 1997.

Grisez, G. "Natural Law, God, Religion, and Human Fulfillment." *American Journal of Jurisprudence* 46 (2001): 3–36.

Grisez, G., J. Boyle, and J. Finnis. "Practical Principles, Moral Truth, and Ultimate Ends." *American Journal of Jurisprudence* 32 (1987): 99–151.

Gutmann, A., and D. Thompson. *Democracy and Disagreement.* Cambridge, MA: Harvard University Press, 1996.

Haack, S. "Confessions of an Old-Fashioned Prig." In *Manifesto of a Passionate Moderate: Unfashionable Essays,* edited by S. Haack, 7–30. Chicago: University of Chicago Press, 1998.

Habermas, J. *Structural Transformation.* Translated by T. Burger. Cambridge, MA: Harvard University Press, 1989.

Hellman, S., and D. S. Hellman. "Of Mice But Not Men: Problems of the Randomized Clinical Trial." *New England Journal of Medicine* 324 (1991): 1585–89.

Howsepian, A. A. "Who, or What Are We?" *The Review of Metaphysics* 45 (1992): 483–502.

Hughes, J. *Citizen Cyborg: Why Democratic Societies Must Respond to the Redesigned Human of the Future.* Cambridge, MA: Westview, 2004.

Hynes, W. J., and W. G. Doty, eds. *Mythical Trickster Figures: Contours, Contexts and Criticisms.* Tuscaloosa: University of Alabama Press, 1997.

Isikoff, M., D. Klaidman, and M. Hirsh. "Torture's Path." *Newsweek* 145 (2005): 54–55.

Jaki, S. L. *Road of Science and the Ways to God.* Edinburgh: Scottish Academic Press, 1980.

James, W. "The Will to Believe." In *Essays on Pragmatism,* edited by A. Castelli, 88–109. New York: Harner, 1951.

Johnson, M. "Delayed Hominization: Reflections on Some Recent Catholic Claims for Delayed Hominization." *Theological Studies* 56 (1995): 743–63.

Jones, H. J. *Bad Blood: The Tuskegee Syphilis Experiment.* New York: The Free Press, 1993.

Joy, B. "Why the Future Doesn't Need Us." *Wired.* http://www.mindfully.org/Technology/Future-Doesnt-Need-Us1apr00.htm.

Kagan, S. *The Limits of Morality.* Oxford: Clarendon Press, 1989.

Kant, I. *Lectures on Ethics.* Translated by P. Heath and J. B. Schneewind. Cambridge: Cambridge University Press, 1997.

Kitcher, P. *Science, Truth, and Democracy.* Oxford: Oxford University Press, 2001.

Knight, D. "Outsourcing a Real Nasty Job." *U.S. News and World Report,* May 23, 2005. http://www.usnews.com/usnews/news/articles/050523/23rend.htm.

Krakauer, J. *Into Thin Air: A Personal Account of the Mt. Everest Disaster.* New York: Anchor, 1999.

Kraut, R. *Aristotle on the Human Good.* Princeton, NJ: Princeton University Press, 1989.

Krauthammer, C. "Why Pro-Lifers Are Missing the Point: The Debate over Fetal-Tissue Research Overlooks the Big Issue." *Time,* February 12, 2001, p. 60.

Kurzweil, R. *The Age of Spiritual Machines: When Computers Exceed Human Intelligence.* New York: Viking, 1999.

Kurzweil, R. *The Singularity Is Near.* New York: Viking, 2005.

LaMay, C., ed. *Journalism and the Debate over Privacy.* Mahwah, NJ: Lawrence Erlbaum Associates, 2003.

Larsen, W. *Human Embryology.* New York: Churchill Livingstone, 1997.

Lee, P. "A Christian Philosopher's View of the Abortion Debate." *Christian Bioethics* 10 (2001a): 7–31.

Lee, P. "Germain Grisez's Christian Humanism." *American Journal of Jurisprudence* 46 (2001b): 137–52.

Levinson, S., ed. *Torture.* Oxford: Oxford University Press, 2004.

Levy, N. "In Defense of Entrapment in Journalism (and Beyond)." *Journal of Applied Philosophy* 19 (2002): 121–30

Lewis, A. "The Right to Be Let Alone." In *Journalism and the Debate over Privacy,* edited by C. LaMay, 61–68. Mahwah, NJ: Lawrence Erlbaum Associates, 2003.

Lewis, C. S. *The Abolition of Man,* London: Geofrey Bless, 1962.

Lewis, C. S. "Vivisection." In *On Moral Medicine,* 2nd ed., edited by S. E. Lammers and A. Verhey. Grand Rapids, MI: Eerdmans, 1998.

"Lift Off for Enterprise." *The Economist.com,* June 21, 2004. Online. http://www.economist.com/agenda/displayStory.cfm?story_id=2765230.

Lithwick, D., and J. Turner. "A Guide to the Patriot Act, Part 1." *Slate,* September 8, 2003. Online. http://www.slate.msn.com/id/2087984.

Locke, J. *Essay Concerning Human Understanding.* Edited by P. Nidditch. Oxford: Clarendon Press, 1975.

Lynch, M. T. *True to Life: Why Truth Matters.* Cambridge, MA: MIT Press, 2004.

May, W. F. *The Physician's Covenant: Images of the Healer in Medical Ethics.* Louisville, KY: Westminster John Knox Press, 2000.

MacIntyre, A. *After Virtue.* 2nd ed. Notre Dame: University of Notre Dame Press, 1984.

MacIntyre, A. *Whose Justice, Which Rationality.* Notre Dame: University of Notre Dame Press, 1988.

MacIntyre, A. "Truthfulness, Lies, and Moral Philosophers." In *The Tanner Lectures on Human Values,* Vol. 16, edited by G. B. Peterson, 307–61. Salt Lake City: University of Utah Press, 1995.

MacIntyre, A. "Plain Persons, and Moral Philosophy: Rules, Virtues and Goods." In *The MacIntyre Reader,* edited by K. Knight, 136–52. Notre Dame: University of Notre Dame Press, 1998.

MacIntyre, A. *Dependent Rational Animals.* Chicago: Open Court Press, 1999.

Maynard-Moody, S. *The Dilemma of the Fetus: Fetal Research, Medical Progress and Moral Politics.* New York: St. Martin's Press, 1995.

McDowell, J. *Mind and World.* Cambridge, MA: Harvard University Press, 1994.

McFall, L. "Integrity." *Ethics* 98 (1987): 5–20.

Merricks, T. *Objects and Persons.* Oxford: Oxford University Press, 2003.

Merritt, D. "Public Journalism: What It Means, How It Looks." In *Public Journalism: Theory and Practice,* edited by J. Rosen and D. Merritt, 19–28. New York: Kettering Foundation, 1994.

Merton, R. K. "The Normative Structure of Science." In *The Sociology of Science: Theoretical and Empirical Investigations*, edited by R. K. Merton, 67–86. Chicago: University of Chicago Press, 1973a.

Merton, R. K. *The Sociology of Science: Theoretical and Empirical Investigations*. Chicago: University of Chicago Press, 1973b.

*Michael A. Newdow v. US Congress et al*. June 26, 2002. Online. http://news.findlaw.com/hdocs/docs/conlaw/newdowus62602opn.pdf.

Milgram, S. *Obedience to Authority*. New York: Harper & Row, 1974.

Miller, F., and H. Brody. "A Critique of Clinical Equipoise: Therapeutic Misconception in the Ethics of Clinical Trials." *Hastings Center Report* 33 (2003): 19–28.

Moodley, K. "HIV Vaccine Trial Participation in South Africa—An Ethical Assessment." *Journal of Medicine and Philosophy* 27 (2002): 197–215.

Moore, K., and T. V. N. Persaud. *The Developing Human: Clinically Oriented Embryology*. 6th ed. Philadelphia: W. B. Saunders, 1998.

Murphy, M. *Natural Law and Practical Rationality*. Cambridge: Cambridge University Press, 2001.

Newman, J. H. *The Idea of a University*. New York: Holt, Rhinehart and Winston, 1966.

Newman, J. H. *Apologia Pro Vita Sua*. New York: W. W. Norton, 1968.

Nozick, R. *Anarchy, State, and Utopia*. Oxford: Basil Blackwell, 1968.

Oderberg, D. *Moral Theory: A Nonconsequentialist Approach*. Oxford: Blackwell Press, 2000.

Olson, E. *The Human Animal*. Oxford: Oxford University Press, 1997a.

Olson, E. "Was I Ever a Fetus?" *Philosophy and Phenomenological Research* 57 (1997b): 95–110.

O'Neill, O. "Some Limits of Informed Consent." *Journal of Medical Ethics* 29 (2003): 4–7.

O'Rahilly, R., and F. Muller. *Human Embryology and Teratology*. New York: Wiley-Liss, 1994.

Orlans, F. B. "Ethical Themes of National Regulations Governing Animal Experiments: An International Perspective." In *The Animal Ethics Reader*, edited by S. J. Armstrong and R. G. Botzler, 285–91. New York: Routledge, 2003.

Peirce, C. S. "The Scientific Attitude and Fallibilism." In *Philosophical Writings of Peirce*, edited by J. Buchler, 42–59. New York: Dover, 1955.

Peirce, C. S. "The Fixation of Belief." In *Essays in the Philosophy of Science*, edited by V. Tomas. New York: The Liberal Arts Press, 1957a.

Peirce, C. S. "How to Make Our Ideas Clear." In *Essays in the Philosophy of Science*, edited by V. Tomas. New York: The Liberal Arts Press, 1957b.

Peirce, C. S. "Lessons from the History of Science." In *Essays in the Philosophy of Science*, edited by V. Tomas. New York: The Liberal Arts Press, 1957c.

Pelikan, J. *The Idea of the University; A Reexamination*. New Haven, CT: Yale University Press, 1992.

Pellegrino, E., and D. C. Thomasma. *For the Patient's Own Good: The Restoration of Beneficence in Health Care*. New York: Oxford University Press, 1988.

Pieper, J. *Leisure: The Basis of Culture*. South Bend, IN: St. Augustine's Press, 1998.

Piliavin, J. A., and I. M. Piliavin. "Effect of Blood on Reactions to a Victim." *Journal of Personality and Social Psychology* 23 (1972): 353–61.

Pistone, J. *Donnie D. Brasco: My Undercover Life in the Mafia*. New York: Signet, 1997.

Plato. *Republic*. Translated by C. D. C. Reeve. Indianapolis: Hackett, 2001.

Pope John Paul II. "Message to the Pontifical Academy of Sciences." October 22, 1996. Online. http://www.cin.org/users/james/files/message/htm.

The President's Council on Bioethics (PCB). *Human Cloning and Human Dignity: An Ethical Inquiry.* July 2002. Online. http://www.bioethics.gov/reports/cloningreport/index.html.

The President's Council on Bioethics (PCB). *Beyond Therapy: Biotechnology and the Pursuit of Happiness.* Washington, DC: PCB, 2003.

Queen, W. *Under and Alone: The True Story of the Undercover Agent Who Infiltrated America's Most Violent Outlaw Motorcycle Gang.* New York: Random House, 2005.

Ramez, N. *More Than Human: How Biotechnology Is Transforming Us and Why We Should Embrace It.* New York: Random House, 2004.

Rawls, J. *A Theory of Justice.* Cambridge, MA: Belknap Press, 1971.

Rawls, J. *Political Liberalism.* New York: Columbia University Press, 1996.

Rawls, J. "The Idea of Public Reason Revisited." In *The Law of Peoples,* edited by J. Rawls. Cambridge, MA: Harvard University Press, 1999.

Raz, J. *The Morality of Freedom.* Oxford: Clarendon Press, 1986.

Regan, T. "The Case for Animal Rights." In *What's Wrong? Applied Ethicists and Their Critics,* edited by D. Boonin and G. Oddie. New York: Oxford University Press, 2005.

Reichberg, G. "*Studiositas:* The Virtue of Attention." In *The Common Things: Essays on Thomism and Education,* edited by D. McInerny, 143–52. Washington, DC: The Catholic University of America Press, 1999.

Resnick, D. *The Ethics of Science.* New York: Routledge, 1998.

Resnick, D. "Biomedical Research in the Developing World: Ethical Issues and Dilemmas." In *Research Ethics,* edited by A. S. Iltis. New York; Routledge, 2006.

Richards, D. A. J. *Sex, Drugs, Death, and the Law.* Totowa, NJ: Rowman & Littlefield, 1982.

Richardson Lear, G. *Happy Lives and the Highest Good.* Princeton, NJ: Princeton University Press, 2004.

Roco, M. C., and W. S. Bainbridge, eds. *Converging Technologies for Improving Human Performance.* Washington, DC: National Science Foundation, 2002. Online at http://www.wtec.org/ConvergingTechnologies.

"Roe v. Wade" (January 22, 1973) Online. Available at http://www.caselaw.lp.findlaw.com/scripts/getcase.pl?court=US&vol=4108&invol=113.

Safire, W. "The Telltale Heart." *New York Times,* November 30, 2000, p. A35.

Sandel, M. "The Case Against Perfection: What's Wrong with Designer Children, Bionic Athletes, and Genetic Engineering." *The Atlantic Monthly,* 293 (April 2004): 50–60.

Sandel, M. *The Case Against Perfection: Ethics in the Age of Genetic Engineering.* Cambridge, MA: Belknap Press, 2007.

Sartre, J. P. *Existentialism and Human Emotions.* New York: Citadel Press, 1984.

Scheffler, S., ed. *Consequentialism and Its Critics.* Oxford: Oxford University Press, 1988.

Searle, J. R. "Politics and the Humanities." *Academic Questions* 12 (1999): 45–60.

Shea, C. "Don't Talk to the Humans." *Lingua Franca* 10 (2000): 26–34.

Shue, H. "Torture." *Philosophy and Public Affairs* 7 (1978): 124–43.

Sidgwick, H. *The Methods of Ethics.* 7th ed. London: Macmillan, 1907.

Silver, L. *Remaking Eden: Cloning and Beyond in a Brave New World.* New York: Avon Books, 1997.

Singer, P. *Practical Ethics* (extracted). In *The Animal Ethics Reader,* edited by S. J. Armstrong and R. G. Botzler. New York: Routledge, 2003.

Slade, F. "*Was Ist Aufklarung?* Notes on Maritain, Rorty, and Bloom with Thanks but No Apologies to Immanuel Kant." In *The Common Things: Essays on Thomism and Education,* edited by D. McInerny, 48–68. Washington, DC: The Catholic University of America Press, 1999.

Smith, B., and B. Brogaard. "Sixteen Days." *The Journal of Medicine and Philosophy* 28 (2003): 45–78.

Smolla, R. "Law Breaking and Truth Telling: Formal Legal Doctrine and the Imbalance Between Intrusion and Revelation Claims." In *Journalism and the Debate Over Privacy*, edited by C. LaMay, 89–106. Mahwah, NJ: Lawrence Erlbaum Associates, 2003.

Society of Professional Journalists (SPJ). "Code of Ethics." Online. 1996. http://www.spj.org/ethics_code.asp.

Solzhenitsyn, A. *The Gulag Archipelago*. Vol. II. New York: Harper & Row, 1974.

Soyfer, V., L. Gruliow, and R. Gruliow, R. *Lysenko and the Tragedy of Soviet Science*. New Brunswick, NJ: Rutgers University Press, 1994.

Sperber, M. *Beer and Circus: How Big-Time College Sports Is Crippling Undergraduate Education*. New York: Owl Books, 2001.

Stuart, G. L. *Miranda: The Story of America's Right to Remain Silent*. Phoenix: University of Arizona Press, 2004.

Taylor, C. "Liberal Politics and the Public Sphere." In *Philosophical Arguments*, edited by C. Taylor. Cambridge, MA: Harvard University Press, 1995a.

Taylor, C. "Cross-Purposes: The Liberal Communitarian Debate." In *Philosophical Arguments*, edited by C. Taylor. Cambridge, MA: Harvard University Press, 1995b.

Thomas, C. "War Is No Time for Interrogation Etiquette." *The Star Ledger*, May 5, 2000, p. 19.

Thomson, J. J. "Abortion." *Boston Review*. Vol. 20. Online. 1995. http://www.bostonreview.mit.edu/BR20.3/thomson.html.

Thompson, M. "The Representation of Life." In *Virtues and Reasons: Philippa Foot and Moral Theory*, edited by R. Hursthouse, G. Lawrence, and W. Quinn, 247–97. Oxford: Clarendon Press, 1996.

Titus, S. L., and M. Keane. "Do You Understand? An Ethical Assessment of Researchers' Description of the Consenting Process." In *Research Ethics: Text and Readings*, edited by D. R. Barnbaum and M. Byron. Upper Saddle River, NJ: Rowman & Littlefield, 2000.

Tollefsen, C. "Sidgwickian Objectivity and Ordinary Morality." *Journal of Value Inquiry* 33 (1997): 57–70.

Tollefsen, C. "Journalism and the Social Good." *Public Affairs Quarterly* 14 (2000): 293–307.

Tollefsen, C. "Managed Care and the Practice of the Professions." In *The Ethics of Managed Care*, edited by W. B. Bondeson and J. W. Jones, 29–40. Dordrecht, Netherlands: Kluwer, 2002.

Tollefsen, C. "Experience Machines, Dreams, and What Matters." *Journal of Value Inquiry* 37 (2003a): 153–64.

Tollefsen, C. "Justified Belief." *American Journal of Jurisprudence* 48 (2003b): 281–96.

Tollefsen, C. "Institutional Integrity." In *Institutional Integrity*, edited by A. S. Iltis. Dordrecht, Netherlands: Kluwer, 2003c.

Tollefsen, C. "Basic Goods, Practical Insight, and External Reasons." In *Human Values: New Essays on Ethics and Natural Law*, edited by T. Chappell and D. Oderberg, 32–51. New York: Palgrave, 2004.

Tollefsen, C. "MacIntyre and the Moralization of Enquiry." *International Philosophical Quarterly* 46 (2006a): 421–38.

Tollefsen, C. "Persons in Time." *American Catholic Philosophical Quarterly* 80 (2006b): 107–23.

Tollefsen, O. "Practical Solipsism and 'Thin' Theories of Human Goods." *Proceedings of the American Catholic Philosophical Association* 61 (1987): 191–98.

Tooley, M. "Abortion and Infanticide." *Philosophy and Public Affairs* 2 (1972): 37–65.

Tutu, D. *No Future Without Forgiveness*. New York: Image, 2000.

van Inwagen, P. *Material Beings*. Ithaca, NY: Cornell University Press, 1990.

Veatch, R. *The Patient as Partner*. Indianapolis: University of Indiana Press, 1987.

Wager, E., P. J. H. Tooley, M. B. Emmanuel, and S. F. Wood. "Get Patients' Consent to Enter Clinical Trials." In *Research Ethics: Text and Readings*, edited by D. R. Barnbaum and M. Byron. Upper Saddle River, NJ: Rowman & Littlefield, 2000.

Walzer, M. "Political Action: The Problem of Dirty Hands." *Philosophy and Public Affairs* 2 (1973): 160–80. Reprinted, abridged, in Levinson, *Torture*, pp. 61–75.

Warner, M. *The Letters of the Republic*. Cambridge, MA: Harvard University Press, 1990.

Warren, S. D., and L. D. Brandeis. "The Right To Privacy [the Implicit Made Explicit]." In *Philosophical Dimensions of Privacy: An Anthology*, edited by F. Schoeman. Cambridge: Cambridge University Press, 1984.

Watson, J. *The Double Helix*. London: Weidenfeld and Nicolson, 1968.

Wiggins, D. *Sameness and Substance*. Oxford: Blackwell Press, 1980.

Wilkinson, T. M. "Individualism and the Ethics of Research on Humans." *HEC Forum* 16 (2004): 6–26.

Williams, B. A. O. "A Critique of Utilitarianism." In *Utilitarianism: For and Against*, edited by B. A. O. Williams and J. J. C. Smart. Cambridge: Cambridge University Press, 1973.

Williams, B. *Truth and Truthfulness: An Essay in Genealogy*. Princeton, NJ: Princeton University Press, 2002.

Wilson, S. "Indirect Duties to Animals." *The Journal of Value Inquiry* 36 (2002): 15–25.

Wolf, P., and S. Lurie. "Unethical Trials of Interventions to Reduce Perinatal Transmission of the Human Immunodeficiency Virus in Developing Countries." *The New England Journal of Medicine* 337 (1997): 853–56.

Zagzebski, L. T. *Virtues of the Mind*. Cambridge: Cambridge University Press, 1996.

# Index

The Political Economy of the Eurion

To Mary and Muireann

# The Political Economy of the European Union
## An Institutionalist Perspective

DERMOT MCCANN

polity

First published in 2010 by Polity Press

Polity Press
65 Bridge Street
Cambridge, CB2 1UR, UK

Polity Press
350 Main Street
Malden, MA 02148, USA

ISBN-13: 978-0-7456-3890-4
ISBN-13: 978-0-7456-3891-1(pb)

A catalogue record for this book is available from the British Library.

Typeset in 9.5 on 13 pt Swift Light
by Servis Filmsetting Ltd, Stockport, Cheshire
Printed and bound by MPG Books Group, UK

The publisher has used its best endeavours to ensure that the URLs for external websites referred to in this book are correct and active at the time of going to press. However, the publisher has no responsibility for the websites and can make no guarantee that a site will remain live or that the content is or will remain appropriate.

Every effort has been made to trace all copyright holders, but if any have been inadvertently overlooked the publisher will be pleased to include any necessary credits in any subsequent reprint or edition.

For further information on Polity, visit our website: www.politybooks.com

# Contents

# Acknowledgements

I would like to thank Maurice Glasman for many stimulating political conversations, all the more useful as they were rarely about the EU. I would also like to thank Pauline and Joe for their patience and perseverance. Muireann remained ever tolerant, if a touch perplexed as to why it took so long. She was not the only one. Mary was as supportive and helpful as ever.

# Tables and Boxes

# Abbreviations

| | |
|---|---|
| ALMP | active labour market policies |
| BDI | Federation of German Industries |
| BEPGs | Broad Economic Policy Guidelines |
| CAP | Common Agricultural Policy |
| CBI | Confederation of British Industry |
| CDOs | Collateralized Debt Obligations |
| CEEP | Centre Européen des Entreprises Publique |
| CEN | European Committee for Standards |
| CENELEC | European Electrical Standards Coordinating Committee |
| CFI | Court of First Instance |
| CME | coordinated market economies |
| DG EcFin | Economics and Finance Directorate General |
| ECB | European Central Bank |
| ECGN | European Corporate Governance Network |
| ECJ | European Court of Justice |
| ECMR | European Community Merger Regulation |
| Ecofin | Council of Finance and Economic Ministers |
| EDP | Excessive Deficit Procedure |
| EEC | European Economic Community |
| EES | European Employment Strategy |
| EGLs | European Employment Guidelines |
| EMCO | Employment Committee |
| EMF | European Metalworkers' Federation |
| EMS | European Monetary System |
| EMU | European and Monetary Union |
| ERM | Exchange Rate Mechanism |
| ESD | European Social Dialogue |
| ESM | European Social Model |
| ETUC | European Trade Union Confederation |
| EWC | European Works Council |
| FSAP | Financial Services Action Plan |
| FSU | Finnish Seamen's Union |
| IPO | initial public offerings |
| ISD | Investment Services Directive |
| ITF | International Transport Workers' Federation |

| | |
|---|---|
| LME | liberal market economies |
| MBR | Mandatory Bid Rule |
| MiFID | Markets in Financial Instruments Directive |
| MMC | Monopolies and Mergers Commission |
| MNCs | multinational corporations |
| NAIRU | non-accelerating inflation rate of unemployment |
| NAP | National Action Plan |
| NCAS | National Competition Authorities |
| NTBs | non-tariff barriers to trade |
| OFT | Office of Fair Trading |
| OMC | Open Method of Coordination |
| PECs | pacts for employment and competitiveness |
| QMV | Qualified Majority Voting |
| SEA | Single European Act |
| SGP | Stability and Growth Pact |
| SMEs | small and medium-sized enterprises |
| TEU | Treaty on European Union (Maastricht Treaty) |
| UEAPME | Association of Craft and Small and Medium-sized Enterprises |

# Introduction

The European Union (EU) embodies a remarkable experiment in inter-state cooperation. In the 50 odd years since its inception, it has evolved from a small community of six West European countries to encompass the great majority of European states, stretching from the Atlantic isles to the Russian border and from the Arctic Ocean to the Mediterranean Sea. At the same time, its policy remit has greatly expanded. Although it was founded as a customs union, by the early twenty-first century questions of immigration, asylum, anti-terrorism cooperation, foreign and defence policy had forced themselves to the centre stage of EU politics to an extent that would have been inconceivable in earlier decades. Though progress has been unsteady and the direction of development strongly contested, integration has persisted even as the international political and economic landscape that shaped its early development has been transformed by the end of the Cold War and the rise of new economic powers.

Unsurprisingly, the political dynamics of this remarkable process of integration have attracted considerable attention. The factors that have persuaded national states to accede to it, the nature and power of the Union's governing institutions and, of course, the ways in which policy is made have all been the subject of extensive analysis. Perhaps equally unsurprisingly, these literatures have generated profound disputes concerning the very nature of the process. Thus, for example, where some analysts perceive in integration the partial transcendence of the nation-state in the international arena, others argue that its progress further demonstrates the innovative capacity of such states to devise new institutional structures to satisfy national interests. Similarly, where some view EU institutions as powerful actors capable of shaping the direction of integration, others regard them as servants of the member states labouring faithfully to implement the deals that they have agreed among themselves. At issue are fundamental questions concerning the power and status of nation-states in the context of the most ambitious experiment in cooperative regional integration yet witnessed.

However, an understanding of the implications of European integration for member states requires more than simply an assessment of the degree to which they dominate its decision-making procedures. It is also necessary to consider the extent to which 50 years of European law and policy have served to change their internal institutional character. How transformative for states is membership of the EU? This question is no more pertinent than in relation to the economy. The core business of European integration has been economic integration. The commitment inscribed in the Treaty of Rome to realize the 'four freedoms' of movement in goods, services, capital and people has provided the political impetus and legal basis for a vast array of subsequent policy initiatives. Barriers to trade in goods and services have been stripped away. The free circulation of capital and people has been substantially realized. A new currency has been established, removing one of the most powerful instruments of economic management available to states. How has all of this activity affected the role and character of domestic political economic institutions in member states?

Recognition of the importance of this question has been sharpened by recent studies in comparative political economy, which have attested both to the often subtle institutional diversity of capitalism across states and to the economic and political significance of these differences. From financial to labour markets, from the role of the state to the collective representative organization of business and labour, national 'models' or 'varieties' of capitalism have evolved highly distinctive governing institutions. These institutions profoundly influence the productive strategies of firms and the distribution of power and resources among socioeconomic actors. Systems of corporate law and finance shape how corporations are owned and governed. Competition policies, labour market rules, social policy rights, etc. affect the terms upon which the factors of production can be acquired and 'mixed' in any given economy. Together, these institutions largely determine the capacity of actors, ranging from workers to capital investors, to protect and advance their interests. To the extent that the EU's pursuit of 'ever closer union' impinges substantially on these properties, the fundamental political economic character of member states may be significantly altered.

The case for characterizing the EU as an agent of national political economic transformation is predicated on a number of closely related arguments. Firstly, European integration is understood to embody a commitment not only to market liberalization but also to the institutionalization of a European system of liberal market governance. Without the creation of such a regulatory system, the benefits to be derived from opening up cross-border trade would, in practice, be undermined by the persistence of national legal and administrative bias. Genuine market liberalization requires the establishment of a liberal European governance system. Secondly, the establishment of such a governance system at the European level is seen to present a profound challenge to the sustainability of national institutional arrangements in a substantial number of member states. This reflects the fact that, in many such states, non-liberal institutional forms play a central role in economic governance. Liberal Europe looks to markets to coordinate economic activity and seeks to protect and enhance competition as the best means of achieving economic efficiency and development. The role of the public authorities is to uphold this system. For states such as Britain, this project tends to work with the grain of established national practice. In contrast, however, markets in 'non-liberal' or 'illiberal' economies are supplemented by a high level of non-market coordination between stakeholders, and a large amount of public intervention in private decision-making over finance, investment and consumption is common (Streeck, 2001: 4). Moreover, employment and welfare protection weigh more heavily as policy objectives than they do in liberal economies. Thus, in Germany, Austria and the Netherlands, it is frequently the case that creditor banks sit on the governing boards of debtor firms; that business associations play a central role in managing inter-corporate relations; and that employees enjoy substantial representation rights within the firm. In France, Italy and Spain, the state continues to exercise a powerful influence over corporate investment and restructuring decisions in key economic sectors, particularly when national corporate actors are threatened by foreign-owned ones. For these systems of 'organized' capitalism, European liberal market governance presents a potentially transformative threat (Höpner and Schäfer, 2007: 5–6).

Finally, it is contended that this conflict between the creation of a truly liberal European economy and the maintenance of illiberal national institutional structures is intensifying. In particular, it is suggested that economic integration is now entering a 'new, post-Ricardian phase in which it systematically clashes with national varieties of capitalism' (ibid.: 6). The Union and, above all, powerful elements within the European Commission are accused of seeking to enforce the dominance of liberal principles of economic governance through a convergence of national institutional structures. Recent European Court of Justice (ECJ) decisions on issues ranging from firm incorporation rules to collective bargaining rights have served to deepen this challenge. Integration 'asymmetrically targets the institutions of organised capitalism and, therefore, results in a "clash of capitalisms"' (ibid.). EU policy initiatives designed to institutionalize a liberal market in Europe pose an ever greater threat to the integrity of the political economic order in a substantial number of member states.

None of these contentions is unproblematic. The existence of the Common Agricultural Policy alone would suggest that the description of European integration as liberal economic in nature needs some qualification. More broadly, Europe has been characterized for much of its existence by quite a shallow form of economic integration that has impinged only to a limited extent on national regulatory arrangements. In addition, the supposed more recent triumph of liberal economic principles in the EU needs careful assessment. The presence of a substantial element of support for 'organized' or 'regulated' capitalism' within the EU has been widely noted (Hooghe and Marks, 1999). Treaty negotiations are frequently marked by a conflict of 'liberal' and 'regulated' visions of capitalism (Pollack, 1998). Recent initiatives pursued by the Commission on the welfare rights of part-time workers hardly conform with liberal economic prescriptions favouring labour market flexibility as a means to improve growth and employment performance in Europe (Wallace, 2004: 115–16). Moreover, the extent to which the building of a truly liberal Europe requires the reconfiguration of many deeply rooted national institutions, and the economic and political relations that they embody, is also open to dispute. More sanguine views suggest that national systems can effectively adapt to the changing European context while retaining the essential features of their national institutional arrangements (Schmidt, 2002b). Substantial change in economic conditions is not a new phenomenon, and national varieties of capitalism have frequently demonstrated a capacity to absorb these pressures while retaining their distinctiveness (Hall, 2007: 41). The irreconcilability of liberal Europe and non-liberal national institutional arrangements cannot be assumed.

Furthermore, even if such irreconcilability did obtain, there is reason to question the capacity of the EU to force through radical changes in national systems. By their nature, these systems are deeply embedded both politically and socially. National administrative and/or private actors may well be able to resist in full or in part the imposition of what they perceive to be undesirable changes. More broadly, national governments often baulk when the full implications of the commitments they have made become apparent. Since his election in 2007, the French President Nicolas Sarkozy has repeatedly and forcefully reasserted the right of the nation-state to intervene in the process of industrial change, notwithstanding EU rules. Though the rhetoric in other states may be less confrontational in tone, practice reflects a similar perspective. Thus, for example, an attempt by American interests to buy Italia Telecom in 2007 was repelled by a domestic coalition of industrial and financial actors orchestrated by the Italian state. A bid by a German firm to purchase the Spanish energy group Endesa in the same year was so delayed by Spanish government interference that it ultimately failed. The prevalence of defensive nationalism in Europe does not invalidate the 'clash of capitalisms' thesis. Indeed, it suggests that many member states perceive a genuine and substantial threat from EU policy to their established arrangements and practices. However, the nature of their response also indicates that they may yet retain both the will and the capacity to shape their own destinies and to resist wholesale incorporation into a new, more liberal, Europe.

This book will evaluate these sharply contrasting perceptions of the EU's economic project. Using the conceptual tools of comparative institutional political economy, it will examine the impact of EU policy on the political economic governance of member states. Is the effort to realize fully European market and monetary integration enforcing a fundamental transformation of their institutional governance? Are the EU's initiatives particularly challenging to non-liberal, organized political economies? Has the EU's liberal ambition taken a more aggressive form in recent years? In addressing these questions, the analytical focus will be on those domains of economic governance that comparative institutional political economy has identified as constitutive of national capitalisms: product, financial and labour markets. How does EU policy challenge national patterns of governance in these crucial areas? How effective has it been in implementing its policies and how successful have these policies been in achieving their objectives? Though there will be some consideration of those states that have recently joined, the overwhelming focus of attention will necessarily be on the pre-2004 member states, the so-called EU15. These are the countries that have been most fully and extensively exposed to the EU. These are the states whose well-entrenched institutions of capitalist governance often present the greatest obstacles to the realization of the EU's liberal ambitions. It is through the examination of the nature and extent of change in these countries, and most especially the extent of change evident in those most marked by non-liberal institutional practices, that the transformative power of the EU can be gauged most accurately.

## Organization of the Book

The examination of these issues is conducted in two broad stages. The first stage is concerned with conceptual clarification and historical contextualization. Chapter 1 will examine the conceptual underpinning of an institutionalist approach to the examination of the impact of the EU on national political economies. What are economic governance institutions and why do they matter? What do concepts of national 'varieties' or 'models' of capitalism mean? How do they differ across the member states of the EU and with what consequences? In what ways and through what mechanisms does the process of European economic integration challenge or threaten these institutions? Chapter 2 will then provide a broad historical survey of the breadth, depth and progression of integration. In terms of market building, what have been the principal objectives and instruments of EU policy? Is it correct to construe the central thrust of European market-building as a liberal economic enterprise? How has this project evolved over time? In particular, how precisely does the advent of the single market and single currency challenge the integrity of national institutions of economic governance in product, financial and labour markets?

The following five chapters will then examine the specific development of EU policy in relation to product, financial and labour market regulation and its implications for established national institutions. Can its policies be properly characterized as embodying a liberal, transformative project in respect of national political economies and their governance institutions? To what extent is the EU capable of achieving its objectives? Is there evidence of substantial change in the institutional character of domestic systems? Can the extent of change that is evident be justifiably described as transformational? Chapter 3 will examine the nature and impact of the EU's competition policy on the governance of product markets. Chapter 4 will examine EU initiatives relating to corporate law and financial market regulation and, specifically, the challenge that they present to established national systems of corporate ownership and governance. Chapter 5 will deepen the analysis through the examination of the impact of these initiatives on patterns of corporate owner-ship and control in Germany and Italy. Both countries possess institutional arrangements that differ substantially from the Anglo-American norms informing much of the EU's reform programme in the area of finance and cor-porate governance. An understanding of the extent and dynamic of change in these national systems will offer considerable insight into the transformative capacity of EU policies. Finally, chapters 6 and 7 will examine the evolution and impact of EU policy in relation to labour markets. Chapter 6 will focus on EU social policy and, especially, employment policy. Chapter 7 will then exam-ine the EU's developing industrial relations role and its impact on national systems. General conclusions will then be drawn in the final chapter.

1

# Economic Governance, National Models of Capitalism and the Challenge of European Integration

## Introduction

The examination of the European Union's role in reshaping economic governance in member states is essentially an exercise in institutional analysis. National political economies are composed of institutions that structure and regulate economic activity, delimiting how actors can behave and interact. The challenge presented by the EU stems from the impact of its policies on these institutional systems. In what ways and to what extent does it necessitate their reform? Before these questions can be properly examined, however, two key issues must be addressed. Firstly, the nature and significance of national institutional systems must be clarified. What constitutes an institution of economic governance? In what way do institutional systems structure the functioning of economies? How are we to distinguish liberal from non-liberal institutions? What does it mean to speak of national 'models' or 'varieties' of capitalism? Secondly, it is necessary to clarify how EU policy affects these institutional systems. What are the linking mechanisms between EU initiatives and national institutional reforms? An appreciation of the challenge presented by EU policy to national systems requires the analysis of the dynamic of 'Europeanization', the process whereby state practices are brought into conformity with EU legal and policy prescriptions, as much as it does the exploration of the policies themselves. How effective is the EU in enforcing change in member states?

## Social Embeddedness and Institutional Governance

The constitution and governance of market economies is a subject that has attracted considerable attention from comparative political economists in recent years. While conceptualizations of the issues and problems involved vary greatly, two core contentions are commonly shared. Firstly, it is argued that far from being universal in nature, capitalist economies are deeply enmeshed in the wider institutional structures of the society in which they operate. Economic activity is embedded within a specific social context and is mediated and shaped by the particular institutions that exist there (Coates, 2005, Jackson and Deeg, 2006: 11). Consequently, the functioning of economies inevitably differs significantly across social contexts. It is neither possible nor legitimate 'to observe a single institutionalized market' or to conclude that 'similar arrangements will have the same consequences' across cases (Zysman, 1994: 256). The functioning of a particular political economy will always be partly determined by social specificity. Secondly, it is contended that the principal social context within which capitalisms develop and operate is the nation-state. While institutions may occasionally be localized within sub-national regions or display some element of sectoral variation, comparative analysis has overwhelmingly identified the state as the key political and social framework within which they evolve and function. This is not because of any inherent affinity between institutional analysis and the nation-state; it simply reflects the historical reality that capitalism was mainly organized and regulated by the nation-state in the twentieth century (Crouch and Streeck, 1997: 2). Tellingly, where the governance of particular industry sectors has been examined, it was found that 'national differences produce different governance regimes within sectors . . . [while] differences in governance within sectors are often recognizable as national differences in that they follow a similar logic across sectors' (Hollingsworth et al., 1994: 272). It is predominantly national social contexts within which capitalism is socially embedded and, therefore, contrasting systems are characterized as 'national models', or 'varieties', of capitalism.

The conception of institutions that underpins this perspective is broad, stretching from formal legal rules through less tangible systems of informal rules or social norms to organizations understood as 'durable entities with formally recognised members' (Hall and Soskice, 2001a: 9). Formal rules encompass the full panoply of legal regulation of economic activity, covering issues ranging from contract law, through the legal definition of the structure, rights and duties of the firm to competition policy, financial market regulation, etc. Informal rules or social norms include conceptions of 'fairness', 'legitimacy', 'social obligation', etc. that may impinge on and structure economic activity. The marked variation in corporate executive pay levels evident across the US, Britain, Germany and Japan, for example, is at least partly the product of differences in prevailing conceptions of 'fairness' and 'acceptability'. Informal rules may also constitute 'common knowledge' that informs how actors choose to interact with each other even though feasible alternative options exist (ibid.: 13). Finally, organizations, whose rules may contribute to the institutions of political economy, come in a wide variety of types running from regulatory agencies to employers' associations and trade unions. Together, these systems of formal rules, informal social norms and organizations constitute a national system of institutional governance.

Though these institutional systems are concerned with the governance of the economy, both their origins and effects are deeply political in nature. Different types of institutional governance 'reflect a politically constructed mix', with elite groups seeking to gain control over 'the strategic levers of the economy and the state at politically opportune moments' (Hancké et al., 2007:

17). Inevitably, this process of construction is frequently attended by conflict, with the institutions that emerge embodying a 'specific social compromise' between competing economic interests (Amable, 2003: 10). This conception of the political origins of institutions has three fundamental implications for our understanding of contemporary varieties of capitalism. Firstly, the political settlement embodied in institutions serves to shape significantly the capacity of actors to secure their interests in the future. Thus, for example, the functioning of labour markets was the object of intense conflict between capital and labour. The institutionalized legacy of this clash, in the form of labour market rights and industrial relations practices, continues to condition deeply the relative bargaining strength and negotiating strategies of employers and employees. Institutions embody and serve to perpetuate a set of power relations. Secondly, distinctive models or varieties of capitalism 'develop from economic and political competition between different kinds of social actors and are always subject to further conflicts' (Whitley, 1999: 19). Though institutions serve to structure economic behaviour, they do not eliminate the potential for political and social conflict between different groups, particularly at times when the relative strength of these groups may shift as a consequence of wider processes of change in the economic and/or political system. Thirdly, there is no assumption that the institutions that develop are economically efficient. Thus, for example, the provision for labour representation in corporate boardrooms that exists in some states reflects the balance of 'power relations at decisive historical moments' (Höpner, 2007: 7). Whether these arrangements are the most economically efficient possible is a separate question.

It is certainly the case, however, that, whatever their historical origins, political character or economic efficacy, these institutional structures will have a major impact on the development and functioning of the economy. Their particular nature will inform and shape the behaviour of economic actors and, by extension, the functioning of the economy as a whole. Specifically, the particular institutional mix in a given state effectively determines 'the incentives and constraints that will lead agents to invest in certain assets, acquire certain skills, cooperate or be opportunistic' (Amable, 2003: 4). Thus, for example, where institutions facilitate collective action by firms, the development of effective employee training programmes becomes more practicable and the development of productive strategies requiring highly skilled labour becomes more feasible. Where such institutions are absent, firms will be loath to invest in expensive training when there is every possibility that competitors who have contributed nothing to cover its cost will reap the benefit by offering marginally higher wages to the newly skilled worker. In such a context, the formulation of a low-cost/low-skill production strategy by firms is more likely. In short, the type of institutions that exists will strongly influence how economic actors interact and coordinate activity in pursuit of their objectives. How they interact and coordinate activity will inform the productive strategies that they adopt (Hall and Gingerich, 2004: 10). All firms need to finance their operations, hire and train labour, acquire technologies and sustain relationships with suppliers and competitors. The particular form of labour or financial market institutions that exists delimits the range of possible solutions open to them and shapes the strategies that they develop to achieve their objectives (Hall and Soskice, 2001a: 15). Economic actors adjust their behaviour to the particular mix of incentives and constraints that a given institutional system embodies.

Finally, it is a core contention of this perspective that, though the product of complex processes of political and economic development across a broad range of areas, 'national economies are characterised by distinct institutional configurations that generate a particular systemic logic of economic action' (Jackson and Deeg, 2006: 6). While economies are complex, there is a fundamental coherence in national institutional governance. Moreover, this coherence is not simply a consequence of the fact that similar sorts of institutional arrangements are found across a wide range of economic activity. Rather, it is argued that these institutions are complementary in nature, with the existence of a particular set operating in one field of activity improving the effective functioning of others in related fields (Hall and Gingerich, 2004: 22). Thus, for example, systems of finance and corporate governance that provide 'patient capital' to management may 'enhance the efficiency of institutional practices in the sphere of labour relations that provide high levels of employment security . . . as well as forms of wage-setting that revolve around strategic interaction between employers associations and trade unions' (ibid.: 22–3). In contrast, systems more reliant on raising capital from demanding, 'impatient' stock markets may be more compatible with fluid, flexible labour markets that facilitate rapid responses to changes in economic opportunities (Hancké et al., 2007).

## Varieties of Institutions

Though the institutional approach is highly sensitive to the significance of territorial and historical specificity in the formation of economic governance mechanisms, analyses of contemporary national systems in Europe demonstrate the operation of a fairly restricted range of institutional types. Thus, all systems rely to a very major extent on the classic liberal economic governance institutions of the market and corporate hierarchy to coordinate the interaction of economic actors in an efficient and stable way. In markets, coordination is achieved through the self-interested behaviour of a myriad of actors engaging in the exchange of goods and services in decentralized arm's-length bargaining underpinned by formal contracting (Hollingsworth and Boyer, 1997: 7). In response to price signals generated by these exchanges, actors adjust their willingness to supply and demand goods and services (Hall and Soskice, 2001a: 8). At least in its purest form, no durable relation between economic actors is observed, and the only purpose of market adjustments is 'to make on-the-spot coherent, instantaneous transactions without any concern for future strategy' (Hollingsworth and Boyer, 1997: 7). In practice, in contemporary capitalist economies the functioning of markets has invariably been supplemented by the development of corporate hierarchies. Some exchanges are internalized within the firm and subject to authoritative management control. This internalization serves to minimize the opportunism inherent in exchange relations, thereby reducing transaction costs (ibid.).

However, analysis of contemporary national systems has also identified the operation of a number of other institutional arrangements that do not conform to liberal economic precepts. In many instances, 'firms develop relationships with other firms, outside actors and their employees that are not well described as either market-based or hierarchical relations but are better seen as efforts to secure cooperative outcomes among the actors using a range of institutional devices that underpin credible commitments' (Hall and Soskice, 2001a: 14). Perhaps the most radically non-liberal institutional form is 'community governance'. In contrast to the self-interested motivations of economic agents that characterize market exchange, community governance is based on the feelings of trust, reciprocity or obligation that exist between the participant actors (Hollingsworth and Boyer, 1997: 10). In contrast to the impersonal relations of the market, which rely on formal contracts to secure reliable behaviour, it is the closeness and nature of the social bonds between economic agents that are key factors determining the form of their engagement. Such bonds enhance the capacity of actors to make 'credible commitments' to each other, thereby reducing the level of transaction costs and opening up opportunities to develop forms of economic activity that would be too costly in a market system. However, they also prohibit the pursuit of economic strategies that simply reflect the 'pure selfish computation of pleasures and pains' (ibid.). Though rare, such systems of governance can be found within tightly knit regions or among ethnic groups.

Markets and communities are at opposite ends of the liberal/non-liberal spectrum, both in terms of their capacity to build long-term relations and in the extent of their dependence on pre-existing social bonds between economic agents in order to operate. In contrast, associational and network forms of institutional governance occupy intermediate positions. Associational governance occurs where representative organizations seek to establish and sustain cooperative relations between particular groups of economic actors as a supplement to, or substitute for, market or corporate managerial forms of coordination. In the case of business and/or employers' associations, for example, collective solutions to the problems of wage-bargaining, research and development or marketing may be developed. These activities reflect the belief that, in certain circumstances, cooperation can improve on the outcomes achievable through individual firm action and market coordination. Associational activity is often characterized by mixed actor motivations, with self-interest frequently augmented by some sense of social obligation (ibid.).

This is most apparent, perhaps, in trade unions, where the objective of driving up individual wages is often mixed with a commitment to social solidarity.

Network governance involves arrangements in which actors coordinate their activity through loose but significant cooperative relationships. Typically established through repeated exchanges, these long-term links enable the participants to collaborate effectively with each other in the pursuit of their respective goals (ibid.: 8). The precise form of these relationships is extremely variable. In some cases, they may be given a formal expression through the establishment of cross-shareholding arrangements between participant firms or by the creation of 'inter-locking' boards, whereby managers of one company take a seat on the board of another, and vice versa. In many other cases, no such formal links emerge. However, as in the case of associations, networks are characterized by a blend of self-interest and social obligation (ibid.: 10). Firms may enter into joint ventures or develop innovation networks for self-interested reasons, but social obligational rules concerning acceptable and 'reasonable' behaviour often develop. In such cases, what actors do is not shaped solely by the calculation of immediate market advantage but also by longer-term considerations of reciprocity and dependence.

The final governing institutional type is the state. This cannot be characterized as intrinsically liberal or non-liberal in nature. In key respects, the state stands behind all other forms of governance. Their functioning is partly dependent on its support. Thus, for example, it is the state that provides the framework of contract law and systems of enforcement without which the market could not function. Similarly, the capacity of associations to assume a governance function is partly dependent on state policy. Without a supportive legal framework, trade unions cannot effectively organize and function, and, therefore, cannot develop the representative and bargaining strength necessary to play a significant role in governing labour market interactions. Again, in the case of networks, the feasibility of building cooperative inter-firm relations is partly dependent on the provisions of competition law. In short, the effective functioning of markets, corporate hierarchies, associations, networks and communities requires the state to assume an appropriately permissive stance.

The role played by any given state will reflect its particular ambition as it has developed over time. Where it seeks merely to perform a regulatory role, the possibility of liberal supporting behaviour is open. Its task is to create and sustain the context within which liberal governance systems can operate effectively. However, where a state seeks to intervene directly in economic activity, either through public ownership and control of industries or through the management of the credit system, it becomes an economic actor with unique properties. A substantial politicization of economic decision-making is unavoidable and the relationship of economic actors is heavily mediated by politics. In such a context, the possibility that liberal economic governance will develop is sharply curtailed.

## Institutional Diversity Illustrated

Across Europe, the practical consequences of operating different governance systems in product, capital and labour markets is readily apparent. In each of these areas, a different institutional mix can be seen to have a major effect both on the development of economic activity and on the distribution of economic power among socioeconomic groups. Thus, for example, in relation to product markets, countries that favour the dominance of market mechanisms of coordination tend to develop strong competition laws and regard inter-corporate cooperation, at least potentially, as collusive and anti-competitive. In contrast, in other states, such 'collusive' activity may be construed as legitimate and beneficial cooperation. The practical impact of these different approaches may be substantial. Thus, while the capacity of small and medium-sized firms to use strong associational bodies to organize cooperative schemes of research and development has been identified as a key element of the German model of innovation, in Britain the strong commitment to protecting competition combined with the weak development of business associations makes such strategies almost impossible (Hall and Soskice, 2001a: 26).

In the case of financial markets and corporate governance, the degree of variation in practice is equally broad. Conceptions of the firm as either a private (Britain) or public (Germany) entity underpin the relative extent of shareholder and employee rights. In Britain, the firm exists to serve the investors and shareholders. In Germany, the firm is legally constrained to protect the interests of a broader set of stakeholders, including employees, suppliers and managers as well as shareholders. Moreover, the bank-based finance system and the frequency of cross-shareholding between firms in Germany sustain intimate forms of inter-company cooperation and coordination that are practically impossible in a securities market-based system such as Britain's. City of London rules prohibit many of these practices. In Italy, by contrast, although the sovereignty of shareholders is legally entrenched, the regulation of the stock exchange has enabled large shareholders to gain a disproportionate share of corporate proceeds at the expense of smaller shareholders. Furthermore, the relative underdevelopment of the stock exchange, and the correspondingly greater dependence of firms on bank-borrowing for raising external investment funds, have facilitated the development of privileged 'insider' networks between banks and firms to the disadvantage of outsiders, be they small shareholders or foreign investors. Institutional governance mechanisms diverge markedly, with substantial consequences for the distribution of economic power and opportunity.

Similarly, the extent to which states are interventionist and associations developed plays a major role in shaping the functioning of labour markets and the conduct of industrial relations. In respect of employment protection and the hiring and firing of labour, a pro-competition state in Britain has striven to reduce the constraints on market forces. In contrast, the Italian state has established a complex set of employment rights that renders the shedding of labour difficult and costly. With respect to industrial relations, in Britain the state is distant and employers' associations are marginal, with the result that bargaining tends to take place at plant level. In other countries, more powerful associations (Sweden) or more interventionist states (Italy, Ireland) have underpinned the continued importance of centralized bargaining at the sectoral and even national level. Finally, in Germany, agreements reached between powerful employers' associations and trade unions in key sectors, such as engineering, exercise a powerful 'wage leadership' influence over pay-setting in the rest of the economy. The role of markets, states, associations and informal social norms varies and the impact on outcomes is considerable.

## The Prevalence of Non-liberal Institutions in EU Member States

Understanding the extent and nature of the challenge presented by liberal Europe to national systems requires some assessment of the extent of the latter's reliance on non-liberal institutional forms of governance. Table 1.1 provides data concerning both the general character of national systems and the prevalence of non-liberal practices in important aspects of product, labour and capital market regulation. The first column is drawn from the coordination index developed by Hall and Gingerich (2004). This is designed to measure the extent to which individual states display the properties of liberal market economies (LME) or coordinated market economies (CME). In the former, 'the market plays the dominant role in coordinating economic behaviour and the state remains an arm's length enforcer of contracts' (Jackson and Deeg, 2006: 22). In contrast, in CMEs, firms engage in longer-term strategies of interaction that are facilitated by the existence of non-market institutions such as associations, inter-corporate networks or state-supported corporatist cooperation in areas such as industrial relations. The core contention is that 'systems vary systematically according to the balance between strategic and market coordination in the political economy' (Hall and Gingerich, 2004: 14). In practice, across EU15 states, Britain and Ireland are adjudged to be the only LMEs. Germany, the Netherlands, Belgium, Sweden, Norway, Denmark, Finland and Austria are categorized as CMEs. The French, Italian, Spanish, Greek and Portuguese systems are deemed to be 'ambiguous' (Hall and Soskice, 2001a: 19–21). The number of ambiguous cases does suggest some conceptual weaknesses within the LME/CME classification. In particular, the 'ambiguity' of these cases largely derives from the central role played by the state in these countries, a dimension underplayed by Hall and Soskice (Hancké et al, 2007: 24–5). Indeed, the role of the state in Italy, Spain, Greece and Portugal is deemed to be so important that some analysts have accorded them their own distinct category, the 'Mediterranean' model, largely in recognition of this fact (Amable, 2003). What is indisputably the case, however, is that like CME states, they too fall well outside the parameters of the LME model.

**Table 1.1** Member states and institutional governance: liberal/non-liberal

| Country | Hall and Gingerich coordination index(1) From most to least liberal | Product-market regulation(2) Summary Indicators Point scale | State control(3) Summary Indicators Point scale | Employment protection(4) Summary Indicators Point scale | Employee co-determination at board level 1990s and 2000s index(5) |
|---|---|---|---|---|---|
| Britain | .07 | 0.5 | 0.6 | 0.5 | 1 |
| Ireland | .29 | 0.8 | 0.9 | 1.0 | 1 |
| Spain | .57 | 1.6 | 2.6 | 3.2 | 1 |
| Netherlands | .66 | 1.4 | 2.3 | 2.4 | 3 |
| France | .69 | 2.1 | 2.6 | 3.1 | 2 |
| Sweden | .69 | 1.4 | 1.5 | 2.4 | 3 |
| Denmark | .70 | 1.4 | 2.5 | 1.5 | 3 |
| Portugal | .72 | 1.7 | 2.8 | 3.7 | 1 |
| Finland | .72 | 1.7 | 2.7 | 2.1 | 3 |
| Belgium | .74 | 1.9 | 2.8 | 2.1 | 1 |
| Italy | .87 | 2.3 | 3.9 | 3.3 | 1 |
| Germany | .95 | 1.4 | 1.8 | 2.8 | 4 |
| Austria | 1.0 | 1.4 | 2.1 | 2.4 | 3 |
| Greece | NA | 2.2 | 3.9 | 3.5 | NA |

Notes

(1) This index is based on a factor analysis of shareholder power, dispersion of corporate control, the size of the stock market, the level of wage coordination, labour turnover and the degree of wage coordination (Hall and Gingerich, 2004: 12–13).

(2) Drawn from OECD Economics Department Working paper no. 226, Nicoletti et al., 2000: 80, table A3.7. This summarizes data concerning the barriers to entrepreneurship, barriers to trade and investment, economic regulation and administrative regulation. It runs from low (liberal) to high (non-liberal).

(3) Drawn from OECD Economics Department Working paper no. 226, Nicoletti et al., 2000: 80, table A3.7, Summary Indicators. This summarizes data concerning both public ownership and state involvement in business such as price controls or the use of command-and-control regulation. It runs from low (liberal) to high (non-liberal).

(4) Drawn from OECD Economics Department Working paper no. 226, Nicoletti et al., 2000: 84, table A3.11. This table summarizes data concerning direct costs of dismissal delays, direct costs of dismissals, and procedural inconveniences under both temporary and regular employment contracts. It runs from low (liberal) to high (non-liberal).

(5) Drawn from Höpner, 2007: 14–15. Index of mandatory employee co-determination rights at the board level of large companies. 1 = no co-determination rights; 2 = participation without voting rights; 3=participation (including voting rights) up to one third of board seats; 4=participation (including voting rights) larger than one-third of board seats.

General classifications of national systems clearly indicate the ubiquity of non-liberal institutional practices among EU15 states. More specific evidence in relation to key aspects of product, capital and labour market regulation confirms and details this conclusion. Indicators of product-market regulation, employment protection and the extent of employee co-determination at board level in member states reveal a widespread tendency to rely on non-market institutions to govern activity. In many countries, barriers to trade and investment are high, administrative regulation heavy, restrictions on employers' dismissal rights severe, employee representation rights in the boardroom extensive. That said, the indicators also reveal the need to be sensitive to the variability of practice within national systems. Thus, it is clear that while Britain is consistent in its liberal character across all the key domains, in most states there are substantial differences in the extent of reliance on non-liberal institutions, depending on the area in question. Thus, for example, while Spain scores quite low on Hall and Gingerich's coordination index, being as close to liberal Britain as to decidedly non-liberal Austria, it does display a marked propensity to deploy employment protection measures that strongly inhibit the operation of market forces in the labour market. In contrast, while Austria scores highly on the coordination index, it has a relatively liberal system of product-market governance. In seeking to assess the extent and nature of the threat presented by the EU to national institutional practices, the most fruitful strategy will be to focus on the implications of its actions for the particular characteristics of product, capital and labour markets. It is on the basis of the evidence gleaned from these specific analyses that a general judgement of the nature of the threat presented by the EU to the sustainability of national models can be made.

## European Integration and National Capitalisms

In seeking to evaluate the nature and the extent of the challenge presented by EU policies to the sustainability of national political economic governance institutions, some preliminary consideration needs to be given to the mechanisms through which such policies impact upon member states. Clearly, it is not within the remit of the EU to seek to reconfigure national institutional systems as a whole. There can be no full frontal assault on national models. However, it is equally clear that in the course of constructing a genuinely integrated European market, measures are taken that do affect the governance of national product, financial and labour markets. What is uncertain is whether the impact of these initiatives is sufficiently powerful to alter substantially national institutional arrangements. A core theme of the seminal work by Hall and Soskice (2001b) on varieties of capitalism is the robustness of national systems in the face of economic globalization pressures. They anticipate that states, and the firms within them, will respond to new externally generated challenges by adapting rather than transforming established institutions. Though not particularly concerned with the EU, the logic of their analysis would predict a similar degree of resistance to European-led liberal transformation. In contrast, other analysts perceive in the EU a political actor possessed of both the necessary ambition and the capacity to overcome such national institutional entrenchment. As European market and monetary integration deepens, a 'clash of capitalisms' inevitably develops (Höpner and Schäfer, 2007). Through an examination of these contrasting perspectives, some preliminary understanding of the extent and the political dynamics of the European challenge to national systems can be gained.

### The transformationalist perspective

European policy affects national institutional systems through both indirect and direct mechanisms. From a transformationalist perspective, the indirect impact largely stems from the simple competitive dynamics of the increasingly open market that the EU has created. This new market transforms the context within which economic actors and national regulatory authorities must operate. For producers in Europe the EU has become the 'home' market. This extends their trading opportunities and expands the number of their competitors. It also opens up the possibility of developing new productive strategies by facilitating access to additional non-national sources of finance, labour, management expertise, etc. As a consequence of this deepening engagement with international markets, it is anticipated that firms tend to outgrow their 'domestic' capitalism. National rules that once appeared to be workable and acceptable will increasingly be perceived as unreasonable fetters on activity. Moreover, national policymakers will have to respond to these shifting perceptions. They must adapt to the fact that in an integrated European market, greater opportunity for mobility strengthens the bargaining position of economic actors. Those who are dissatisfied with some aspect of public policy can either leave the jurisdiction of the offending state or leverage the threat of exit to pressurize policymakers to change tack. Workers can go in search of better jobs, welfare and healthcare. Capital can move to minimize taxation or escape regulation. While mobility is neither a costless option nor one that is equally practicable for all economic actors, where the threat is plausible states must accommodate these pressures or risk relative economic disadvantage. A government that does not respond to these threats through deregulation and tax reduction will 'be limited in its general economic policy by the threat of capital flight, the long-term erosion of its tax base, and its inability to attract internationally dynamic firms and sectors to locate there' (Cerny, 1997: 180).

Such market developments will also serve to generate greater political mobilization in pursuit of substantial policy reform. Economic actors attracted by new opportunities for profitable trade will have a strong incentive to coalesce to press for regulatory reforms that will facilitate their exploitation. This may not be a straightforward, conflict-free matter. Trade theory suggests that regional market integration, like economic globalization more generally, will have a differential impact on the interests of economic actors and, above all, on business interests. At its most basic, the thesis is that the process of market integration benefits those who export and those who consume imports, while hurting those who compete with imports (Frieden and Rogowski, 1996). This fundamental division of economic experience and opportunity will feed into and structure the process of public policy reform. However, it is anticipated that those who see significant potential benefit from further integration will have an incentive to defect from established systems and practices that inhibit market liberalization, and to mobilize politically to press for reform. Moreover, as economic integration develops, the proportion of the economy that will benefit from liberalization will expand and the number of economic actors with an incentive to press for reform will grow. The process of market integration will generate the development of a reformist coalition committed to driving through facilitating regulatory change.

These indirect market pressures for reform are not inconsiderable. However, the strongest source of transformative power available to the EU derives from the strength of its central institutions and its legal system. Its impact on national systems is not just, or even principally, felt through changing competitive market dynamics, but directly through European law and policy. In respect of a broad range of matters, the EU enjoys substantial rights to police the behaviour of national economic policymakers and regulatory authorities. A cursory glance at its policies confirms that many of the EU's activities impinge on the domains that are central to the functioning of national capitalisms. Its competition policy directly addresses the structure and operation of product markets. Efforts to integrate the financial service industry in Europe have profound implications for national systems of finance and corporate governance. Considerable controversy has attached to Commission initiatives and European Court of Justice (ECJ) judgments in the area of corporate law. Labour-market regulation and related social policies have been a growing preoccupation of the Union, especially since the adoption of the Lisbon economic reform strategy in 2000. Central to the transformationalist perspective is the belief that the ECJ and the Commission now 'directly target member states' institutions and aim at transforming them, even in situations in which no other country's economic activities are involved at all' (Höpner and Schäfer, 2007: 21). Such is the authority of the EU that it can enforce a substantial transformation in national governing institutions that do not embody its liberal economic preferences.

### The accommodationalist perspective

The accommodationalist viewpoint does not deny the existence or importance of EU authority and changed market dynamics. However, it argues that those who anticipate transformation in response to them both underestimate the durability of established national institutions and oversimplify the process whereby market liberalization induces economic actors to organize politically to press for reform. Durability is partly attributed to the deep social embeddedness of national capitalisms. As noted above, the latter are the product of long-term historical development and radical change is likely to be difficult, if only because their agents and beneficiaries will strongly oppose it. Partly, however, the expectation of durability reflects the core assumption of the institutionalist perspective. While some see 'institutional economies' as vulnerable to regional and global market integration (Crouch and Streeck, 1997: 12–14), others hold that institutions should not be viewed as obstacles to efficiency, but, rather, as potential sources of competitive advantage for industries and firms in any given national system. They can, in fact, be a source of *comparative institutional advantage* (Hall and Soskice, 2001a: 37). Economic agents have adapted their behaviour to the pattern of incentives and constraints that specific institutional systems create. These adaptations may take the form of investments in particular types of productive strategies or the forging of particular types of relationships with competitors, financiers, labour, etc. A radical departure from these arrangements would involve considerable economic cost and risk. Economic agents would not merely have to learn new ways of producing goods and services; they would have to build new types of relationships with each other. Rather than abandon this source of advantage, greater competition is likely to intensify their dependence upon it. As Franzese and Mosher point out, where comparative advantage exists, the standard model of trade theory anticipates its durability in the face of intensifying competition. Trade 'spurs production specialization according to comparative advantage' and this is likely to bolster rather than undermine 'the diversification of institutional and policy configuration' (Franzese and Mosher, 2002: 179). Such 'path-dependent' effects have led many to predict that national economies will continue to operate and perform differently, with convergence in institutional structure a highly unlikely outcome (Coates, 2005: 17). Where capitalism is practised has a major influence on how it is practised. How it is practised will significantly constrain how it is likely to be practised in the future.

It is also suggested that the political impact of market liberalization is less predictable than the transformationalist perspective suggests. In practice, it is argued, the costs of achieving policy change are often more immediately apparent than the benefits. Identifying a set of reforms and mobilizing a reforming coalition presents a major challenge when the scale of the benefit is frequently less than certain and the temptation to free-ride is substantial. Moreover, it is likely that negatively affected interests will be better placed to mobilize in defence of the status quo. The threat presented by a reform to established interests is often more immediately apparent and the political task of mobilizing resistance is correspondingly less demanding. In short, even if the economic calculus makes change appear an attractive option to many actors, the political costs of persuading others to accommodate the new approach could be substantial. Indeed, as Franzese and Mosher (2002) have argued, the general economic benefits accruing from a process of trade liberalization may actually undermine the incentives to form reform coalitions. If integration is delivering growth, this may offset the cost burdens stemming from the operation of inferior national institutions and reduce short-run pressures for reform (ibid.: 180).

The feasibility of building a successful reform coalition is also strongly conditioned by local political factors. These are partly related to differing national political cultures. At least in some cases, the defenders of the status quo, or the advocates of non-market priorities in policy formation, may be able to assume the mantle of national champion. Economic nationalism is a powerful political weapon, though the extent of its availability varies considerably across states. More broadly, however, the capacity to achieve institutional reform through mobilizing political coalitions is substantially influenced by national political institutional structures. In a simple pluralist model of reform, the tipping point between policy continuity and significant change will come when the potential beneficiaries outweigh the likely losers from reform. However, this model is clearly overly simple. The capacity of even the most powerful reforming coalition to effect change is greatly dependent on the nature of political institutions (Garret and Lange, 1996). Thus, for example, in consensual political systems, typically marked by decentralized power and multi-party coalition government, there are multiple 'veto points'. The opportunities to resist, dilute or redirect reforms that they provide may be considerable, irrespective of the extent of the clamour for change induced by market integration. In majoritarian systems, in contrast, where power is centralized and the impact on government composition of a small shift in votes may be considerable, radical reform may be a far more feasible option (Gourevitch, 2003a: 319). The consequences of a given set of market pressures for policy reform will greatly depend on the political culture and institutions of each country.

If the impact of indirect market pressures on national institutions is unpredictable, recent studies of 'Europeanization' suggest that the EU's effectiveness in enforcing reform directly through legal instruments is also much more problematic than might initially appear to be the case. This uncertainty is a product of the nature of EU policy. Though it is active across a very broad range of economic policy areas, the EU rarely 'prescribes an institutional model to which domestic arrangements have to be adjusted' (Knill and Lehmkuhl, 2002: 257–8). Beyond the areas of consumer rights, environmental policy, and health and safety at work, where states have only limited discretion when deciding how to comply with EU law, the coercive content of EU initiatives diminishes, in some cases to little more than exhortation. Its most common strategy is to focus on striking down 'national barriers to the emergence of European markets without prescribing models' (Radaelli, 2003: 42). The objective is to remove barriers to trade, investment and to the establishment of businesses in other member states. Thus, the EU often simply 'sets targets for the date, kind, and amount of liberalization of a formerly highly regulated sector such as telecommunications or electricity, but leaves the country to specify many of the details of liberalizing policies and regulatory arrangements' (Schmidt, 2002a: 897). This leaves each state with a considerable degree of leeway to shape the new regulatory order in whatever way is deemed most beneficial to national interests. In other areas, moreover, the coercive powers of the EU are even more modest. Thus, where policy is formulated through the 'open method of coordination' (OMC), implementation is effected through 'soft' instruments rather than 'hard' law. The strategy is to achieve reform through the generation of a process of 'mutual leaning' among member states, relying on practices such as 'benchmarking' and the identification and sharing of best practice. In such cases, Europeanization's impact on member states 'does not denote adaptation to vertical pressures, but more subtle impacts of socialization processes, ideational convergence, learning, and interpretations of policy paradigms and ideas' (Radaelli and Pasquier, 2007: 38). The EU may generate major change in national policy and institutions, but in many areas of economic and social policy it will not do so through hierarchical, coercive means.

The modesty of its coercive, prescriptive power means that, to a considerable extent, the precise impact of EU initiatives will be shaped by the uncertain dynamic of domestic politics and policymaking within member states. EU action can change the domestic policy agenda. Moreover, its intrusion into national politics may alter the balance of power between domestic actors, with some gaining 'additional resources to exert influence', while others see a substantial weakening of their position (Börzel and Risse, 2000: 8). Ultimately, however, its success in achieving the reforms it seeks depends on the relative power of domestic actors, their respective political skill and the political institutional context within which they must operate. EU pressure becomes a significant part of the domestic political game, but it does not determine how it plays out. On the basis of such observations, some analysts have concluded that, in many instances, 'domestic politics and the domestic polity serve as forces of inertia and explain the resilient or "sticky" responses to Europeanization' (Bulmer, 2007: 48). Though this may not always be so, it is clear that the opportunity for defenders of national varieties of capitalism to resist the European liberal challenge is much more extensive than might initially appear to be the case.

### FURTHER READING

Hall and Soskice (2001b) offer the clearest statement of the varieties of capitalism thesis. Useful critiques can be found in Coates (2005) and Hancké et al. (2007). For Europeanization, Graziano and Vink (2007) provide a comprehensive and up-to-date discussion.

2

# The European Union and the Evolution of Liberal Europe

## Introduction

The establishment of a European Economic Community (EEC) in 1957 presented a clear challenge to national markets and regulatory institutions. A new European body endowed with substantial legal authority was charged with overseeing the functioning of key aspects of national economic systems. National sovereignty was to be limited in important ways. The broad liberal thrust of the new European project was also clearly evident. Building on earlier initiatives in relation to the coal and steel industries, the fundamental purpose of the new organization was to integrate national markets and facilitate greater cross-border trade. However, while the general policy orientation of the EEC/EU was evident from its inception, its full potential as an agent of national political economic transformation only gradually became apparent. From modest beginnings, the depth and breadth of its liberal ambition, the willingness of members to accommodate its activities and the effectiveness of its policy implementation have evolved significantly over the course of its 60-odd years of existence. An understanding of the extent and limits of the EU's challenge to national governance institutions in product, financial and labour markets requires an appreciation of the broad course of this evolution.

Analysis of the EU's developing role can be usefully and justifiably divided into two distinct phases. The first runs from the foundation of the EEC in 1957 to the early 1980s, during which time a real but heavily circumscribed form of liberal market integration was achieved. The second phase runs from the early 1980s to the present, when a relaunch of the integration project initiated an extended period of institutional and policy innovation that has served to deepen market integration in Europe. By tracing the contours of the EU's development as an economic policy actor during these periods, the broad nature of its challenge to national institutions of political economic governance can be more clearly grasped.

## Qualified Liberalism: 1957–1980

The general intent of integration was clearly expressed in the Treaty of Rome, the instrument of the EEC's creation.[1] In the context of its time, it was a strikingly liberal economic document. Article 2 stated that 'by establishing a common market and progressively approximating the economic policies of member states', it would seek to 'promote throughout the Community an harmonious development of economic activities, an increase in stability, an accelerating raising of the standard of living and closer relations between the States belonging to it.' In order to achieve this outcome, all qualitative restrictions on trade between them was to be abolished, a common external tariff was to be established, a common commercial policy vis-à-vis third countries was to be formulated and 'obstacles to the free movement of goods, persons, services and capital' were to be eliminated (Article 3). Any form of discrimination based on nationality was to be suppressed (Tsoukalis, 1993: 19).

The principal strategy of integration was negative in nature. The overwhelming focus was on the removal of obstacles to the functioning of an effective market. Article 3(f) enshrined the commitment that 'competition in the common market is not distorted'. To this end, member states were to 'approximate' their domestic laws 'to the extent required for the proper functioning of the common market'. Articles 85–94 (now 81–9) gave a legal basis for European institutions to adopt measures to combat restrictive practices; to monitor and control state aids to industry; and to eradicate dumping. Commercial behaviour that distorted free competition between member states was deemed to be 'incompatible with the common market'. While the creation of a European Investment Bank and the European Social Fund was designed to allow a degree of positive intervention to aid development in Italy's Mezzogiorno, the poorest region of the six founding states, there was no provision for the development of common industrial or regional policies (Tsoukalis, 1993: 20). Europe was to integrate through building markets rather than correcting them. Of the 128 clauses in the treaty not concerned with institutional and administrative design or synoptic overviews, 73 were concerned with issues of free movement of goods, persons and capital or with rules designed to eliminate distortions to competition (Gillingham, 2003: 62).

The extent of the EEC's success in integrating its members into a common, liberal market in its first two decades was not insubstantial. Internal tariffs and quotas were completely removed by 1968. A common external customs policy was agreed and a common commercial policy established. This latter was principally concerned with collectively structuring relations between the new regional customs union and world free-trade agreements, and between the member states and their numerous ex-colonies (Bartolini, 2005: 180). The openness of member states to trade, measured in terms of the exports of goods and services as a percentage of GDP, rose substantially between 1960 and 1980 from 39 per cent to 57 per cent in Belgium, 14 to 20 per cent in France, 13 to 22 per cent in Italy and 19 to 26 per cent in Germany (Tsoukalis, 2003: 17). Moreover, the rate of trade growth between members substantially exceeded that between them and the rest of the world. However, there were also severe limits to this success. While the move towards the removal of tariff and quota barriers and the completion of a customs union was achieved ahead

of schedule, non-tariff barriers largely remained in place and efforts to harmonize regulatory standards soon ran into strong national resistance (Dinan,
2004: 114). While workers had the right to move freely between member states,
practical obstacles such as the recognition of foreign qualifications were not
effectively addressed. While competition policy was applied with some success
in the area of restrictive practices, price-fixing, etc., it had far less success in
addressing state subsidies, mergers policy or the abuse by large companies of
their dominant market position (Butt Philips, 1986: 8). Perhaps most tellingly,
while trade in goods developed rapidly, capital markets remained subject to
tight national control (Dinan, 2004: 114). Member-state economies remained
deeply national in many aspects of management and regulation.

The limited nature of integration partly reflected the fact that the liberal
commitment of the signatories to the Treaty of Rome was far from unquali-
fied. Many of the market-making provisions agreed were subject to restrictive
qualifications or lacked specificity. Thus, state subsidies were exempt from
competition policy rules (Scharpf, 1999: 51). Provisions to eliminate the
innumerable non-tariff barriers to trade were often unspecific. For example,
the clarity of the commitment to the elimination of tariffs and qualitative restrictions on imports contrasted with the rather vague prohibitions
against national regulation, most of which were further qualified by 'public
interest' exemptions (ibid.). These qualifications reflected the broader desire
of the member states to protect their freedom to develop independent industrial and welfare policies. As Tsoukalis has argued, the 'influence of Keynes's
ideas meant that governments were keen on retaining direct control over
fiscal and monetary policies to be used for the attainment of the objective
of full employment at home' (1993:21). The common market in Europe was
to be an important adjunct to domestic full employment policies. Where
these policies come into conflict, the activities of the EEC would have to be
curtailed.

Similarly, in the social policy field, the signatories of the Treaties of Paris
(ECSC) and Rome had no intention of surrendering their national prerogatives. On the contrary, the creation of a common market and the corresponding enhancement of the opportunities for international trade were viewed
as necessary in order to provide the means for the further development of
national welfare regimes. Neither the founding fathers of the Community nor
the governing elites of the member states challenged a division of purpose
that has been characterized by Milward (2000) as a 'European rescue of the
nation-state'. The welfare state was seen as a desirable institution that should
remain the preserve of the national state. Community and national leaders
favoured 'social protection, high labour standards, and full employment
objectives, whose national scope and closure preconditions were taken for
granted' (Ferrara, 2005: 92). The common market would generate the necessary resources for its development, though 'in no case should it be allowed
to weaken social standards through regulatory competition' (ibid.: 93). This

general perspective was reflected in the very limited competence in these areas assigned to European institutions by the treaty.

It is evident, then, that though the liberal promise of the Treaty of Rome was genuine, it was also heavily qualified and somewhat contradictory in nature. The signatory states combined a commitment to liberalize external trade with a strong desire to build a mixed economy domestically, involving strict regulation of capital and labour markets and the development of welfare systems. The European market was conceived principally as a means to link consumers and producers beyond the national borders without challenging national productive or social organization in any substantial way. Moreover, in practice, even this limited goal quickly became bogged down in political and bureaucratic wrangling. Thus, for example, the harmonization of prod-uct standards in order to facilitate cross-border trade was frequently stymied by conflicts between entrenched national interests. As technology advanced, the necessary technical or legal requirements associated with new products 'tended to be agreed at the national level, reflecting the interests of the national industry(ies) concerned' (Armstrong and Bulmer, 1998: 16). Barriers to trade grew rather than diminished. These limitations were compounded by the failure to address differences in the regulation of corporate governance or to initiate a substantial liberalization of the financial services sector. In effect, corporate ownership structures were protected from unwelcome foreign incursion and both creditors and debtors remained locked into the national economy. Commission initiatives designed to unravel these arrangements were regularly obstructed in the Council of Ministers, with the unanimity decision-making rule severely limiting the feasibility of substantial reform.

This combination of 'Keynes at home and Smith abroad' initially proved economically successful in broad terms. The early years of the integration coincided with the so-called 'golden age' of post-war European capitalism. However, the arrangement came under increasing pressure when the dynamic expansion of these years began to falter and the multiple economic crises of the 1970s gained intensity. Faced with slowing growth, increasing unem-ployment and rising inflation, the response of member states was to develop independent national strategies that profoundly challenged the liberal prin-ciples and policy practices of the EEC. Thus, they reacted to the intensifying competition not by removing existing non-tariff barriers to trade (NTBs), but by instituting new ones. The development of national champion firms in high-tech sectors and the deployment of discriminatory subsidies or credit breaks that disadvantaged firms from other member states became common. The dominant instinct informing national reactions to the deteriorating eco-nomic conditions was protectionism. Against the rising tide of 'restructuring agreements, concentration and protectionist national subsidies, all of which made a mockery of attempts by the DGIV to implement its policy effectively', the Community in general offered little resistance (Cini and McGowan, 1998: 27). Indeed, the Commission itself became directly involved in some of these restructuring efforts, leading crisis cartels in the steel industry, operating complex production-allocation regimes in textiles and managing decline in shipbuilding. While these actions were justified as alternatives to outright protection, the Commission could reasonably be accused of, in effect, subverting the operation of a liberal market it was charged with establishing and policing (Gillingham, 2003: 130). By the end of the 1970s, it appeared that the broad, if never pure, liberal impetus of the Treaty of Rome had been overwhelmed by the national protectionist impulses of the member states and the harsher climate of international economic competition.

### The Common Agricultural Policy

Perhaps the clearest and most significant demonstration of the limits of the EEC's liberal commitment could be found in its agricultural policy. The importance of the agricultural sector in the early decades of the Community's existence reflected a variety of factors. Firstly, there was a genuine concern about food security. In the light of the post-war experience of food shortages and rationing in many states, it is perhaps unsurprising that matters of food supply should exercise political leaders so greatly. Secondly, agriculture contributed substantially to overall national economic income, rising from a low of 8.8 per cent in Belgium in 1950 to 12.3 per cent in Germany and almost 30 per cent in Italy (Ackrill, 2000: 17). Its condition was of general economic significance. Thirdly, the sheer size of the agricultural labour force in many of the founding member states inevitably meant that the sector's problems were of general political significance. While the percentage of the population active in agriculture in 1950 only touched 11.9 per cent in highly industrialized Belgium, it rose to 23 per cent in Germany, 30.9 per cent in France and a staggering 44.4 per cent in Italy (Rieger, 2005: 163). Fourthly, the socioeconomic importance of agriculture was sharpened by its very particular economic condition. As an industry, agriculture was in the midst of a secular decline that had been ongoing for well over half a century. Relative to other sectors, per capita income levels were substantially and persistently low. In 1970, for instance, agricultural incomes in Belgium only reached 74 per cent of the level enjoyed by workers in other sectors. The comparable figure in the Netherlands was 61 per cent, in Italy 51 per cent, in France 44 per cent and in Germany 34 per cent (ibid.: 168).

Given these circumstances, it is no surprise that the principal goal of agricultural policy in the 1950s was to achieve a substantial rise in farm incomes (Fennell, 1997: 7). However, the realization of this objective within the context of a competitive market would inevitably require a radical restructuring of industry, including large-scale consolidation of small farms. The fact that in Italy alone there were approximately 2.5 million farms of less than five hectares occupying about 75 per cent of utilized agricultural land illustrates the extent of the economic and political challenges that such an approach would involve (Ackrill, 2000: 18). Abandoning the sector to the logic of market forces would be a decidedly risky strategy; in fact, it was not seriously contemplated by any West European state. Across the continent, and indeed the wider world, it was generally accepted that agriculture merited special economic treatment (Grant, 1997: 64). As a consequence, the terms of the Treaty of Rome exempted agriculture from the pro-market, 'negative integration' approach adopted in respect of the rest of the economy. In order to secure the support of farmers and farmworkers for European integration, they were to be treated to a very particular version of it. The objective of European policy was to preserve a sector regarded as possessing distinctive institutional and social features deemed to be 'incompatible with the principles of industrial production and competitive markets' (Rieger, 2005: 162).

The form of special treatment to be accorded to agriculture was not imme-diately apparent. While recognizing the sector's special nature, the Treaty of Rome failed to offer any clear guidance on how it should be accommodated. The five principles adumbrated in Article 39 (now 33), setting out the basis of an agricultural policy for the Community, were vague, aspirational and, in many respects, practically incompatible. Thus, for example, the injunction to ensure fair prices for consumers was matched by a commitment to ensur-ing 'a fair standard of living for the agricultural community, in particular by increasing the individual earnings of persons engaged in agriculture'. There was no acknowledgement of the potential tension that existed between these objectives. Moreover, there were substantial differences of interest among member states over pricing policy. Most importantly, Germany was extremely concerned that a harmonized European market would leave its farmers unable to compete with lower-cost producers in countries such as France (Ackrill, 2000: 32). However, by the mid-to-late 1960s, a Common Agricultural Policy (CAP) was agreed and implemented. This policy unam-biguously committed itself to the protection of agriculture and agricultural incomes in the face of any and all competitive pressures. It was effectively a policy against the market. It established a complex system of price support to ensure that farmers' incomes were protected from the vagaries of fluctuations in output and prices. Product prices were to be agreed annually by national agriculture ministers in the Council of Ministers. The Commission was then charged with ensuring that prices did not fall below the agreed level. If this did occur, it moved to drive up prices by employing agents to buy the product concerned. The relationship between the Community and world markets was to be governed by the principle of 'Community preference'. This meant, in effect, 'that producers inside the Community should always be more favour-ably placed than competing overseas suppliers' (Grant, 1997: 68). Thus, levies were imposed on imported products to ensure that they did not undercut European producers. In addition, export bounties were paid to European producers who sold abroad to cover any gap between the price they achieved for their sale and the guaranteed CAP price. The CAP system was effectively designed to override the market in relation to the level and distribution of agricultural incomes.

A more thoroughgoing rejection of liberal market principles than the CAP system would be difficult to conceive of – short of centralized planning. Moreover, the depth of member states' commitment to its maintenance – notwithstanding differences of interest between them in relation to the details of its structure and operation – is remarkable. One undeniably damaging consequence of the regime was that it favoured the expansion of output irrespective of the level of demand, as farmers could be certain that they could sell at or above the administratively set price. Consequently, the costs of supporting this system grew dramatically, rising from approximately 28 per cent of the total Community budget in 1965 to 70 per cent in 1985 (Reiger, 2005: 165). Judged as a welfare policy, its performance was equally poor. The rise in farm incomes did not reflect the scale of the transfers from taxpayers and consumers that the policy effected, largely because of marketing costs and administrative inefficiencies (Ackrill, 2000: 202). Moreover, in supporting prices, the system inevitably paid the biggest subsidies to the largest producers, still leaving many smaller farmers with barely enough to survive (Fennell, 1997: 409–10). Yet it was only in the early 1990s that significant structural reform was agreed.

## Deepening Liberalism: 1980s to the Present

Any judgement made at the end of the 1970s would have had to conclude that the EU had demonstrated little inclination or capacity to challenge the operation of national institutions of economic governance. Indeed, in the eyes of many, it looked as if the high water mark of integration had been reached and the most likely development in future years would be a deepening nationalization of economic organization across Western Europe. However, a number of fundamental developments combined to confound this expectation. The first relates to the consolidation of the EU institutional and legal system. Notwithstanding its poor policy performance in many areas, the EU did gradually succeed in establishing its own credibility and effectiveness as a political and administrative organization. Most importantly, its ongoing legal consolidation during the 1960s and 1970s served to provide a sounder basis for future policy initiatives. With the adoption of the doctrines of the supremacy of European over national law and the principle of direct effect, a new European order was created that gradually empowered European institutions to restrict member states' capacity to evade treaty commitments to market liberalization. The effective 'constitutionalization' of treaty law meant that the principles enshrined in the Treaty of Rome gradually gained a pre-eminent status; member states became trapped by the legal implications of their initial great bargain, as these were progressively established and elucidated by ECJ judgments.

One consequence of this process of legal consolidation was the effective 'constitutionalization of competition law' that it effected (Scharpf, 1999: 54). Protecting competition gained a privileged quasi-constitutional status that other aspects of economic management and regulation did not enjoy. The Commission successfully exploited the opportunity to enhance its own power by manipulating 'the appeals procedure to its own advantage so as to build up competition precedents and consolidate its legal base' (Cini and McGowan, 1998: 28). A second key example of its impact on the course of integration came in the *Cassis de Dijon* judgment handed down by the ECJ in 1979. In its ruling, the Court first asserted its right to adjudicate what constituted a legitimate 'public interest' restriction of competition. It was a matter for the European legal system. It then gave legal substance to the view that the freedom to sell and to consume had achieved constitutional protection. Furthermore, this status could not be overturned by the political judgement of democratically legitimized national legislatures (Scharpf, 1999: 56). The Court's decision established the principle of 'mutual recognition' of national regulatory standards. Rather than having to harmonize standards and rules across member states, the satisfaction of one set of national standards enabled producers to distribute and sell their product in all member states (Schmidt, 2007: 673). What was good enough for one member state was good enough for all. There were legal and practical limits to the applicability of this principle. Exemptions were allowed for national restrictions that could be justified for reasons relating to public morality, the protection of humans, animals and plant health and safety (Young, 2005: 103). Moreover, the generalizability of mutual recognition across the full range of EU competence was far from automatic. In its reasoning, the ECJ did not offer an 'injunction to recognize' but a 'road map' for future legislation (Nicolaïdis and Schmidt, 2007: 721). However, the political implications of the principle were substantial. Even as the implementation of competition policy fell into disarray in the 1970s, the legal basis for the enforcement of a more rigorous and effective policy by the Commission was being established. Even as member states' commitment to the implementation of their initial bargain reached its lowest ebb, the threshold for gaining political agreement to overcome regulatory barriers to trade was effectively being lowered. Through a set of largely unanticipated developments, the protection of economic freedom was accorded quasi-constitutional status, while the capacity of states to obstruct its enforcement was severely curtailed.

The second crucial development that served to re-energize the integration project was political in nature. There was a renewed commitment by many member states to the realization of the core objectives set out in the Treaty of Rome. This renewal was most clearly manifested in the adoption of a new treaty, the Single European Act (SEA), in 1986. At the heart of this treaty lay a collective agreement to reinvigorate the process of market construction. To facilitate this task, the SEA introduced a number of institutional changes, the most notable of which concerned decision-making rules. Member states agreed to abandon the unanimity rule and adopt a system of Qualified Majority Voting (QMV) in respect of measures designed to implement the single market programme. Moreover, this process of renewal did not end with the SEA and the single market. In 1991, the Maastricht Treaty (formally, the Treaty on European Union, or TEU) was agreed. Though it too introduced important institutional changes, including broadening the application of QMV and strengthening the role of the European parliament, its greatest significance lay in its provision for the creation of a single European currency to complement the single European market.

The sources of this political reinvigoration are a matter of some dispute. The failure of the nationalistic policies of the 1970s and a deepening sense of anxiety about the growing challenge from the dynamic economies of the Far East certainly played a significant part. Yet precisely why and how these general developments were transformed into the specific commitment to a single market and a single currency has generated considerable debate. Disagreements rage over the role and relative importance of domestic political factors and state strategies, the rise of neo-liberal economic ideas, the demands of multinational corporations and the consequences of policy entrepreneurship on the part of the European Commission (see, for example, Sandholtz and Zysman, 1989; Moravscik, 1998; Sandholtz and Stone Sweet, 1998; van Apeldoorn, 2002). However, the concern here is not with the explanation of this European 'relaunch', but with its character and the nature of its impact on member states. In the 1980s, the EU returned to the liberal vision that shaped its foundation and pursued it with a renewed vigour. Where 1957 was conceived as a means 'to connect consumers and producers beyond national borders within established productive structures', the single market programme sought 'to modify the productive structures themselves' (Bartolini, 2005: 181). If the Treaty of Rome sought to encourage monetary policy coordination, the single currency project sought to transcend national authority and render monetary policy control a supranational matter. It is undeniably the case that, as a consequence of these initiatives, a new phase of integration was initiated that presented a much more profound challenge to the integrity of its member states' political economic institutions.

### The single market project

The principal objective of the single market project was to realize the commitment to the creation of a genuinely common European market inscribed in the Treaty of Rome. The strategy was developed in the Commission's 1985 White Paper, *Completing the Single Market*. It set out to overcome the myriad legal, political and administrative obstacles to the realization of a truly common market that had emerged over the previous three decades or so. Thus, firstly, it sought to remove the physical barriers to trade. These largely concerned administrative controls at frontier crossings. Secondly, it sought to overcome technical barriers, most of which involved differing national requirements for the sale of goods and services. These barriers could either assume a legal character or involve technical standards agreed by responsible national agencies. Whatever the form, their common effect was to fragment markets and inhibit integration by, in many cases, preventing goods sold in one country from being eligible for sale in another (Armstrong and Bulmer, 1998: 23). Thirdly, it sought to eliminate fiscal distortions stemming from differing rates in excise duties, indirect taxation and aspects of corporate taxation. These distortions served to inhibit economically rational trade and investment decision-making and undermine efficiency. Though the political and administrative challenge of removing these barriers varied greatly from one area to another, it was anticipated that the collective effect of their removal would be to catalyse a far more profound integration of markets than had hitherto occurred.

In order to overcome the implementation and enforcement problems that had long plagued the common market project, the Commission pursued two broad strategies. The first was to minimize the necessity for regulatory harmonization, which so frequently proved slow and exhausting, if not fruitless. This was to be achieved partly by delegating responsibility for developing detailed product standards to private European standard-making bodies such as the European Committee for Standards (CEN) and the European Electrical Standards Coordinating Committee (CENELEC). The growing effectiveness of these bodies counteracted the nationalistic tendencies that had characterized the 1960s and '70s in this field. By the early twenty-first century, approximately 80 per cent of standards were the product of European or international rather than national standard-making bodies, an almost exact reversal of the situation obtaining a decade and a half earlier (Tsoukalis, 2003: 99). Even more significant, however, was the decision by the Commission to generalize the application of the principle of mutual recognition to as many areas as possible. If a good satisfied the required standards in one member state, it could be sold in all others regardless of the particulars of local national regulations. Thus, the need for harmonization across a wide range of areas was simply sidestepped. It has been estimated that by the 1990s, approximately 50 per cent of intra-EU trade was accounted for by goods subject to mutual recognition (Young, 2005: 102). Moreover, even where there remained a need for a minimum level of harmonization, the introduction of QMV in the Council of Ministers significantly eased the task of achieving agreement. In the financial services sector, for example, although firms were allowed to sell products in all states if they adhered to their 'home country' regulation, some agreement on the minimum requirements of national standards was necessary to ensure a basic credibility for products. QMV enabled the Commission to successfully pass a facilitating directive in a relatively short period of time.

The second strategy pursued by the Commission to achieve and sustain a genuine common market was to enhance its own policing powers. While the White Paper focused attention on removing the technical and physical

barriers to trade, it also aimed 'to eliminate the very causes of those obstacles at source, namely the distortions and barriers created by government
intervention in the market in all its infinite variety' (Hancher, 1996: 55).
Among the principal weapons deployed to achieve this was competition
policy. Buttressed by ECJ judgments and the terms of the SEA, the rigour and
breadth of its application was to be greatly reinforced. State aids were subject to control from the late 1980s. National public procurement processes
were to be policed by the Commission. Responsibility for controlling merger
activity was added in the early 1990s while, from the mid-to-late 1990s, the
Commission assumed a central role in the liberalization of the utilities sector
(Wilks, 2005a). Within a decade, the Commission's capacity to police Europe's
integrated market was transformed from minimal to formidable. The EU was
given the tools to enforce more effectively provisions of the Treaty of Rome
that had long been ignored. The ability of the member states to evade the
requirements of EU policy or reserve whole swathes of economic regulation
to national control was substantially curtailed. Policy instruments that were
central to the operation of the mixed economy at national level were undermined and the ability of national governments to influence the allocation of
resources within countries was restricted (Hancher, 1996: 11). Moreover, with
firms increasingly structuring their investment and productive operations on
a pan-national basis, matters such as the rules on corporate takeovers, which
had traditionally been purely national concerns, now assumed a far greater
salience at the European level (Martin, 2007: 117). Through the enhancement
of EU authority and the deepening of market integration, the challenge of
Europe to national economic institutions in the key institutional domains
of product markets, financial markets and corporate governance was greatly
intensified.

### Monetary union

The EU's deepening challenge to national systems of institutional governance in product, financial and labour markets is perhaps best exemplified by
the decision to establish a European monetary union. The objective of this
union was to achieve 'the full liberalization of capital circulation, the full
integration of financial markets, the total and irreversible convertibility of
currencies and, eventually, their institutionalization in a single currency'
(Bartolini, 2005: 195). Its achievement would transform the economic context
within which national public and private actors had to pursue their objectives. By eliminating exchange-rate risks and enhancing the comparability
of prices and wages across the member states of the Union, it would greatly
facilitate capital mobility, intensify price competition and pressurize firms
to contain their labour costs (Dølvik, 2004: 281). Furthermore, designed as
it was to secure and extend the single market, the form of monetary union
adopted served to create a powerful new European actor and entrench a set of

fundamental economic policy choices that can legitimately be characterized as neo-liberal in nature.

The agreement of monetary union represented a major recasting of the original European bargain. Though the Treaty of Rome had provided for the formation of a Monetary Committee as a device to coordinate monetary policies, the EEC's role in relation to monetary policy was extremely marginal for the first decade of its existence. Currency relations among its members were managed as part of the wider post-war Bretton Woods system centred on the US dollar (Verdun, 2007: 197). It was only following the destabilization and ultimate collapse of this system that, as a result of the effective withdrawal of the US from its pivotal role, monetary policy emerged onto the EEC's agenda. European leaders feared that the unstable currency exchange rates that followed the ending of Bretton Woods would disrupt trade and undermine growth in the Community by making it harder for traders to set prices and negotiate contracts (McNamara, 2005: 143). A variety of attempts to manage these perceived problems were made. The first of these was the Werner Report (1970), which proposed the creation of a European economic and monetary union. Although the report was endorsed in March 1971 by the member states, only one substantial aspect of its proposals was ever implemented. This related to the creation of an intra-EEC exchange-rate regime, termed the Snake (Dinan, 2004: 133–4). This sought to establish a mechanism that could substitute for Bretton Woods in terms of stabilizing exchange rates among member states. Participants committed themselves to maintaining their currency's value in a narrow band of plus or minus 2.25 per cent relative to each other, deploying the monetary and capital controls necessary to do so (Bladen-Hovell, 2007: 250). The history of the Snake was one of turbulence and failure. Britain withdrew shortly after its establishment and Italy soon followed. Neither could bear the economic pain of staying within the narrow exchange-rate band that had been set. Despite a series of reformulations and relaunches, the French too had withdrawn by 1974 (McNamara, 1998: 109). This failure was partly a product of fundamental differences in approach among the member states in relation to the management of economic crises and inflation. For some, the economic costs of remaining in the system were deemed to be too high. Most typically, the monetary tightening required to arrest a decline in the value of the national currency was judged to be too damaging to growth and efficiency. It was also partly a product of the unique position of the Deutsche Mark in the global monetary system. Germany's currency, supported by the country's strong economy and its central bank's (the *Bundesbank*) unrivalled anti-inflationary credentials, experienced an ongoing process of appreciation. In order to remain within the Snake band, other currencies had to match this appreciating Deutsche Mark. However, few could do so without causing considerable damage to their domestic producers. By 1974, what was left of the Snake had effectively become a Deutsche Mark zone, entirely composed of states that had abandoned any pretence to running an independent monetary policy (Verdun, 2007: 202).

Despite the severity of the challenge, the desire to stabilize exchange rates was sufficiently strong for a second attempt to be launched in 1978, with the establishment of the European Monetary System (EMS). As in the case of the Snake, its purpose was to stabilize exchange rates in order to facilitate trade and investment activity within the common market. However, it sought to overcome the limitations of its predecessor by spreading the cost of stabilizing rates among all participants, with both the weak and the strong members having to intervene when currencies began to diverge from the agreed central rate (Gillingham, 2003: 271–2). Yet it quickly became apparent that the new system was 'more like the Snake than not' (McNamara, 1998: 128). In practice, the *Bundesbank* determined monetary policy for the Deutsche Mark on the basis of a sound money policy for Germany, and other states were required either to take the necessary steps to match this policy or to exit the system. Ultimately, what distinguished the EMS from the Snake, and underpinned its relative success, was the preparedness of the participating states to bear the costs necessary to accommodate themselves to the *Bundesbank*'s actions. For complex reasons, domestic policy priorities had altered in many countries. Though Britain remained outside the Exchange Rate Mechanism (ERM) of the EMS for a decade, most other EU states fought strongly to remain members of the ERM, compromising their traditional Keynesian strategies when it was necessary to do so (McNamara, 1998: 128). The cost of importing German inflation levels through the EMS, in terms of lost growth and higher unemployment, was a price that many states were now prepared to pay. As a result, the 1980s witnessed a substantial reduction in exchange-rate volatility among European currencies, and a rise to dominance of anti-inflationary, stability-oriented monetary policies effectively overseen by the German *Bundesbank* (Bladen-Hovell, 2007: 253).

The experience of the EMS both reflected and furthered the rise of a new monetary policy paradigm that embodied a neo-liberal, anti-inflationary perspective. This paradigm emphasized the necessity of focusing on the creation and maintenance of freer markets and greater price stability. If these conditions were achieved, economic and employment growth would follow as a by-product. These priorities, and the intellectual rationale underpinning them, exercised a growing influence among policymakers in member states, especially among central bankers (McNamara, 1998: 6). Yet the EMS was not itself regarded by many states as a satisfactory mechanism for furthering these policy goals or for solving Europe's monetary problems. This scepticism partly reflected pragmatic concerns about its sustainability. As demonstrated by the periodic realignments and crises that occurred, the longer-term stability of the system could not be assumed. With the rapid growth of private capital flows in the 1980s, the degree of stability achieved from mid-decade was becoming increasingly difficult to sustain (Evans, 2009b: 45). Moreover, the commitment of member states to liberalize capital movements as part of the single market project only served to accentuate these pressures. However, the desire to push on from the EMS to full monetary union was also partly the product of political concerns felt by many member states. Most basically, the design of the system afforded a dominant role to the Deutsche Mark and Germany's *Bundesbank* that was difficult for other states to endure. It embodied a Germanization of European monetary policy, with a German institution effectively setting interest-rate policy for Europe on the basis of German economic needs. The difficulties that this presented to members of the EMS were further exacerbated in the early 1990s when the cost of German unification began to drive up interest rates across Europe. In this context, the argument that a move to fully Europeanize monetary policy would actually serve to repatriate to member states a degree of monetary control was plausible. A European bank would be constrained to set policy on the basis of collective, European requirements. Moreover, member states could expect a seat in the governing councils and a role in policymaking. Neither could ever be achieved while the *Bundesbank* retained its dominance.

How the ambition to create a European monetary system came to be realized is a complex question that need not detain us here. The ultimate prize of wresting control of Europe's monetary policy from the *Bundesbank*'s grip had appeared unfeasible, with even French pressure being rebuffed by Germany. Undoubtedly, the combination of the new policy paradigm and fortuitous changes in the geopolitical context played a major role in altering this situation. The willingness of the German government (if not the *Bundesbank*) to consider the virtues of Europeanizing monetary policy grew as its need for the agreement of its fellow EU member states to the realization of its most profound political ambition – unification – became more urgent (for details, see Dyson and Featherstone, 1998; Moravscik, 1998). But whatever the precise causation, the agreement of monetary union undeniably represented a significant deepening of Europe's economic integration. What is of more concern here is the policy principles that the new system embodied. In this respect, it is ironic that while the *Bundesbank* was hostile to a project that threatened its predominant influence in European monetary policy under the EMS system, the terms of monetary union set out in the TEU amounted to little less than the apotheosis of its structures and practices. Thus, the core policies and institutional features of the new system were modelled closely on German practice, despite the best efforts of France to craft a broader form of economic governance (Pisani-Ferry, 2006: 827). Firstly, and most crucially, the arrangements agreed in the TEU embodied the triumph of a 'sound money' policy in Europe. Such a policy 'privileges price stability as a special economic policy objective' (Dyson, 2000: 27). Price stability was defined as the 'primary objective' of the new European Central Bank (ECB). Moreover, the treaty left it to the ECB itself to determine what constituted price stability. It chose to commit itself to maintaining inflation below 2 per cent per annum. Though charged with supporting 'the general economic policies in the community' and a 'high level of employment and social protection' (Article 3 and Article 105), where these objectives clashed with price stability the latter objective was to take precedence (Martin and Ross, 2004: 8). Indeed, as the new Bank strongly tended to the view that, in the medium to long term, inflation is a monetary phenomenon and that price stability is neutral with respect to growth and employment, it effectively denied its responsibility for encouraging growth and focused its attention squarely on price stability (Dyson, 2000: 27).

The second key characteristic of EMU was the degree of independence granted to the ECB and national central banks (Artis, 2007: 266). This embodied a commitment to depoliticize monetary policy. National acceptance of this disjunction between monetary policy and politics was a precondition of membership of the Eurozone. Neither the ECB nor national central banks were 'to seek or take instructions from any EU bodies or member state governments'. In turn, these bodies had to undertake 'to respect this principle and not seek to influence the decision-making bodies of the ECB or of national central banks' (Martin and Ross, 2004: 8–9). Indeed, such was the strength of the guarantees of central bank independence provided by the treaty that it was more securely entrenched in Europe than it had ever been in Germany prior to EMU (Dyson, 2000: 13). Moreover, the treaty status of these provisions means that they can only be altered in the unlikely circumstance that all 27 member states agree to it in a new treaty.

Some aspects of the German system could not be so readily replicated, however. The success of the *Bundesbank* in the past 'cannot be understood in isolation from the way in which the German political system functioned . . . including relations between government, business and organized labour' (Tsoukalis, 2003: 156). In contrast, the third key characteristic of EMU was the disjunction it established between a Europeanized monetary policy and other areas of economic policy. Effective economic management typically requires the deployment of a range of monetary, fiscal and structural policies (e.g. labour market, regional, etc.), in order to achieve a balanced outcome between the objectives of price stability, employment and growth. By shifting monetary control to a new independent European institution while leaving fiscal responsibility and wage-setting at national level, EMU made policy coordination extremely difficult. Moreover, its terms established a new hierarchy between these areas of policy. Price stability was entrenched at the European level, with national fiscal and wage-setting arrangements forced to accommodate themselves to the unbending demands of the ECB's sound money policy.

Efforts to overcome the coordination deficit have been made, yet they are all predicated on this basic policy hierarchy. Thus, for example, the Stability and Growth Pact (SGP), designed to ensure the compatibility of European monetary and national fiscal policies, clearly placed the burden of accommodation on the latter. Created at Germany's insistence, the terms of the SGP were strongly supported by the ECB and the Commission (Verdun, 2004: 91). The concern was that individual member states might pursue irresponsibly lax fiscal policies, running up excessive deficits that could force up interest rates for all other participating states. An excessive annual deficit was defined as one that exceeded 3 per cent of GDP. The enforcement of the Pact was to be overseen by the Commission. It would conduct annual surveys of member states' fiscal policy, issue early warnings if governments were deemed likely to breach the 3 per cent ceiling and, where such governments failed to make the necessary adjustments, it could initiate an Excessive Deficit Procedure (EDP) (Morris et al., 2007: 298). Ultimately, this process could result in the imposition of punitive fines on the offending state if the Council of Finance and Economic Ministers (Ecofin) chose to act on the Commission's recommendation. Though control of fiscal policy remained at the national level, governments had to ensure that its broad parameters conformed to the requirements of European monetary policy.

Other forms of coordination were also developed. Article 99 of the Maastricht Treaty committed the Council to agreeing 'broad guidelines on the economic policies of member states and the community'. In fulfilment of this requirement a system was devised to establish a set of Broad Economic Policy Guidelines (BEPG) for each member state annually. The guidelines were formulated by the Commission and approved by the Council. Though they were without legal force, the process of their formulation entailed an unequalled degree of scrutiny of national public finances. National policymakers were chivvied, called to account and pressurized in a wholly original fashion. Similar coordination arrangements were developed in relation to the reform of product and capital markets (the Cardiff process), labour market reform (the Luxembourg process), and wage-bargaining (the Cologne process) (Sbragia, 2004: 54). Through collective analysis and discussion, and the shared understandings of problems and solutions that this might produce, the hope was that these processes would generate a substantial degree of cross-national coordination. However, the ECB is exempt from the need to demonstrate flexibility and a willingness to adjust to the actions of others. In practice, national fiscal policy and cross-national coordination must adapt to its policy priorities.

The effectiveness of these mechanisms of coordination has been the subject of considerable scepticism. The brief history of the SGP has tended to validate those critics who argued that its design was neither politically sustainable nor economically desirable. When France, Germany and Italy exceeded the 3 per cent deficit limit in 2003, Commission efforts to impose sanctions foundered on these states' capacity to dissuade Ecofin from acting on its recommendation. Tellingly, this exercise in political strong-arming provoked little reaction in the financial markets, suggesting widespread scepticism about the Pact's value (Leblond, 2006). Reforms agreed in 2005 did increase the flexibility of the SGP (Morris et al., 2007: 301). The time between the diagnosis of a violation and its punishment was lengthened considerably. Moreover, states could avoid censure completely if they mustered a sufficiently convincing economic case for breaching the deficit limits (Chang, 2009: 76). Yet while the terms of the pact have been softened, there is little to suggest that its effectiveness as an instrument of coordination has been significantly enhanced.

There is also scepticism about the BEPG and related processes of 'soft' coordination. Their economic rationale and analytical basis have been characterized as 'fuzzy' (Pisani-Ferry, 2006: 836). They have little coercive power and their effectiveness in shaping national fiscal strategy has yet to be demonstrated. It can be readily imagined that governments may choose to endure the condemnation of national policy by European institutions rather than introduce deeply unpopular domestic reforms. Indeed, when the Commission first sought to call a member state to account on the basis that it had breached the terms of its BEPG in 2001, the country in question (Ireland) refused to alter its policies and stoutly asserted its economic sovereignty (Hodson and Maher, 2004). There is little evidence to suggest that subsequent efforts to modify these mechanisms by incorporating them into broader National Reform Programmes has done much to bridge the 'competency gap' that has emerged in the management of EU economies (Chang, 2009: 151). The institutional provisions for EU-level economic policy coordination are markedly weaker than those established to support central bank independence and price stability (Pisani-Ferry, 2006: 828). The close interlinkage of monetary, fiscal and wage-setting policies that has long been central to the operation of national political economies in Europe is now much more difficult to develop and implement at any level. National capacity has been lost without the creation of an effective compensating European mechanism (Dyson, 2000: 45).

The general challenge presented by monetary union to national product and financial markets is clear. At a stroke, the elimination of exchange rates removed one of the greatest obstacles to closer integration across national borders (Jappelli and Pagano, 2008: 5). However, the form of monetary union adopted presented particularly severe challenges to many national labour market institutions. The effect of the weak policy coordination mechanisms that have been established is to shift the burden of adjusting to economic shocks from macroeconomic and exchange-rate policies to other areas. It is much more likely that demand or supply shocks that previously might have been managed through 'national budgetary, fiscal or incomes policies . . . , will have to be met through the harsher mechanism of recession and employment adjustment (unemployment, mobility of labour and wage flexibility)' (Bartolini, 2005: 197). In the midst of the severe financial crisis and economic downturn in the summer of 2008, the ECB President, Jean-Claude Trichet, gave clear expression to its perspective on the necessary dynamics of adjustment. The 'only goal of the ECB is to ensure price stability in the medium term', while 'responsibility for solving specific economic problems confronting individual euro area members rests with national governments, parliaments and social partners'.[2] What this means in practice is indicated by the frequency with which both the ECB and the European Commission have sought to deflect criticism of the Eurozone's monetary policy regime by insisting that it is overly regulated labour markets that are the genuine inhibitors of economic growth and employment expansion. Together, they have advocated fundamental changes, with the ECB repeatedly calling for 'greater wage differentiation, more latitude for employers in allocating work time, shaping unemployment benefits so as to encourage great labour force participation and . . . a lessening of employment protection' (Sbragia, 2004: 62). For the ECB, effective management of the single currency regime requires the 'disorganization' of key institutional aspects of national political economies. Though neither the Bank nor the Commission has the legal authority to enforce these reforms, the effect of the monetary policy regime that has developed has been to intensify greatly the impact of European integration on long-established national labour market institutions and related industrial relations and welfare arrangements.

### Lisbon

The EU's drive towards a deeper form of liberal market integration did not end with the establishment of monetary union in 1999. The adoption of the so-called 'Lisbon Agenda' in 2000 reflected a determination to press ahead with structural economic reform. Famously, and certainly foolishly, its declared objective was to create 'the most competitive and dynamic knowledge-based economy in the world, capable of sustainable economic growth with more and better jobs and greater social cohesion' by 2010.[3] Substantively, it was 'essentially an attempt to replicate US success' by copying key features of its economic model (Block and Grahl, 2009: 143). The agenda had two principal strands. The first focused on social policy and, in particular, employment policy. The reference model for reform was the US, perceived to have performed much more successfully than Europe in relation to employment growth. The thrust of the proposals was to 'modernize' the so-called 'European Social Model' by reforming national systems of labour market regulation and social protection (Wallace, 2004: 113–15). Europe's excessively 'rigid' labour markets would be rendered more flexible and responsive to changing market conditions through the adoption of 'best practice' policies. In order to identify and disseminate 'best practice', member states were to be drawn into a complex Commission-orchestrated process of cooperation, 'mutual learning' and review. While states would retain their sovereign power to decide in such matters, labour market regulation and related social policy provisions were increasingly incorporated into a European policy community, with the effective Europeanization of national policy as its ultimate goal.[4]

The second major strand of the Lisbon agenda sought to exploit the opportunity presented by the creation of the euro to push forward the integration of EU financial markets. Integration would intensify competition and greater competition would enhance efficiency (ibid.: 105). The core objective was to enable Europe to match the lower capital costs and greater innovative

capacity that the US was perceived to enjoy (Grahl, 2009b: 117). It was anticipated that the scale and dynamism of an integrated European market would
facilitate the development of more open patterns of corporate ownership and,
ultimately, the emergence of a 'share-owning democracy'. European finance
would be substantially remodelled along Anglo-Saxon lines. The realization
of this goal would require a fundamental re-regulation of national financial systems, the great majority of which were bank- rather than securities
market-based in structure. The struggle to replicate the USA's performance
was deemed to necessitate profound institutional change, with all its attendant implications for the structure of corporate ownership and governance in
Europe. If successfully implemented, such a programme would deeply undermine the sustainability of established national models of capitalism in many
member states.[5]

## Limits of Liberalism

While recognizing the liberal deepening that has occurred since the 1980s, an
analysis of the challenge presented by the EU to national governance institutions must also take account of the ambiguities and contested nature of significant aspects of the project. In some policy areas, the effects of significant
countervailing influences on European activity are apparent. In relation to
labour market governance, for example, while the social policy strand of the
Lisbon reform programme may reflect the growing impact of the US example
on European policymakers, EU social policy also embodies the influence of
non-liberal perspectives. It is notable that for Jacques Delors, the activist and
influential Commission President who had driven the single market forward,
the creation of 'social Europe' was necessary precisely to counterbalance
'market Europe' (Dinan, 2004: 225). Most member states signed up to a charter
that sought to establish an irreducible and substantial core of social rights
that the single market would have to respect. The development of 'regime
competition' between national standards that might serve to drive down
levels of protection was deemed to be undesirable. The SEA (1986) provided
for the agreement of new common health and safety standards by Qualified
Majority Vote. The Commission enthusiastically exploited this provision over
the next decade to push through major initiatives relating to working time
and maternity rights (Johnson, 2005: 29). In addition, the anti-discrimination
aspect of European law was broadened significantly in this period. Equal pay
provisions had formed an aspect of the Treaty of Rome. Successive treaties now
strengthened and broadened such social rights. Gender and national equality
protection was given a firm treaty basis in the TEU. The Treaty of Amsterdam
in 1997 extended anti-discrimination rights to cover race, religion and belief,
disability and sexual orientation. Some of these measures had more symbolic
than legal significance (Purdy, 2007: 214). Frequently, the Council of Ministers
shied away from enacting substantial social policy measures (Wallace, 2004:

111). However, it is telling that Margaret Thatcher rejected many of them precisely because they embodied a betrayal of the liberal single-market deal in 1986, and both she and her Conservative successor, John Major, forcefully resisted their introduction (Leibfried, 2005: 248).

Developments in the CAP since the 1980s reflect a similarly complex mix of liberal reform and non-liberal continuity. Thus, on the one hand, changes were introduced during this period that greatly strengthened the impact of market forces on agricultural output. In 1992, reforms introduced by the then Agricultural Commissioner, Ray MacSharry, reduced the guaranteed price level across a wide range of commodities (Ackrill, 2000: 66). Subsequent reforms in 2003 not only further reduced the level of price support, but also provided for the complete 'decoupling' of CAP farm support from output (Colman, 2007: 98–9). As a consequence, food production and prices once more became subject to the laws of supply and demand. On the other hand, this 'market-turn' had very strict limits. While the mechanisms employed to achieve it were radically recast, the commitment to the protection of farm incomes irrespective of market conditions was upheld. Whether farmers chose to continue or cease to produce food, they were guaranteed a payment based on their historical output level. While production and subsidy were 'decoupled', the reliance on historical output data to calculate the level of subsidy per farm perpetuated the unfairness of a system that subsidized larger, and frequently wealthier, producers more than small ones. Though part of the motivation in reforming the policy was to accommodate the enlargements of 2004 and 2007, which would bring in 12 new states, many of which had very large agricultural sectors, the extension of the CAP apparatus to incorporate these new members can be seen as a further entrenchment of the CAP within the life of the EU (Rieger, 2005). While reform was partly driven by the need to accommodate international trade pressures for a reduction in 'market-distorting' agricultural policies, the goal was mostly defensive in nature (Colman, 2007: 98). Moreover, though the reforms largely eliminated the beef mountains and wine lakes, there was no significant reduction in the CAP budget as direct farm payments replaced intervention costs. Indeed, total CAP spending rose from 45.2 per cent of the total EU budget in 1999 to 48.2 per cent in 2004 (European Commission, 2006b: 68). Aspects of agriculture were 'marketized' to some degree in order to save CAP from a more thoroughgoing liberal reform.

These manifestations of equivocation reflect fundamental disagreements amongst member states over how far to press the liberal-reform agenda. Some states continue to favour strongly a liberal vision of Europe in which EU institutions confine themselves to overseeing and sustaining open markets and free competition; others favour a more 'regulated' vision in which the EU acquires the capacity to intervene in markets, redistribute resources and foster close relationships between public and private actors (Hooghe and Marks, 1999: 86). The depth of these divisions strongly informs the dynamics of treaty negotiations and places limits on the innovative capacity of the EU (Pollack, 1998). Moreover, this fundamental difference in aspiration between states also finds reflection within European institutions. Most notably, within the Commission itself there are sharp differences in perspective between those directorates responsible for competition policy and the single market and those responsible for matters such as social affairs and regional policy. Where the former are imbued with a strong liberal economic mindset, the latter typically favour the adoption of positive, 'market-correcting' policies. Such is the distribution of power between states and within European institutions that it is difficult for either side to force through their favoured reform agenda.

The potentially disruptive impact of these divisions on the progress of liberal integration is perhaps best illustrated by the fate of the 'Bolkestein' Services Directive, which came to general public attention during 2005 and 2006. Its purpose was to open up member states' service sectors to cross-border competition by applying the principle of mutual recognition. The proposals provoked great controversy. The issues in dispute partly revolved around the directive's coverage. With the Commission pressing for the most inclusive approach possible, critics feared that it might enforce the liberalization of services with a 'social purpose', thus threatening key aspects of national welfare systems. Reflecting such concerns, France and Germany took the lead in blocking the directive's applicability to healthcare provision. Even more controversial, perhaps, was the proposal to apply the 'country-of-origin' principle to the regulation of services (Nicolaïdis and Schmidt, 2007: 722). If accepted, this would have allowed companies and individuals to provide services throughout the EU while subject only to the laws and regulations of their home country. Pressed strongly by Frederik Bolkestein, the Commissioner responsible for the single market, and his successor Charlie McCreevy, the proposal provoked a storm of criticism from trade unions and left-leaning governments. They feared that it would generate a 'race to the bottom' in social standards, with service providers from those countries with the least onerous regimes enjoying a substantial cost advantage over their more heavily regulated competitors. The issues became highly politicized in the French referendum in 2005 on the proposed Constitutional Treaty, with the 'Polish plumber' coming to symbolize all that was most feared about the increasingly liberal and 'Anglo-Saxon' orientation of EU policy (ibid.: 725–6). In the event, the Commission was forced to compromise and the 'country-of-origin' principle was removed from the directive to be replaced by the less threatening requirement that member states actively facilitate freedom of services by removing or simplifying the administrative obstacles inhibiting foreign service providers (Johnson, 2007: 262). The EU's capacity to enforce the liberal reform of national governance institutions is at least partly constrained by the wider political dynamics of EU lawmaking.

**Table 2.1** Exports of EU15 to other EU members as a percentage of each country's total exports: 2005

| Country | % of total exports |
|---|---|
| Belgium | 76.4 |
| Denmark | 70.5 |
| Germany | 63.4 |
| Ireland | 63.4 |
| Greece | 52.9 |
| Spain | 71.8 |
| France | 62.6 |
| Italy | 58.6 |
| Luxembourg | 89.4 |
| Netherlands | 79.2 |
| Austria | 69.3 |
| Portugal | 79.8 |
| Finland | 56.0 |
| Sweden | 58.4 |
| Britain | 56.9 |

*Source:* Eurostat

## Conclusion

Following the relaunch of integration in the 1980s, the EU really began to make good on the Treaty of Rome's liberal promise. The ambition of its policymakers grew, implementation became more rigorous and fewer areas were exempted from the application of European liberal market rules. For all her subsequent Euroscepticism, an avowed neo-liberal such as Margaret Thatcher could trumpet the single market project as a major victory for economic freedom (Hancher, 1996: 53). Moreover, as a consequence of these developments, European economies were markedly more open, competitive and consumer-oriented by the early twenty-first century than they had been in the 1950s. Cross-border trade, investment and competition had grown considerably. In every instance, the majority of goods and services exported by EU15 states were consumed by other member states. Production and marketing had increasingly become organized on a continental rather than a national level. The degree to which domestic producers were favoured by national public authorities at the expense of foreign competitors had been substantially curtailed. While these changes were not solely the product of EU policy, its creation and development were undoubtedly major contributing factors to this outcome. Member state economies were opened up, cross-border trade was facilitated and a greater degree of competition was encouraged.

The challenge presented by the EU to the sustainability of established national systems of institutional governance has undoubtedly been deepened by the progress of these liberal reform measures. The strengthening of EU competition policy, the commitment to the reconfiguration of the European financial system and the development of new European social, employment and monetary policies clearly impinge significantly on national institutional arrangements in product, financial and labour markets. However, an assessment of whether these European initiatives have enforced a substantial liberal transformation of national systems will require a much more detailed examination of the policies, their implementation and the response of the member states. This task will be undertaken in the chapters that follow.

### FURTHER READING

Dedman (2010) offers a good historical introduction. Gillingham (2003) is an interestingly polemical work. Chang (2009) offers a good overview of the operation of monetary union while Martin and Ross (2004) offer more detailed case examinations of its key policy implications.

3

# National Capitalisms and EU Competition Policy

## Introduction

Liberal systems of political economic governance are predicated on a belief in the superior power of markets to coordinate economic activity efficiently. Effective regulation of the economy requires the state to build and protect free markets. The more successfully this is done, the better the economy will perform. At the heart of any such system of regulation lies competition policy. Free and open competition is central to the efficient functioning of liberal market economies. Measures designed to oversee and uphold competition in the face of attempts to subvert it are vital for good governance. Thus, great importance is attached to the prevention of anti-competitive collusion between private firms, and the restriction of state intervention favouring particular activities or specific actors.

Among West European states, the commitment to protecting and enhancing market competition in the post-war period was partial, at best. In many countries, market coordination of economic activity was not thought to be invariably superior to alternative arrangements. Competition was perceived to be just one of a number of economic virtues, along with stability, long-term investment, the development of cooperative relations between economic actors, etc. Across Europe, public ownership of financial and industrial companies was common and competitor or potential competitor firms often found their operations restricted by laws and regulations (Nicoletti et al., 2000: 38). Administrative or licensing requirements were frequently exploited to favour domestic over foreign firms. The formation of cooperative 'networks' of firms in the same industry was often viewed benignly. In many countries, prohibitions against the formation of private cartels were quite minimal (Martin, 2007: 107). Direct subsidizing of private firms by the state was common practice. It is the case that in Britain and Germany there was a greater commitment to establishing and sustaining competitive market structures. Both countries designed explicit, focused 'competition policies' that sought to identify and eliminate practices restricting trade and competition. This was demonstrated most clearly in the establishment of public agencies empowered to combat market-fixing activities by firms (Eyre and Lodge, 2000). However, even in these states, the opportunity to grant 'exemptions' from the law or to exercise political 'discretion' on the grounds of protecting 'the public interest' was extensive. The regulation of product markets in Western Europe fell a long way short of the liberal economic ideal.

Clearly, these practices and perspectives presented a major obstacle to the creation of a common European market. Public intervention by states frequently favoured local economic agents. Private, collusive anti-competitive behaviour is typically directed against both consumers and new entrants in the market. The persistence of such practices would inhibit the sort of dynamic economic changes that were necessary if genuine European market integration was to be achieved. That the founding member states recognized this problem is indicated by the inclusion in the Treaty of Rome of provisions for regulating competition as it affected cross-border trade. Thus, for example, Article 81 prohibited all agreements and concerted practices between firms affecting trade between states that 'have as their objective or effect the prevention, restriction or distortion of competition within the common market'. At the same time, however, the caution of the founding states in challenging their own practices too radically was also evident. The same article went on to allow for exemptions in respect of agreement or concerted practices that contributed 'to improving the production or distribution of goods or to promoting technical or economic progress'.[1] The proper basis of this distinction between legitimate and illegitimate practices was left unstated. The treaty recognized the existence of a competition problem, provided for action at the European level, but largely left unspecified the nature of that action or the principles that should underpin it.

The substantiation of these treaty provisions has been the work of half a century of activity by the European Commission and the European Court of Justice (ECJ). Ultimately, this effort has proved remarkably fruitful in terms of establishing the Union's power and authority in relation to these matters. Modest early achievements contrast with the contemporary global impact of EU decisions. Corporate giants such as Microsoft have been forced to change their business practices in important ways in order to satisfy Commission demands (Martin, 2007: 117). A major merger between General Electric and Honeywell collapsed in the face of a ruling by the Commission, despite the fact that both companies were incorporated in the USA and had the support of the relevant US regulatory authorities (Cini and McGowan 2009: 127). Member states have been prevented from subsidizing important national companies that were in serious difficulty. Anticipating the likely response of 'Europe' has become a central element of corporate decision-making in respect of major initiatives in inter-firm collaboration or merger-and-acquisition activity. The breadth and impact of European competition policy has reached undeniably impressive proportions.

What is less clear, however, is the effectiveness of EU competition policy in enforcing a liberal transformation in the product-market governance of member states. Has the protection of competition become the overriding principle shaping public policy in this field? To answer this question, it is necessary to examine the ambition and reach of EU policy, the principles that inform its operation and the mechanisms of its implementation. What objectives did policy privilege? How thoroughgoing was the commitment to liberal market principles? Have the highly disparate practices of member states been effectively Europeanized? This chapter will first examine the evolution of the policy from the Treaty of Rome to 2003. It was during this period that its fundamental ambition, legal basis and implementation strategy were developed. It will then examine the process of Europeanization. To what extent has EU policy penetrated national systems of governance and enforced substantial liberal reform? Finally, a major reform of competition policy was introduced in 2004. What was the nature and objective of this reform? Has it deepened or moderated the challenge presented by the EU to national systems of product-market governance?

## European Competition Policy: 1957–1986

It is frequently remarked that the economic power and authority of the EU, and particularly that of the European Commission, are most evident in relation to its competition policy. In its conduct, the European Commission enjoys an exceptional degree of autonomy. It has extensive powers to investigate, determine and punish instances of illegal practice (Hix, 2005: 243). It is the College of Commissioners that decides whether to impose a fine on firms that are in breach of European competition rules or to block a merger on the grounds that it diminishes competition. There is no requirement for its actions to be confirmed by the Council of Ministers. Of course, its behaviour is subject to European law, and it has been the case that on occasion the ECJ has overturned its decisions.[2] However, if the Commission conducts its investigations properly and follows the correct procedure in accordance with the law, it can expect that its action will be upheld. For these reasons, it has been argued that 'competition policy has represented the best example of a genuinely supranational policy, and one that actually possessed "federal" implications for the future administrative and political structure of Europe' (McGowan, 2005: 988).

This pre-eminence did not, however, spring automatically into being on the basis of the provisions of the Treaty of Rome. In the early years of the EU's existence there 'was very little inclination in Brussels to apply the competition articles and no sense of how it was to be done' (Wilks, 2005b: 433). It was not until 1962, with the agreement of Regulation 17, that some flesh was put on the bones of the treaty articles. Moreover, if in retrospect it is evident that the consequence of 17/1962 was to place the Commission at the centre of economic regulation, empowered to determine the permissibility of the great array of intercorporate cooperation agreements affecting cross-border trade, its importance was not immediately appreciated. For the first two decades of the system's life, the political climate was such that the Commission typically adopted a permissive stance towards the strategies of firms and the potential significance of the regulation lay largely unrealized, 'like a ticking time bomb' (Wilks and Bartle, 2002: 164).

Notwithstanding these caveats, however, by the mid-1960s the principles that would inform European competition policy for the next 40 years were taking shape. The central objective of policy would be to protect and enhance the open, competitive character of European markets. However, the precise understanding of competition embodied in this policy was substantially influenced by German 'ordo-liberal' (constitutional liberalism) conceptions of markets and capitalism. These ideas reflect a basic perception that markets are fundamentally fragile. Free-market capitalism is inherently unstable and, left to its own devices, it will degenerate and undermine the conditions necessary for its own survival (Budzinski, 2008: 305). Competition is a vital condition, but it is also self-destructive. In consequence, in order to preserve open and free economic life, public intervention designed to constitute and sustain competition is necessary (Wigger and Nölke, 2007: 491). European practice did not rigidly follow German principles. However, the conception of competition as a product of public action was reflected in the notification system adopted by regulation 17/1962. This required firms to inform the Commission of all proposed inter-company agreements. Until explicitly approved by the Commission, all of these agreements should be considered illegal.

By the same logic, the Commission also took on responsibility for enforcing policy. In contrast to the reliance on private action in the courts to punish anti-competitive practice, which predominated in the US, in the German tradition it was the role of the public agency charged with investigating possible anti-competitive behaviour also to prosecute those responsible. Anti-competitive behaviour was a matter of public rather than private interests and needed to be addressed as such. Moreover, in relation to substantive matters, the Community imbibed 'ordo-liberalism's' distrust of high levels of industry concentration and shared its commitment to achieving economic development in balance with the furtherance of broader social objectives. Thus, the Commission's approach to implementation manifested a belief in the need to reconcile competition concerns with a variety of long-term, developmental goals. It adopted a multi-goal strategy that revealed itself in its willingness to grant so-called 'block exemptions', which defined acceptable agreements that could be made in areas such as technology cooperation or joint initiatives in relation to research and development (Wilks, 2005a: 119). It also allowed the favourable treatment of small and medium-sized firms and facilitated the creation of crisis cartels in industries undergoing traumatic change such as coal, steel and automobiles. Taken together, these provisions generated 'a high degree of legal certainty and public support for the pursuit of long-term strategies' (Wigger and Nölke, 2007: 495). There was a willingness to accommodate the sort of 'non-liberal' forms of inter-firm collaboration that were common in organized systems such as Germany. The policy clearly presented a challenge to many member states in which the protection of competition was a low-priority concern of public policy. However, the nature of this challenge represented a particular, significantly qualified form of liberalism.

## The Single Market and Beyond: 1986–2003

The first substantial toughening of the EU's competition policy began in the 1980s and 1990s, with the launch of the single market programme. This initiative embodied a decisive push to create a liberal, integrated European market; its architects understood that an effective competition policy would be central to its realization. Thus, the Commission White Paper setting out the programme for the market's realization, *Completing the Internal Market*, states that 'as the Community moves to complete the Internal Market, it will be necessary to ensure that anti-competitive practices do not engender new forms of local protectionism which would only lead to a re-partitioning of the market' (European Commission, 1985: 3). The adoption of the single market project saw a growing assertion by the Commission of its prerogatives and a greater determination to acquire the instruments for their effective application. Administrative procedures were overhauled to improve the capacity of the directorate responsible for competition policy within the Commission, DG Comp (until 1999 known as DGIV), to identify and focus on the important cases. Substantial efforts were made to act effectively in previously neglected fields such as state aid. New powers were acquired in the area of cross-border merger control. Though not formally a part of competition policy, the Commission increasingly sought to exploit its authority to liberalize heavily protected sectors such as telecommunications, energy and transport. Indicative of the Commission's growing confidence in this area was the invocation of Article 9 of the Treaty of Rome, which allowed the Commission to issue directives without recourse to the Council of Ministers (Schmidt, 2005: 161). The use of this measure in relation to the telecommunications industry demonstrated a new assertiveness that was upheld by the ECJ in a subsequent judgment. Buttressed by the favourable political climate and the appointment of a series of capable and economically liberal Commissioners to oversee competition policy, European policy evolved substantially across four key sectors.

### Anti-trust: restrictive practices policy and abuse of market dominance

Articles 81 and 82 of the Treaty of Rome afforded the Commission a role in overseeing and protecting the competitiveness of the European market. Article 81 focused on restrictive practices, explicitly prohibiting the direct or indirect fixing of purchase or selling prices; the limitation or control of production, markets and technical development; the sharing out of markets or sources of supply; and the application of dissimilar conditions to equivalent transactions

> **Box 3.1: Competition policy: key treaty and legislative provisions**
>
> **Treaty Provisions**
> *Article 81*
> Restrictive Practices Policy: prohibits agreements or concerted practices between firms which are likely to prevent, restrict or distort trade within the Community.
>
> *Article 82*
> Monopoly Policy: seeks to prohibit 'abuses of dominant position' by companies within a market where this behaviour is likely to affect trade between member states.
>
> *Articles 87–89*
> Prohibits subsidies granted by national or sub-national authorities if they are likely to distort competition between member states. Exceptions are made in certain circumstances relating to social, regional or competitiveness-supporting policies.
>
> **Regulations**
> *Regulation 17 (1962)*
> Sets out the key mechanisms for the implementation of Articles 81 and 82, including: notification requirements; fines and penalties; conditions for exemptions.
>
> *European Community Merger Regulation 1990 (updated 2004)*
> Empowers the Union to regulate mergers between companies over a certain size in order to prevent the development of excessive concentrations of economic power that may have an adverse affect on competition.
>
> *Sources:* Treaty of Rome; Rodger and MacCulloch, 2004

with other trading parties. Essentially, this was a policy aimed at eliminating the formation of cartels among competitors that were designed 'to create or protect a collective monopoly and to make excess profits' (Wilks, 2005a: 119). Article 82 empowered the Commission to take action against undertakings which abused a dominant position in the market by raising prices, restricting output, adopting unfair discounting practices, etc. (Rodger and MacCulloch, 2004: 83). Such monopolistic behaviours were to be subject to sanction.

In the 1960s and 1970s, the enforcement of these provisions was minimal. This was partly owing to difficulties in gathering evidence and poor legal definition. Thus, for example, in relation to one particular form of restrictive practice, namely the abuse of a dominant market position by a small number of firms through oligopolistic behaviour, the Commission frequently struggled to prove its suspicions of collusion (Martin, 2007: 109). In relation to monopolistic behaviour, the Commission found it extremely difficult to establish a clear definition of what constituted abuse and dominance (Cini and McGowan, 2009: 98). However, attempts at effective enforcement were also undermined by the supportive attitude taken by many member states towards the emergence and development of 'national champion' firms. National governments often viewed the behaviour of these firms in a positive light, regarding them as national standard bearers in the global economic market. They were, consequently, reluctant to see their competitive strength on the global stage curtailed by the vigorous application of the norms of European competition policy. Whatever its legal powers, the Commission had to remain sensitive to the balance of political opinion at national governmental level if it was to avoid a powerful backlash against its authority.

In the 1980s and 1990s, this relationship between policy practice and political context began to work much more in the Commission's favour. Emboldened by the member states' renewed commitment to the completion of the single market, it began to adopt a far more vigorous approach to implementing its restrictive practices policy. Under the tenure of Sir Leon Brittan (1988–93), cartel-busting was pursued with enthusiasm, and the imposition of very heavy fines, frequently amounting to many millions of pounds, became much more common. Successful cases were brought in the packaging, steel, cartonboard, cement, shipping, glass-making, plasterboard and brewing industries, amongst others. In 2007 alone, Dutch brewers were fined €273.3 million, manufacturers of gas-insulated switchgear €750 million and 'flat glass'-makers €489 million (Cini and McGowan, 2009: 85). From 1996, the Commission sought to improve its detection rate by offering the possibility of amnesty to firms involved in illegal cartels if they were prepared to betray their fellow-conspirators (Clarke and Morgan, 2006a: 128). In relation to Article 82, in the mid-1980s, the Commission successfully took a case against IBM on the grounds of abuse of a dominant market position in the computer industry (Büthe, 2007: 183). In 2006, it effectively used the threat of multi-million euro fines to force Microsoft to share key technical information with rival firms (Martin, 2007: 117). The renewed liberal commitment of the member states, manifested in the single market project, enabled the Commission to implement the treaty's anti-trust provisions with a new vigour.

### Merger policy

The importance of the single market project as a catalyst for enhancing the competition policy role of the Commission is also clearly evident in respect of merger-control policy. The Treaty of Rome had not provided for such a policy. In the context of the 1950s and 1960s, industry concentration was widely viewed by national governments as necessary in order to reap economies of scale (Büthe, 2007: 186). None of the founding states had national merger policies, with Germany the first to acquire one in 1973. Though this relaxed, permissive attitude at national level did alter in the light of experience, member states were not prepared to countenance the Commission gaining the authority to act in this area, and its attempt in 1973 to introduce a regulation to cover mergers was rebuffed (Cini and McGowan, 2009: 129). However, with the adoption of the SEA the situation changed. The number of cross-border mergers in the EU had grown from 115 in 1982–3 to 622 in 1989–90

(Tsoukalis, 1993: 103). With the establishment of a genuine single market this trend would certainly intensify. Given their restricted jurisdictions, national authorities were poorly placed to police this activity effectively (Morgan, 2006: 79). In consequence, member states were constrained to acquiesce in the formation of a European policy, though the precise nature of this policy was the subject of intense political conflict. Some states were very concerned about the threshold level set for allocating responsibility to national authorities or the Commission. Others were particularly preoccupied by the degree of discretion left to the Commission in coming to a final decision on cases. Perhaps of greatest concern were the criteria for determining whether a concentration was anti-competitive or not. In particular, France pressed for account to be taken of industrial policy considerations, such as the creation of powerful 'Euro-champion' firms that could take on their Japanese and American counterparts on the world stage. Negotiations threatened to drag on indefinitely. However, legal developments helped to truncate debate. An ECJ judgment on a case involving Philip Morris appeared to open up the possibility that Article 82 could be applicable to some mergers (Rodger and MacCulloch, 2004: 205). If states failed to agree a merger policy, they risked Commission and ECJ activism generating a de facto system over which they exercised little or no influence.

The European Community Merger Regulation (ECMR), which was finally agreed in December 1989, was the result of compromise between competing national and European concerns. Thus, on the one hand, it succeeded in establishing a strong policy with responsibility for all mergers with a 'community' dimension. These were defined as mergers between firms with an aggregate turnover of more than €5 billion worldwide and €250 million within the EU. Where 'more than two-thirds of turnover fell within the respective territory' and turnover figures failed to meet the threshold, national law was applicable (Budzinski and Christiansen, 2005: 315). Article 2 of the ECMR clearly stated its purpose, declaring that 'a concentration which creates or strengthens a dominant position as a result of which effective competition would be significantly impeded in the common market shall be . . . incompatible with the common market'.[3] In addition, the terms of the regulation served to secure the powerful institutional position of the Commission itself. It gained the right to investigate, accuse, decide and sanction. On the other hand, the thresholds triggering Commission involvement were set at a high level, ensuring that the national authorities would retain control over all but the largest cases. Moreover, in response to German pressure, the regulation provided for investigations to be referred back to national authorities where the proposed merger threatened to affect significantly competition within a particular member state (Rodger and MacCulloch, 2004: 212).[4] However, notwithstanding these features, the ECMR clearly marked a substantial advance in the Commission's authority over the regulation of competition in the single market.

The operation of this policy has been heavily criticized for the opacity and highly politicized nature of decision-making. It is the College of Commissioners

that makes the final determination on whether a merger can proceed. Critics argue that, too often, the concerns of Commissioners have reflected the interests of their respective home governments rather than the need to uphold the principles of liberal market competition (Hix, 2005: 245). In the case of a proposed takeover of Perrier by Nestlé, for example, the Commission demonstrated a sensitivity to its implications for local concerns that was condemned by supporters of a more robust competition approach (Cini and McGowan, 1998: 126). Defenders of the Commission's record can point to major decisions it has taken in the teeth of industrial and national governmental resistance. Thus, the Commission blocked a proposed merger between General Electric and Honeywell that had the approval of the US authorities in one instance, while, in another, it prevented the merger of aircraft manufacturers Aérospatiale and de Havilland, in spite of very active lobbying by the French and Italian governments in its support (Cini and McGowan, 2009: 154). Suffice to say that the nature of the College of Commissioners leaves it open to political influence, but its record does not support the claim that sectional, state interests always, or even often, determine outcomes.

### State aid

The European Union's policy on state aid represents a direct challenge to the close relations between state and business that exist in many member countries. Its objective is to control the activities of governments through a process of external review and, as such, it is an inherently supranational policy (Büthe, 2007: 189). The basis of the Commission's authority in this field was laid down in the Treaty of Rome. Article 87 (Consolidated Treaties) stated that: '[A]ny aid granted by a Member State or through State resources in any form whatsoever which distorts or threatens to distort competition by favouring certain undertakings or the production of certain goods shall, in so far as it affects trade between Member States, be incompatible with the common market.' Though the treaty did not offer a precise definition of state aid, the policy has come to encompass a very broad range of state actions in relation to tax policy, public holdings in firms, the provision of state guarantees to firms or industries, the preferential provision of goods and services to particular firms or industries, and direct subsidies to firms, industries and regions. Provisions for exemptions to these restrictions were also made in Article 87. Aid may be legitimate if it is designed to overcome market failures. Paragraph 3 provides for discretionary exemption where it is intended to 'promote the economic development of areas where the standard of living is abnormally low'; to facilitate 'the development of certain economic activities or of certain economic areas'; to 'promote the execution of an important project of common European interest or to remedy a serious disturbance in the economy of a Member State'. The opaqueness of these provisions led to considerable uncertainty about what did or did not constitute legitimate state support. In practice, the definition of state aid has frequently been the product of Commission decisions or ECJ rulings 'that fine-tune, or sometimes radically extend, the range and type of measures that are subject to control' (Wishlade, 2006: 232). In the absence of substantial legislation, EU institutions have enjoyed a considerable freedom to press forward with their own agenda.

Some degree of clarity was achieved with the adoption of the 1999 regulation on state aid procedures. It decreed that member states must notify and gain the approval of the Commission before they can implement an aid measure (Martin, 2007: 123). Governments can expect Commission approval where their proposals:

- facilitate innovation, research and development;
- help disadvantaged regions to guarantee cohesion and equal opportunity;
- contribute to the creation of secure, viable, long-term employment for EU citizens.[5]

As a general rule, where aid is 'horizontal' in nature – that is non-discriminatory in terms of individual firms, sectors or regions – the Commission adopts a favourable attitude. However, where this is not the case, the Commission is quite rigorous in its application of social, employment or regional development tests in evaluating the proposals (Wishlade, 2006: 245–50). Moreover, though not formally a part of the state aid policy, the Commission has also sought to prevent the discriminatory use of public procurement programmes. Practices such as outright exclusion of competing firms, domestic content rules or opaque bidding and tendering procedures that favour local, 'insider' firms at the expense of others are forbidden. Much that national governments had done in the past, under the broad rubric of 'industrial policy', is now deemed to be illegal under EU rules.

The Competition Commissioner, Nellie Kroes, has justified the state aid policy on the grounds that it is 'essential to maintaining a level playing field for free and fair competition in the Single Market'.[6] Without such a policy, it is argued, there would be a real possibility that each government would favour its own national firms in order to advantage them vis-à-vis their foreign competitors. Such 'beggar-thy-neighbour' policies would undermine the entire integration project. However, the importance attached to controlling state aid is a relatively recent phenomenon. Until the completion of the customs union in 1968, the issue was largely irrelevant. In the 1970s, when states frequently offered enormous subsidies to national firms and industries in order to ameliorate the impact of successive recessions on jobs and prosperity, the political climate was utterly uncongenial to the Commission's development of a forceful policy on state aid. Rather, as noted in chapter 2, the Commission itself toyed with proposals for an interventionist European industrial policy that could supplement, if not supplant, national efforts. As in so many other areas of competition policy, the development of a more robust policy had to await the liberal turn by member states in the 1980s. Only then was the political climate conducive to the formulation of an active policy that took as its task the disciplining of the actions of national governments.

### Sectoral liberalization

The final key aspect of the EU's competition regime concerns the liberalization of the so-called 'network' industries of telecommunications, energy, railways and airline transport. Traditionally, these sectors were heavily protected by national governments and often used as instruments rather than objects of public policy. Many were considered to form 'natural monopolies' because the technical requirements for their operation, such as networks of wires or pipes, were too costly for potential competitors to duplicate. In consequence, it was deemed necessary to create a single operator, often publicly owned. Moreover, the provision of energy, transport or a universal postal system was frequently conceived to be a matter of 'public interest', different in nature from ordinary economic activity and, therefore, exempt from standard regulatory rules. This special status served to remove them from the remit of European competition policy. However, from the 1980s, a combination of technological and political change has transformed this situation (Thatcher, 2004: 766). New networks or network-sharing technologies have undermined the claim of many such industries to be 'natural' monopolies (Jordana et al., 2006: 443). Simultaneously, in many countries a mixture of the desire to stimulate service improvements, reduce public financial commitments and enhance efficiency has weakened their politically protected status. As a result, they have become increasingly subject to competition constraints imposed and policed by independent regulatory agencies in accordance with EU law. Rules on accounting transparency, market access, price-setting in monopolistic situations and state subventions have all served to open up traditionally close, if not fetid, relationships between service providers, equipment suppliers and governments. The consequences have been significant. In a comparative study of Britain, Germany and France, Thatcher concludes that all three countries have moved 'towards a competitive regulated market', weakening in the process the role of non-market coordination mechanisms that have traditionally been particularly influential in France and Germany (2007a: 167).

The earliest and most substantial liberalization initiative concerned the telecommunications sector. The task facing liberalizers was immense. Until the 1980s, member states' telecommunications systems were generally characterized by publicly owned operators enjoying a monopoly control over supply, the distributional network and almost all services (Thatcher, 2001: 561). The EU's attempt to restructure these systems was initially quite tentative. Acting on Commission proposals, the Council of Ministers adopted a set of non-binding *Recommendations* that encouraged the harmonization of telecommunications standards across national systems and the introduction of competitive tenders into the process of public procurement for at least 10 per cent of equipment orders (ibid.: 562–3). This initiative was followed by similar attempts to ensure common specification of equipment and shared technological developments. However, in the late 1980s and early 1990s, more robust liberalizing measures were passed. New directives ended the right of member states to have legal monopolies over the supply of advanced services such as fax, email, etc. The 1990 Public Procurement Directive enforced public competitive tenders in supply contracts for telecommunications. The 1990 Open Network Directive laid down a set of principles governing access to the telecommunications infrastructure with a view to reducing the control of national telecom providers that owned and operated the system (Cubbin, 2006: 184). This pattern of liberalization was extended in the mid-to-late 1990s to cover newly emerging services such as satellite and mobile telecoms. Such was the degree of 'normalization' in the sector that, by mid-decade, general competition policy could be applied to the myriad takeovers, joint ventures, and cooperation agreements initiated by increasingly internationally oriented companies such as Deutsche Telekom and France Télécom. In 2002, in an attempt at simplification, the welter of liberalizing directives was incorporated into a new integrated regime that came into effect the following year. These changes served also to strengthen the role of the Commission by requiring national regulators to consult with it more frequently (ibid.).

The extent of liberalization achieved in other network industries has not matched that of telecommunications. In the crucially important electricity-generating industry, for example, a directive (96/92/EC) passed in 1996 simply set out a framework establishing broad principles. Countries were provided with a number of alternative methods of implementing them that, in practice, allowed enthusiastic and reluctant liberalizers to pursue their preferred paths (ibid.: 189). Governments were to move towards liberalization but the precise mechanics of how to do so, the regulatory regime that should be adopted to oversee the new system and the precise date by which the market as a whole was to be fully opened were all left unspecified. Instead, broad targets were set. By 2000, each state had to have opened 30 per cent of the national market to competition. By 2003, that figure had to rise to 35 per cent. States that were more committed to liberalization were free to press forward more quickly, and by 2000 the Commission estimated that some 66 per cent of the overall European market was open.[7] However, the EU regime did allow more restrictive forms of restructuring that were exploited by states less committed to liberalization. Thus, integrated companies with control over transmission and distribution were still permitted, even though this would allow them to dominate the market. Moreover, while new directives set a 2007 deadline for the full liberalization of the electricity market, defined as the right of all consumers to choose their preferred supplier from a range of alternative options, states still enjoyed considerable leeway to determine the structure of the new systems operation. Thus, for example, the French government retained a key ownership stake in EDF and has sought to manage the process of change in order to maximize national advantage (Bauby and Varone, 2007).

Notwithstanding these limitations, the role of the Commission and competition policy in enforcing change has been clearly evident in sensitive economic areas. DG Comp has repeatedly applied its anti-trust and merger power to prevent national attempts to evade the core liberalizing thrust of policy. Thus, for example, in Spain a long-term contract agreed between Gas Natural, a gas supplier, and Endesa, an electricity producer, would effectively have served to close the sector to new entrants. A Commission investigation forced the rewriting of the contract to render it more pro-competitive.[8] In Portugal, a proposed takeover of Gas de Portugal by the local electricity supplier, Energias de Portugal, in alliance with the Italian energy group ENI, was blocked by the Commission on the grounds that it would only strengthen the already substantial dominance of the market by the two Portuguese companies.[9] Moreover, where large and potentially dominant firms have emerged, the Commission has actively sought evidence of price fixing. Thus, in early 2009, Commission officials conducted a surprise inspection at EDF's Paris headquarters in search of evidence of wrongdoing.[10] The energy sector is now an active front in the ongoing conflict between the principles of competition policy and the practice of national industrial policy.

## National Institutions Transformed?

Clearly, the EU has established itself as a major actor in policing competition in the ever more integrated European market. The Commission enjoys an exceptional capacity to control the development and implementation of this policy. Its decisions on mergers have had a major influence on the global evolution of the computing and aviation industries. It has busted cartels in a large number of sectors. Member states are now severely constrained both in the nature and the quantity of aid they can provide to productive enterprises, whether public or private. The development of a European competition policy with clear objectives and powerful instruments of implementation is undeniable. Yet if its triumph is to be complete, it must succeed in transforming national competition policies. Most instances of collusive, anti-competitive behaviour occur within rather than across states. It is national authorities that must investigate, judge and sanction these activities. If the governance of product markets is to be remade on liberal economic principles, national authorities must internalize the norms and practices of EU competition policy. The EU's ultimate challenge is to realize a thoroughgoing Europeanization of national policies and practices.

### Europeanizing at work: National Competition Authorities

There is clear evidence that a substantial Europeanization of national competition regimes has taken place in many member states. In a number of countries where competition had previously hardly figured as a concern of public policy, National Competition Authorities (NCAs) modelled on EU practice have been established. Thus, in the Netherlands, Sweden and Italy, extremely underdeveloped national regimes have been substantially overhauled in accordance with the legal and institutional pattern developed at the European level. In 1993, the Netherlands and Sweden established new competition agencies modelled on DG Comp (Wilks and Bartle, 2002: 150). In 1998, the Dutch switched from an abuse regime, within which restraints of trade were accepted unless it could be demonstrated that they damaged the common good, to a prohibition regime modelled on the EU. Under the new system, the burden of justifying an exemption from the law fell on those who were seeking to restrain trade, and the Netherlands shifted from being a 'cartel paradise' to an ardent implementer of European competition policy norms (van Waarden and Drahos, 2002: 915–17). In the Italian case, the wording of Law 287/1990, which created and empowered the new national competition authority,[11] was taken directly from Articles 81 and 82 of the Treaty of Rome (Giraudi, 2003: 161).

Where national regimes already existed, the challenge of Europeanization differed in nature. Such systems had developed their own institutional structure and operating principles; effective Europeanization required their overhaul or displacement. Thus, for example, competition policy in Britain had developed in the context of post-war reconstruction. The Monopolies and Restrictive Practices Act was passed in 1948 and further developed in 1973 by the Fair Trading Act. Decisions were based on 'case-by-case investigations of specific problems by a panel of experts with reference to the "public interest"' (Eyre and Lodge, 2000: 65). Voluntarism and decision-making discretion lay at the heart of the system. Companies were expected to volunteer information to the authorities but there was no formal notification requirement, in contrast to the developing European system. The decision on whether to refer a case for investigation by the Monopolies and Mergers Commission (MMC), or whether to take heed of its recommendations when it had completed an investigation, was left to the discretion of the Secretary of State for Trade and Industry. It is notable that reforms introduced in 1973, the year of Britain's accession to the EU, only deepened the distinctiveness of this regime. The Office of Fair Trading (OFT) was added to the organizational mix, though the MMC retained its investigative role. Moreover, despite considerable criticism, the Secretary of State continued to enjoy the right to decide on what action to take in the event of a negative finding by the MMC/OFT. Yet despite this heritage, a signifi-cant convergence towards the EU system was initiated in 1998 (Clarke, 2006: 23). The Competition Act shifted the basis of policy from voluntary coopera-tion and decision-making discretion to a juridical and coercive regime that was now much closer in type to that of the EU. The discretionary power of the Secretary of State was eliminated. Firms found guilty of illegal activities faced the possibility of fines of up to 10 per cent of their UK revenues. The public interest criterion was explicitly rejected in favour of a focus on the impact of actions on competition. The act incorporated substantial elements of Articles 81 and 82 of the EC Treaty, prohibiting any agreements that might restrict competition or involve an abuse of a dominant position. Moreover, the Act specified that national decisions 'must have regard to the decisions of the European Commission', suggesting that 'guidance is provided by EU law, not UK law' (Zahariadis, 2004: 57). Convergence with EU practice was not total. Merger control and complex monopolies were excluded from the 1998 act. The new regime was to be operated by the old institutions, albeit in slightly altered form. In certain aspects, most notably pertaining to the criminalizing of competition law enforcement, British policy reflected the influence of US rather than EU practice (Clarke and Morgan, 2006a: 116). However, notwithstanding these qualifications, it is evident that a significant degree of Europeanization has taken place.

In Germany, too, a substantial but not complete process of Europeanization is apparent. Established in the post-war period under the influence of 'social market' thinking and the US military administration, it embodied a rather different approach from that of Britain. In contrast to the latter's voluntarism and flexibility, it operated in a highly juridical way with 'its role to apply and interpret legal norms rather than to consider the "public interest"' (Eyre and Lodge, 2000: 66). Though there was some provision for political discretion in the application of policy, the agency responsible for implementing the policy, the Federal Cartel Office (*Bundeskartellamt*), gained a peculiar status of being 'above' government, charged with safeguarding 'the integrity of the market system itself and not merely to secure particular administrative efficiencies' (Wilks and Bartle, 2002: 162). For many decades, the balance of opinion in Germany was that there was no need to Europeanize this system. As late as 1990, the German government spurned the opportunity to harmonize with European practice when it legislated reform of the national system. However, this stance altered somewhat during the 1990s and a substantial degree of convergence with 'reference model Europe' was proposed (Eyre and Lodge, 2000: 72). The wording of the EC Treaty setting out the prohibition on horizontal agreements was incorporated directly into German law, while its merger provisions were brought more closely into line with those of the EU. The degree of convergence was not total. Thus, for example, while a European 'prohibitive approach' was introduced in relation to 'abuses of dominant market position', a specifically German 'split definition' of market dominance was maintained (ibid.). However, although convergence was less complete than in Britain, overall it is valid to conclude that the German system was subject to a substantial degree of Europeanization.

### Europeanization at work: the power of ideas

Though the process was neither complete nor equally manifest across all member states, national competition regimes had clearly been significantly

Europeanized by the early twenty-first century. The extent of this convergence was all the more remarkable given the absence of any formal legal EU require-ment for member states to introduce such changes. No directive provided for such measures, while the ECJ had never dealt directly with a national competition act (van Waarden and Drahos, 2002: 924). Moreover, there is little evidence to suggest the operation of a dynamic of 'regime competition' in this area. In relation to competition policy, there is little opportunity for firms to 'regime shop'. The only option 'for an enterprise which wants to avoid the cartel rules of, say, Germany is not to do business in Germany' (ibid.: 915). Substantial convergence on EU norms appears to have occurred in the absence of significant coercive or regulatory competition pressures. Understanding the dynamics of change can offer insight into the nature of the EU's challenge to national systems of institutional governance.

A range of alternative explanations of the process of Europeanization has been offered. The producer-group interest approach contends that national systems were reformed in response to the demands of business interests. The shifting perspectives of business led to changes in national regulatory regimes. Certainly, in the British case there is evidence to support such an interpretation. Thus, in 1992, the suggestion in a government White Paper that British law should converge with EU practice was rejected largely as a consequence of the opposition of the Confederation of British Industry (CBI) (Suzuki, 2000: 11). Subsequently, the CBI reversed its stance and, at least partly in consequence, the 1998 reform embodied a substantial shift towards EU norms (Baldi, 2006: 513). However, in many other member states, the influence of business on developments was much less significant. Neither in Austria nor in the Netherlands did business lobbies exercise significant influence over reform. In the Dutch case, business support for adaptation to EU law followed rather than led the decision by government to introduce the prohibition principle (van Waarden and Drahos, 2002: 927). In Italy, business accepted the creation of an anti-trust authority only reluctantly as a necessary price to pay for entry to Europe (Giraudi, 2003: 142). In Germany, the lobby-ing efforts of the Federation of German Industries (BDI) were condemned by critics as an attempt to ease the competition pressures on its members, and its attempts to influence reform were marked by failure (van Waarden and Drahos, 2002: 924).[12] In general, the role of business leaderships in driving the Europeanization of national competition-policy regimes has been marginal.

The extent to which the status quo came to be regarded as unsustainable appears to have been of more importance in shaping the progress of reform. In the case of states where competition policy had been largely absent, the initiation of the single market project and the related strengthening of the European competition-policy regime made it much more difficult to continue ignoring the issue at national level. Change was unavoidable. Once the need for major reform at national level was accepted, the question became: what sort of reform? For countries with little policy tradition in this area, the EU offered a ready-made template to copy. The Italian experience illustrates this dynamic. Anxious to participate fully in the single market and single currency projects, it needed to demonstrate its Euro-commitment. The development of a credible competition-policy regime was a necessary part of this process. Adopting the European model was a relatively quick, easy and effective way to establish the credibility of its pro-integration credentials. Once the initial commitment to strengthening national competition policy was made, the political and practical attractions of incorporating European norms and prac-tices into the new domestic regime were considerable.

Similarly, in the case of states with established competition policies, it was the combination of a de-legitimated status quo and the exemplary power of EU ideas and practices that proved decisive in shaping developments. In both Germany and Britain, the initial momentum for change was triggered by a perception that national systems had failed to fulfil their function effectively. In Germany, serious consideration of convergent reform only emerged in the 1990s, in the context of a deteriorating economic performance. In Britain, the pressures for reform arose 'because of a recognition in the 1980s of the inad-equacies of the existing national competition regime' (Baldi, 2006: 515). Eyre and Lodge argue that by the 1980s, policy was 'held in widespread disrepute and arguments for change were promoted by all actors in the policy domain' (2000: 68). Just as the wholesale borrowing of EU policy norms by states such as Italy reflected the recognition of the inadequacies of the status quo, the initial impetus for reform in Britain and Germany reflected dissatisfaction with established national policy.

However, once reform commenced in Britain and Germany, the role of Europe as a generator of ideas again appears to have been very substantial. In particular, there is evidence that the bureaucratic elites responsible for developing competition policy and operating NCAs in both countries had become increasingly influenced by European perspectives during the 1980s and 1990s. This 'cultural' evolution was at least partly the product of the inter-action between the national agencies and the Commission. In the British case in particular, these contacts appear to have generated the development of an 'epistemic community' possessed of a shared understanding of the problems faced by its members and the appropriate solutions that should be adopted. Thus, in a study of reform in Britain, Zahariadis notes that, despite the fact that merger policy was excluded from the 1998 Competition Act's coverage, European ideas about how best to regulate them 'seeped into the British policy community by way of increasingly more frequent interaction between national civil servants and their EU counterparts and between British and other European firms' (2005: 664). In her study of the same process, Suzuki concludes that reform in Britain was preceded by a 'silent revolution' in the attitudes of competition-policy officials who came to favour the more robust prohibition rules and enforcement procedures of the EU system (2000: 17). As a consequence of these processes, policy elites in both countries shifted from 'a passive symbolic defence of a competitive market economy to an aggressive promotion of market freedoms' (Wilks and Bartle, 2002: 170). More generally, Van Waarden and Drahos have identified a process whereby the internationalization of epistemic communities has led competition officials 'to develop a greater interest in the solutions of their counterparts in other member states and in the cases and solutions of the EU officials' (2002: 931). Ideas developed and diffused through cross-national expert interaction appear to have played a decisive role in shaping events.

Of course, the power of ideas can and has cut both ways. There is no guarantee that all participants in the network will come to share a common view. Thus, in the German case, the reluctance of the Federal Cartel Office to embrace Europeanization wholeheartedly reflected a certain *hauteur* based on a deeply rooted sense of its own success in sustaining the 'ordo-liberal' economic model established in the post-war period (Eyre and Lodge, 2000). It remained unconvinced of the superiority of the European way and this moderated the extent of Europeanization that occurred in Germany. In the British case, whatever the preferences of civil servants or staff of the MMC, attempts at substantial Europeanization were stymied for a long time by the Eurosceptic ideas of the governing Conservative Party. Long after officials at the Department of Trade and Industry and the OFT had come to favour reform, a succession of ministers, stretching from Norman Tebbit, through Nicholas Ridley to Ian Lang, baulked at the prospect of such a Europhile venture. The power of epistemic communities in the competition-policy field to shape reform depended on the emergence of a propitious political circumstance, namely the accession to power of a more Euro-friendly Labour government. However, notwithstanding these caveats, there is substantial evidence to support the contention that, in the area of competition policy, it was the combination of failing domestic institutions and the quality of EU ideas and practices that proved to be the most potent agent of Europeanization.

### The limits of transformation

The development and diffusion of formal competition-policy regimes across member states from the late 1980s clearly demonstrate the EU's ability to effect substantial change in the institutions of national economic governance. Whether through the creation of powerful legal instruments or the more genteel dynamic of elite interaction and epistemic community formation, it provided the context, much of the basic impetus and an exemplary model for change in member states. Ultimately, however, the purpose of competition policy is to strengthen the functioning of markets by restructuring the operation of national economies. Its effectiveness can only be judged on the basis of evidence that EU markets are more liberal and competition more intense. Has it reduced the capacity of producers to gain and exercise 'market power' at the expense of the consumer? Has it served to open up formerly closed sectors to competition? Has it succeeded in transforming national governance institutions and overcoming the tendency of many European governments to favour their own producers at the expense of foreign firms?

While there is evidence of change in the condition of European markets, it is doubtful that this change can be legitimately characterized as radical in degree. Even after decades of European competition policy and significant Europeanization of national regimes, analyses of the intensity of product-market competition reveal that great variation persists across European states. Thus, an OECD study published in 2000 identified a complex pattern of diversity that defied easy generalization. Scoring individual countries according to their product-market regulation, it found that member states varied little in the degree of outward-oriented regulation, affecting barriers to investment and competition from non-member states. The EU does appear to regulate effectively the trading relationship between the member states and the rest of the world. In contrast, however, in respect of so-called 'inward-oriented' regulation, which encompasses such factors as public ownership, bureaucratic barriers to entrepreneurship, etc., substantial diversity among member states persists. In the case of Britain and Ireland, for example, there is relatively low state control and few barriers to entrepreneurship. In contrast, in the case of Italy, it was found that despite privatization and recent regulatory reforms, 'state-controlled enterprises are still numerous and recourse to "command and control" regulations and price controls in competitive industries is frequent relative to other countries' (Nicoletti et al., 2000: 30). Moreover, in many countries access to a large number of industries continues to be 'restricted by laws and regulations that limit the number of competitors' while 'administrative burdens on start-ups remain significant' (ibid.). Where the EU's remit is most developed, liberal-oriented regulation is predominant. However, in respect of inward-oriented policies where domestic regulation remains dominant, the traditional practices of economic governance tend to persist.

More general measures of product-market competition in Europe generate equally mixed conclusions. One approach has sought to identify changes in the pattern of price dispersion. This measure is predicated on the premise that exceptionally high prices in a particular country or commodity may be an indication of the ability of producers to gain 'market power' as a consequence of weak competition. Studies of price dispersion in the EU suggest that while the establishment of the single market did have an immediate and strong effect in the early 1990s, in more recent years the process appears to have lost steam (Gjersem, 2004: 7). A survey produced in 2001 by the European Commission itself found that cross-country dispersion remains on average four times higher than dispersion within countries.[13] While European markets have grown more competitive, they still do not match the degree of integration achieved within national markets. It appears that significant barriers to trade across member states remain.

The extent of illiberal continuity partly reflects persisting weaknesses in the implementation of EU policy. In respect of the state aid regime, for example, the impact on national practice has been very uneven. There have been spectacular cases affecting the British (Rover), French (Renault) and German (Volkswagen) car industries, where Commission rulings have forced firms to repay substantial amounts of aid received from national or regional governments. In general terms, the figures on total state aid provided by member states do suggest a considerable diminution in scale and a shift in composition of state aid between the early 1990s and 2005. Excluding aid to agriculture, fisheries and transport, the total amount provided by member governments has fallen from €75 billion to €52 billion, which represents a decline from 0.84 per cent of total GDP to 0.40 per cent.[14] Furthermore, the overall focus of expenditure has shifted significantly towards the 'horizontal' type approved of by the Commission. Such aid consumed some 79 per cent of total aid in 2003, compared to just 50 per cent in the mid-1990s.[15] At the same time, however, where governments are hostile to its decisions, the Commission has often struggled to enforce them effectively. It is notable that only a small percentage of the aids banned by the Commission are ever recovered (Wishlade, 2006: 237). Moreover, notwithstanding the Commission's hostility towards the use of 'restructuring' aid by member states, considerable amounts of public money are still transferred to support ailing firms in key sectors. Indeed, in many instances the failure of this aid to return the firm in question to profitability has occasioned further grants of public support. The fate of Italy's national airline, Alitalia, which despite the Commission, was repeatedly bailed out until its final demise in 2008, merely represents an extreme example of the process. There is also evidence that the impact of the policy, and the broad liberal values it embodies, has varied greatly across member states, in respect of their propensity both to subsidize and to break EU rules. Thus, figures for the period between 2002 and 2004 show that the Commission approved the provision of state aid by Italy on 349 occasions as opposed to 299 for Germany, 220 for France, 203 for Spain and 156 for Britain. More tellingly, perhaps, the same report recorded 35 negative judgements by the Commission on German aid, compared to 25 in the case of Italy, 12 for France and just 6 for Britain.[16] In respect of public procurement, Eurostat data demonstrates that even after a decade of sustained effort by the Commission, only about 15 per cent of the value of total procurement is advertised throughout the Union, with Germany lagging behind with just 6 per cent (Gjersem, 2004: 31). There is a persisting desire and capacity on the part of many national governments to continue favouring local or national firms at the expense of others.

Even when EU policy appears to have been successful in effecting liberal-oriented reform, on closer inspection the picture often becomes somewhat murkier. In the telecommunications and energy sectors, for example, while the degree of liberalization achieved has been substantial, many regulatory practices have retained a distinctly national character. In case after case economic nationalism has proved a more potent force in shaping the behaviour of economic and political actors than have the norms of EU competition policy. Thus, an analysis of telecoms reform in Spain and Portugal found little to support the contention that new EU-level policies 'constrain traditional mercantilist behaviour by governments and market actors' (Jordana et al., 2006: 446). While new regulatory authorities were established as required by EU policy in both countries, in each case steps were also taken to ensure that 'the ministries kept enough power . . . to protect "national interests" mainly through the promotion of national champions' (ibid.: 448). When the decision was taken to privatize the national post and telegraph utilities, the timing and structure of the process was designed to ensure that the successor companies were strong, capable competitors who could meet any challenge from outside. Moreover, the decision to privatize did not mean that governments eschewed industrial intervention. Thus, in both Spain and Portugal, the state retained so-called 'golden shares', effectively blocking unwanted takeover bids from foreign competitors. The entire process was regarded as an opportunity 'to shape the sector in ways that would have a long-term impact on the extent of competition and on the structure of ownership of the operators' (ibid: 449). European regulatory schemes were exploited to achieve industry modernization, but when they were seen to threaten national interests, 'both liberal and European principles were modified' (ibid.: 445).

Such nationalist motives were by no means confined to the Iberian peninsula. France successfully bartered its acceptance of the EU telecoms regime for the Commission's approval of an alliance between Deutsche Telekom and France Télécom. More broadly and substantially, its support for the general liberalization of telecoms was informed by the opportunity presented for French operators to expand abroad into formerly closed markets. It provided the means to 'attack overseas monopolies and attempts to restrict French suppliers, who have often been larger and better capitalised than other European suppliers, notably in Italy, Spain and Germany' (Thatcher, 2007a: 161). From energy to telecoms, the precise structure of reform was calibrated to ensure that favoured 'national champion' firms would have the financial and technical resources to acquire 'Euro-champion' status. Thus, in the energy field, the introduction of favourable accounting practices in relation to the fixed costs of nuclear stations was designed to enable EDF to export electricity to neighbouring states comparatively cheaply, thereby enhancing its position in the slowly liberalizing European energy market (Bauby and Varone, 2007).

Nor did the establishment of independent sectoral regulators, partly in response to EU requirements, necessarily mark a substantial change of objectives. In Britain, these independent regulatory authorities, such as the telecommunications regulatory Oftel and the electricity regulator Offer, resolutely favoured competition-enhancing and nationality-blind strategies. In France, however, industrial policy considerations strongly informed the actions of the equivalent bodies. Thus, in Britain, a fundamental objective of the system devised to issue licences for the operation of third-generation mobile networks was to enhance competition. Oftel developed an open auction system to achieve this outcome. In contrast, the *Authorité de Régulation des Télécommunications*, the equivalent regulatory body in France, sought to protect existing French suppliers and deter potential foreign investors (Thatcher, 2007b: 11). The system of allocation was contrived to achieve this outcome and would-be new entrants were effectively barred from entering the sector. New regulatory structures established to oversee and protect liberalized markets continued to serve traditional French economic nationalist ends. Deeply rooted national perspectives and patterns of behaviour successfully transcended legal change and formal institutional redesign.

## Competition Policy After 2004

Many of the weaknesses of EU competition policy were recognized by the European Commission itself and in 1999 it published a White Paper entitled *Modernization of the Rules Implementing Articles 81 and 82 of the EC Treaty*, setting out a far-reaching programme of reform. In December 2002, the White Paper's principal proposals were agreed by the Council of Ministers and issued as Regulation 1/2003. Coming into force in 2004, the regulation instituted such significant changes in the operation of competition policy that a former director-general of DG Comp characterized them as amounting to nothing less than a 'legal and cultural revolution' in European competition policy (Ehlermann, 2000: 537). The reforms encompassed substantial shifts both in the principles informing policy and the system of its enforcement. Although they were presented as a technical, efficiency-oriented modernization, their purpose was to strengthen the authority of the Commission and DG Comp, to deepen the liberal economic character of competition policy and to enhance its impact on national economies by developing a more effective strategy of Europeanization.

The principal changes introduced by the new regulation were threefold. Firstly, the notification system was abolished. Under the new regime, it would be up to firms themselves to ensure that the agreements into which they entered did not contravene the provisions of Article 81, or, if they did so, that they met the criteria for exemption. As well as self-assessing the legality of agreements, firms were also encouraged to become enforcers of the rules. It was hoped that they would come to police their competitors, distributors and suppliers by taking anti-trust infringements to court (Wigger and Nölke, 2007: 497). Secondly, the system of enforcing competition rules was decentralized. There were two aspects to this process. At an institutional level, national competition authorities were now required to apply EU Articles 81 and 82 directly at national level (McGowan, 2005: 992; Clarke, 2006: 39). In the event of any ensuing legal action, the case would be heard in national courts. In addition, NCAs also gained the right to assess whether an agreement met the

EU requirements for exemption, a function previously reserved exclusively for DG Comp. Thirdly, the reform package revised the merger regulation. Partly in response to a series of spectacular failures in which Commission decisions were subsequently overturned by the Court of First Instance (CFI), the traditionally highly legalistic approach to the assessment of proposed mergers was to be supplemented by economic analysis (Morgan, 2006: 81). At the same time, procedures were to be clarified and more flexibility introduced into the system of case allocation between the Commission and NCAs (Wilks, 2005b: 434).

At the level of principle, these reforms represented a substantial 'Americanization' of EU competition policy. A former US Deputy Attorney General for Anti-Trust characterized the 2004 measures as being as 'close as it could get to the US style without copying the whole caboodle' (quoted in Wigger and Nölke, 2007: 499). At a general, quasi-philosophical level, they embodied a shift from the pessimistic German ordo-liberal view that capitalism is innately unstable to a more optimistic liberal view that understands markets to be essentially benign, self-correcting institutions, which should be left to function freely in all but the most exceptional of circumstances. More concretely, the changes saw the basis of Commission policy move much closer to US competition-policy norms, which emphasize consumer welfare protection above all other objectives. This is illustrated by a reworded definition of industry concentration or 'dominance' that now emphasizes short-term consumer welfare considerations and marginalizes concerns about industry concentration.[17] The European tradition of pursuing broader goals in competition law enforcement, such as the protection of competitors from the concentrated power of dominant companies, has been correspondingly downgraded (ibid.). Finally, there was an explicit attempt to encourage the development of an American-style private enforcement culture. With the ending of the notification system, it was hoped that legal action initiated by private actors would flourish. Mario Monti, the EU competition commissioner who oversaw the reforms, argued that such actions would prove an effective deterrent to illegality and would contribute to an improvement in compliance with competition law. Indeed, he anticipated that private litigants would take action against infringements that national authorities tended either to ignore or lacked the resources to pursue.[18]

In respect of Europeanization, the reforms embodied a major shift in strategy. The Commission presented the new approach as an exercise in decentralization necessitated by pragmatic considerations. Thus, it argued that the established system of notification overburdened DG Comp, a problem enlargement would exacerbate. Resources expended in processing routine, legitimate agreements would be better deployed in investigating and prosecuting serious cartelistic behaviour. This justification has met with some scepticism. Riley, for example, has questioned whether 'system overload' was really such a problem (Riley, 2003). More importantly, however, the characterization of the reforms as decentralizing in nature has been challenged as misleading. Rather than devolving power to NCAs, in key respects the new system serves to incorporate them more fully into the European regime. Thus, Regulation 1/2003 lays down that national authorities 'must inform the Commission at an early stage of cases that they are investigating under Article 81', thereby affording the Commission a panoramic view of all competition investigations and cases within the Union (McGowan, 2005: 993). Furthermore, when it chooses, the Commission can assume control over any investigation, forcing the NCA concerned to withdraw. Moreover, a European Corporate Governance Network (ECGN) was established, composed of NCAs and the Commission. It was designed to facilitate communication and disseminate information among its participants. Through its creation, the Commission sought to foster the formation of an epistemic community that in time would generate a common set of values and policy orientations among competition-policy officials. In short, elements of genuine decentralization were matched by more centralizing measures. NCAs have gained a greater role but only as part of a wider process of incorporation into a 'transnational agency' that is difficult for individual national governments to influence effectively.

Indeed, the Commission's achievement in gaining the Council's assent for these changes has been termed an 'extraordinary coup' (Wilks, 2005b: 437). Under the guise of modernization and decentralization, it has extended its authority over NCAs to a substantial degree while surrendering little of its own authority or independence of action. Through the extension of its influence and the fostering of private enforcement, it has sought to outflank any persisting tendency or capability on the part of NCAs to give weight in the formulation of their decisions to factors other than those provided for in European competition policy. By exercising greater control over NCAs, and by partially devolving to them responsibility for implementing European law, the Commission more securely integrates them into the European liberal market regime. It compels them to 'apply a free market logic embedded in European competition law, precedent and supervised procedure' (ibid.: 440). Where competition objectives clash with employment, welfare or industrial policy goals, national authorities would be constrained to give them greater weight. Thus, for example, the German government decision in 2001 to allow the merger between E.ON and Ruhrgas, despite the existence of clear anti-competitive elements to the deal, reflected broader national industrial policy considerations (Green, 2007: 16). Under the new regime, it was hoped that such 'nationalistic' decision-making would be curtailed.

The implications of these changes for national models of capitalism remain unclear. Wigger and Nölke perceive in them a direct challenge to the operating principles of 'Rhenish' capitalism (essentially, the German model). By emphasizing 'short-term consumer welfare and private enforcement, the Rhenish focus on long-term strategies and broader conceptions of economic efficiency will be difficult to maintain' (2007: 499–500). In addition, private enforcement promises greater unpredictability, rendering the inter-corporate collaboration strategies, so common in this variety of capitalism, less sustainable. More broadly, the growing emphasis on consumer welfare is likely to challenge the sustainability of many 'exemption' arrangements. In general, exemptions were granted in order to safeguard longer-term economic and social developmental goals.[19] Such measures may be more difficult to justify when the defence of consumer interests is privileged above other considerations.

The precise implication of the reforms for the sustainability of national models is likely to take some time to unfold. Much will depend on the manner of their implementation and here there is a great deal of uncertainty. Whether viewed as a managerialist or a Machiavellian initiative, the reforms' effectiveness is difficult to predict. While the terms of decentralization may have been carefully designed to protect the integrity and extend the reach of European competition norms, the reliance on 27 different national institutions to implement policy still carries substantial risks to the policy's coherence. Though NCAs may be required to enforce European law, and DG Comp may retain powerful oversight rights, distinct national legal and institutional inheritances are likely to have some impact on how policy is implemented. Soon after the regime's institution, the Spanish government agreed a merger between the power-generating company Endesa and Gas Natural that clearly diminished the level of competition in the market. Though subsequently aborted for commercial reasons, the proposed deal demonstrated that 'the attractions of creating a national champion appear to outweigh the advantages of a less competitive home market, [with] the Commission . . . unable to intervene' (Green, 2007: 17). Moreover, with cases to be heard before national courts, long-established and highly diverse legal traditions are certain to influence final determinations. The effectiveness of the new reliance on private enforcement faces similar difficulties. A large number of cases will have to be taken and precedents set before the potential costs and rewards to private actors of pursuing litigation can be known with any degree of certainty. Furthermore, it is far from clear that national judicial systems will interpret the new rules in precisely the same way, a fact that may weigh heavily with any firm or investor considering launching a legal challenge. Where the alleged illegal action is taking place may matter as much as its character. The effect may be to increase divergence rather than convergence in implementation across member states.

## Conclusion

The success of the EU in developing a powerful European competition policy is evident. In the formulation of their collaborative strategies and merger and takeover plans, firms across Europe – and indeed the wider world – must reckon with the powerful presence of European law and DG Comp. States have been constrained to alter substantially their policies of industrial support and development. Formerly closed sectors such as telecommunications or energy generation and distribution are now subject to a sustained liberalizing pressure. It is also apparent that, buttressed by the Lisbon process, the Commission is committed to extending a pro-competition policy into areas that previously had remained largely subject to the control of member states. Moreover, recent reforms appear to embody a significant shift of EU policy towards US norms and procedures. These changes may in time serve to intensify the challenge of European policy to the sustainability of inter-corporate relationships that proliferate in 'organized' or Rhenish forms of national capitalism.

However, the seriousness of this challenge will depend greatly on the nature and effectiveness of policy implementation. As noted above, while competition policy is now a significant component of the governance systems of both the EU and the member states, the extent to which national bodies adhere to the preferred approach of DG Comp in their determination is less clear. Much of the recent 'modernization' was designed to overcome these weaknesses of Europeanization. However, even if NCAs do come to practise what the Commission preaches, evidence from the liberalization of the telecoms and energy sectors demonstrates the extent to which states continue to possess both the will and the capacity to pursue economic nationalist agendas that are clearly in contravention of the spirit and, at times, the letter of European law. While industries are being liberalized, states persist in exercising their authority to structure them in ways that are deemed to serve the national interest. While key institutional features of national models are under pressure, national governments retain a substantial capacity to resist their wholesale reconfiguration.

### FURTHER READING

Cini and McGowan (2009) provide a comprehensive and up-to-date introduction to competition policy. Clarke and Morgan (2006b) offer a more detailed look at many of the major issues. Thatcher (2007b) explores the dynamics of national regulatory reform to illuminating effect.

4

# Finance, Corporate Ownership and Governance in an Integrating Europe

## Introduction

The corporation lies at the heart of modern capitalism. To operate success-fully, an economy is deeply dependent on the performance of the firms that produce and trade within it. The capacity to exercise control or influence over corporate behaviour is a major determinant of an actor's power and wealth. How corporations are structured can vary enormously. Comparative political economic analysis has identified very marked differences across economic systems in relation to corporate financing, ownership and governance. These differences have major implications both for the productive strategies that corporations adopt and for the capacity of different socioeconomic groups to realise their objectives. Thus, for example, the 'financial system is widely regarded as one of the key institutions that distinguish coordinated from market-based capitalist systems' (Deeg, 1999: 2). It strongly influences the extent to which ownership is widely dispersed among many shareholders or 'closely held' by a small group of dominant shareholders. The structure of ownership and control, in turn, has major implications for the degree to which business comes to possess the institutional capacity to engage in coordinated forms of action. Dense cross-shareholding networks facilitate col-lective action. Diffuse ownership patterns tend to sustain impersonal market relationships. For their part, governance rules substantially affect both the objectives that firms pursue and the strategies they adopt to achieve them. In shareholder-oriented systems, the overriding concern of management is with maximizing dividends and share values (Hansmann and Kraakman, 2002: 58). In contrast, in so-called stakeholder systems, the protection of employee, supplier, creditor, etc. interests also becomes a fundamental responsibility of management (Maher and Andersson, 2002: 389). Indeed, in some instances, employees are accorded the right to representation on the governing boards of the company. Unsurprisingly, the pattern of corporate restructuring adopted in the face of economic change often differs between firms subject to shareholding or stakeholding governance regimes. The forms of ownership and control fostered by the financial system and the obligations imposed by corporate governance rules profoundly influence both the nature of the rela-tionship between socioeconomic actors and the operating strategies devised by firms to achieve their objectives.

Given the importance and complexities of these interrelationships, it is evident that substantial changes in relation to banking, financial market regulation and corporate law may have major implications for corporate ownership and its contestability. Moreover, changes in the nature of finance and/or governance rules may fundamentally alter the capacity of shareholders, managers and the workforce to advance their respective interests. That the EU has sought to develop a substantial role for itself in these areas is undeniable. By 2005, it had adopted some 37 directives and 10 regulations in the area of company law (Enriques, 2005: 7). By the end of the 1990s, EU legislation had transformed banking regulation. In the early years of the twenty-first century, a highly ambitious programme of financial market re-regulation was embarked upon. Less clear, however, is the precise objective of all of this activity and its effects upon established national systems. In the Commission's strenuous efforts to institute a European takeover regime, critics have perceived an attempt to establish an Anglo-American-style system of corporate governance that exalts shareholder interests at the expense of other stakeholders (Höpner and Schäfer, 2007). Indeed, the Commission has been quite open about its belief that economic integration and efficiency require the freeing-up of closed national systems of corporate ownership and control (Block and Grahl, 2009). What is less immediately evident, however, is whether the EU's reforms amount to a coherent, unambiguous programme of liberal economic change. Is this a valid characterization of the reforms implemented? Moreover, even if the key elements of such a programme can be discerned, has it been effective? Has the nature of corporate ownership, control and governance in member states been significantly transformed as a consequence of EU action?

This chapter will seek to evaluate the extent to which EU initiatives challenge established national systems of corporate finance, ownership and governance. Firstly, it will examine the diverse nature and interrelatedness of national systems of finance and corporate governance and their implications for ownership and control. What is the extent and significance of the variance evident across member states? Secondly, the nature of EU policy on corporate law and the financial sector will be analysed. How substantial have these policies been and how should they be characterized in terms of their fundamental logic? An evaluation of their success in transforming the nature of national systems will be undertaken in the following chapter.

## The Diversity of Member States

### Financial systems

At the core of any national model or variety of capitalism lies the financial system. It allocates scarce capital to investment alternatives and monitors the performance of those who employ this capital. Its functioning carries important implications both for the general efficiency of the economic system and for the specific opportunities open to different economic actors. Its structure plays a major role in shaping the pattern of corporate ownership and control, and the manner in which such corporate control is transferred. Furthermore, the operation of the financial system may have a considerable effect on the broader social compromises within an economic system through, for example, its impact on the behaviour of economic actors in fields such as wage-bargaining (Grahl and Teague, 2005: 1005).

The core task of a financial system is to channel the assets of savers to those who want to borrow for consumption or investment. Savers may be households, corporate actors or governments, and the same three sets of actors may also be borrowers. The mechanisms linking these two groups are diverse and, frequently, compete with each other. However, two broad channels predominate. In the first, savings are held in 'the form of deposits or alternative types of claims issued by commercial banks, savings organizations, insurance companies or other forms of financial institution' (Story and Walter, 1997: 108). These 'mediating' institutions aggregate savings, match the maturities of savings and investments in order to minimize liquidity problems, and evaluate and monitor investment risks (Jackson and Deeg, 2006: 13). In such systems, it is the bank that is directly liable to its depositors and holds the claim on the ultimate users of the funds. The bank's 'reputation and solidity are the basis of the confidence in the system' (Grahl and Teague, 2005: 1006).

The second channel involves the allocation of savings to purchase securities, such as equities and bonds, issued by companies or governments in the *primary* national or international financial markets. In purchasing these financial instruments, savers directly assume all the risks involved. Confidence in the financial system 'then rests on the ability of the investors to sell their claims (in the *secondary* markets where the shares, bonds and other financial instruments are actively traded)' (ibid.: 1007). In practice, such a direct transfer of funds from the saver to the issuer is relatively rare. Much more frequently, the transfer is done through collective investment mechanisms such as mutual or pension funds. However, though these 'financial institutions' may be large and powerful, they do not mediate the relationship between savers and investors in the manner of banks, as the individual saver remains fully exposed to the risks involved in the transfer. Though highly dynamic, security-markets systems have historically been prone to quite high levels of instability in comparison with bank-based ones (Allen and Gale, 2000: 21).

## Financial systems and corporate control

The relative centrality of banks and securities markets within a particular financial system has important consequences for the nature of corporate control and the distribution of economic power among socioeconomic actors. In a securities market-based system, firms raise the major part of their external funding from capital or corporate bond markets. Shares of corporations are held by the public, either through direct ownership or via financial institutions such as mutual funds, pension funds, etc., and are actively traded. The ownership of companies is typically widely dispersed and relations between owners and their firms are distant and impersonal. Financial transparency is an essential lubricant of the system. Extensive, publicly available information provides the basis on which financial institutions and/or individuals judge which shares to buy and when to sell. It is through the publication of regular and extensive financial information that managerial performance is monitored. It is through the reaction of shareholders to such information that their judgement of managerial performance is conveyed and sanction or reward exercised. In cases of poor performance, unhappy shareholders may sell their shares, thereby driving down the share price and exposing the firm management to hostile takeover bids (Evans, 2009a: 21). Alternatively, if they retain their shares, management must fear their willingness to support any reasonable takeover bid that is forthcoming from a third party. Either way, the extent and nature of corporate restructuring is strongly determined by the operation of the capital market. The operation of an effective market for corporate control becomes a central mechanism through which good management performance can be encouraged. Critics of this system maintain that it leads to 'short-termism', with shareholders impatient for quick returns on investment and managers fearful of the consequences of disappointing them (ibid.: 19). Its supporters contend, however, that the incentives for strong financial performance built into its foundations generate efficiency, to the benefit both of shareholders and customers.

In bank-based systems, in contrast, non-financial firms tend to rely on retained earnings and long-term bank loans for investment finance rather than capital markets. Though these systems differ significantly in detail across countries, in the ideal typical case banks are 'universal'[1] and are legally entitled as well as practically inclined to hold shares in non-financial firms. With such significant exposure to their clients, through both debt and equity, banks must 'exert a vital monitoring role in the management of corporations, including active boardroom participation and guidance with the benefit of non-public (*insider*) information' (Story and Walter, 1997: 141). The reliance on bank finance has major implications for the pattern of corporate ownership. With only a marginal role as a conduit between savers and investors, capital markets inevitably tend to be underdeveloped in such systems, a fact reflected in much lower rates of stock market capitalization to GNP. Smaller and less liquid, these markets are inevitably much less central to the restructuring of corporate ownership and its transferability. Thus, it is far more common in bank-based systems for firms to be closely held, i.e. owned and controlled by a single or very small group of shareholders. Shareholders also differ in type. Rather than investment or pension funds, the key investors tend to be families, other corporations, banks or even the state. Moreover, ownership patterns tend to be more stable, with shareholders much more deeply locked into the company than is the case in capital-market-based systems. One consequence of these structures is that the marginality of capital markets becomes self-reinforcing. With the dominant shareholders enjoying insider access to information, there is little incentive to publish extensive financial information. Company accounts tend to be opaque, designed to satisfy the tax and regulatory authorities rather than 'ordinary' shareholders. Without access to the information enjoyed by privileged insiders, small or foreign investors considering the purchase of shares face great additional risks that frequently prove prohibitive. Indeed, in some bank-based systems, private shareholders prefer to lodge their shares and related voting rights with banks that, as 'insiders', are regarded as better placed to secure their long-term value (Deeg, 1999: 99).

A key consequence of the creation of an insider system is that many of the relationships that are mediated by the market in securities-based systems become personalized. Where problems arise in the performance of firms, voice (directly challenging management) rather than exit (sale of shares) is the banks' most likely recourse. Where corporate restructuring is deemed necessary, this is achieved through personalized contact and negotiation rather than by adversarial takeover actions. Close coalitions of interest between large investors and management frequently emerge and are often extended to employees, suppliers and others (Grahl and Teague, 2005: 1007). Though their precise role varies across states, banks often play a pivotal coordinating role in such systems, thereby contributing more generally to the development and operation of highly coordinated forms of political economic organization. Critics of bank-based systems argue that they favour insiders at the expense of outsiders and are slow to respond to change. Their defenders argue that the sustained and informed relations between financiers, owners and managers which these arrangements generate facilitate the development of economically desirable, long-term, 'patient' investment strategies (Evans, 2009a: 22).

Within the European Union, Britain is the outstanding example of a securities market system. In 1995, its level of stock market capitalization reached 124 per cent of GDP. The comparable figures for Italy were 19 per cent, for Germany 24 per cent, for France 32 per cent, for Denmark 33 per cent, for Belgium 38 per cent, for Sweden 70 per cent and for the Netherlands 73 per cent (Hirst and Thompson, 2000). Of the 1,000 largest firms in Britain in 1996, some 53.8 per cent were listed on stock exchanges. The comparable figures for Germany were 18.9 per cent, France 27.5 per cent and Italy 13.5 per cent (Franks et al., 2008: 27). Institutional investors are the major owners, with their share of equities rising from approximately 30 per cent in 1962 to some 60 per cent by the early 1990s (Stapleton, 1996). However, for a mixture of regulatory and prudential reasons, these institutions tend to take relatively small shareholdings in a large number of firms. Ownership concentration is consequently low (Amable, 2003: 149). A recent study has revealed company ownership in Britain to be very diffuse, with 'a coalition of at least eight shareholders required to reach an absolute majority of voting rights in the average listed company' (Goergen and Renneboog, 2001: 280). Though firm managements tend to devote considerable time and effort to explaining and justifying their actions to institutional investors through regular contacts, the most important messages between the two sets of actors are communicated via the share price. The threat of exit is the greatest sanction available to unhappy shareholders; the possibility that they may exercise it exerts a powerful influence over management strategy.

Within the EU, however, the great majority of member states fall into the bank-based category. Capital markets tend to be underdeveloped, frequently being illiquid and rarely providing a significant source of venture capital (Amable, 2003: 149). In many cases, specialized state-owned or private credit institutions have been developed to provide subsidized long-term funds for different sectors such as agriculture, industry and property. In most, cooperative and savings banks play a central role in the credit system. In addition, the structure of banking tends to be heavily regionalized, with a myriad of relatively small, local banks servicing the requirements of the small enterprises that typically predominate in both agriculture and industry (Molyneux, 1996: 248; Frangakis, 2009a: 65–6). Finally, rather than pensions or mutual funds, the non-bank financial institutions in these systems tend to be insurance companies closely bound to banks through ownership links. They lack the conditions that encourage the growth of a large population of Anglo-American-style financial institutions looking for investment opportunities with a high level of financial return across a wide spread of companies.

Taken together, these properties have generated ownership patterns characterized by high levels of concentration and complex cross-shareholding arrangements. In Belgium, for example, while banks are not major holders of shares in industrial companies, in the majority of cases such companies are controlled by a single large shareholder with an average holding of 45 per cent of the voting rights. The frequent creation of group blocks or coalitions among firms pushes the degree of ownership concentration even higher (Becht et al., 2001: 94). In Austria, highly concentrated ownership is also the norm. However, in this case, banks do play a key direct ownership role in large and small firms alike (Gugler et al., 2001: 58). Similarly, in German companies, voting power is highly concentrated. An analysis of companies listed on the DAX index found them to be generally majority-controlled, either by a single blockholder or by banks via proxy votes (Becht and Böhmer, 2001: 142). Sweden is strongly characterized by closely held, family-dominated governance structures, while a study of Dutch industrial firms listed on the Amsterdam Stock Exchange found that the average stake of the largest blockholder was 27 per cent and that of the top three blockholders stood at 41 per cent (Agnblad et al., 2001: 254; de Jong et al., 2001: 205). None of these countries possessed an active market for corporate control. This is typified by Germany, where only three successful hostile takeovers were mounted between 1945 and 1994. In contrast, a study of Britain found 35 successful bids launched in just a two-year period in the mid-1980s (Allen and Gale, 2000: 100).

There are some important differences between bank-based systems. For example, in relation to the ownership of industrial firms, while the practice does occur in Denmark and Sweden, banks there tend to play quite a passive role and the credit/GNP ratio is quite low.[2] In Germany, France, Italy, Austria, Portugal and Spain, by contrast, the ideal type of the bank-based model finds a clearer manifestation. In these states, the credit/GNP ratio is high, while insurance companies play a major role as institutional investors in non-financial firms (Amable, 2003: 149). Yet, even here, there are substantial differences across cases, with German banks commonly taking ownership stakes in industrial firms in a way that until recently would have been illegal in Italy. Furthermore, the extent of the state's place in the system varies significantly across cases. In some, its impact on how the financial system functions has been very indirect. Thus, in Germany, the state has played a permissive rather than an active role. In Italy and France, by contrast, the state has been far more central in determining how the banking system operates. From the 1930s to the 1990s, by far the greater part of the financial system in Italy was state-owned. For much of this period it was subject to considerable political manipulation, being a central 'resource' for political parties in the development and operation of the wider system of clientelist patronage that has characterized so much of Italian politics (Barca, 1997). In France, although a more mixed pattern of public and private ownership has generally prevailed, the state has assumed a central role in determining decisions concerning the allocation of credit for much of the post-war period (Zysman, 1983).

### Financial regulation and corporate governance

The differing properties that characterize these national systems have deep historical roots. Gerschenkron has famously demonstrated the importance of the timing of industrialization in determining the centrality of banks or capital markets to investment. Most particularly, the demands of late, 'catch-up' industrialization tended to intensify the need for large capital sums, generating a powerful role for banks in supplying finance and a strong role for the state in supporting and guiding the process (Gerschenkron, 1966). Others have demonstrated the relationship between firm size and capital-market development. The existence of a substantial cohort of large firms, which typically are better placed to pay the relatively high costs of issuing equities, tends to support the growth of capital markets. It is also the case that fundamental social policy choices may play an unanticipated but important role in shaping the development of financial systems. In particular, it has been argued that the choice between establishing a private pensions system or a state-run, tax-based 'pay-as-you-go' regime has enormous ramifications. Private pension savings serve to create a set of large financial institutions with both the capacity and the need to seek investment opportunities in financial markets. In the case of tax-based schemes, no such actors emerge (Verdier 2001; Jackson and Deeg, 2006).

However, despite their diverse origins, it is apparent that the operation and sustainability of these systems is greatly influenced by and dependent on the nature of company law and financial regulation. In a market-based system such as Britain, company law, the policy of the Bank of England, rules concerning capital adequacy and stock exchange listing requirements all exercise a powerful influence over the pattern of ownership and control. Thus, for example, mutual investment companies have been legally proscribed from taking large stakes in individual firms. Insurance companies and pension funds operate limits on how many of their assets can be invested in one company, due to fiduciary requirements of liquidity (Story and Walter, 1997: 152). Cross-shareholding arrangements, 'the purpose of which is to prevent the transfer of control of stock', are prohibited under the City Code on Takeovers and Mergers (Allen and Gale, 2000: 90). As a prerequisite to listing on the London Stock Exchange, a company must agree to a set of conditions that preclude effective – and potentially exploitative – company control by a dominant shareholder at the expense of minority shareholders. In such circumstances of dominance, deemed to exist when a shareholder owns more than 30 per cent of the stock, the rules of the exchange demand that the applicant for listing 'must be capable at all times of operating and making decisions independently of any controlling shareholder and all transactions and relationships in the future between the applicant and any controlling shareholder must be at arm's length and on a normal commercial basis' (cited in Wymeersch, 2003: 589). To ensure that companies adhere to such rules, a majority of the directors must be independent of the controlling shareholder. If minority shareholders are not satisfied with these protections, they can choose to exit the company by selling their shares to the controlling shareholder, who is forced to make a fair offer for them under the City Code on takeovers and mergers (ibid.: 590).

In contrast, no such equivalent restrictions are applied in bank-based systems. In Germany, for example, complex cross-shareholding networks proliferate. These are typically 'defensive arrangements whereby two companies buy stakes in each other and senior managers/owners sit on each other's board and vote their shares together defensively' (Grant and Kirchmaier, 2004: 8). They serve to protect the current owners and managers from external predators and marginalize the interests of small shareholders. In states such as Germany, Belgium, Italy and Sweden, the practice of creating group ownership 'cascades' or 'pyramids' is common. Under such arrangements, company 'D' holds a controlling shareholding in company 'E'. In turn, company 'C' holds a controlling stake in company 'D'. This ownership chain links up to the top of the pyramid, where a holding company,

'A', controlled by a particular individual, family or company, presides. Such pyramids serve to spread the rights of minority shareholders out over a large number of firms and concentrate those of the entrepreneurs in the company at the top of the pyramid. This allows the latter 'to obtain control over the greatest possible amount of other people's capital with the smallest possible amount of their own' (Bianco et al., 1996: 13). Such opaque systems of control are typically facilitated by undemanding accountancy practices and relaxed rules on financial transparency that would not be acceptable in the British securities-based system. They are also sustained by prevailing corporate law provisions and patterns of judicial practice in the countries concerned. In many European civil law countries, it has been found that 'the expropriation of minority shareholders by the controlling shareholder in a transaction with a plausible business purpose is often seen as consistent with directors' duties, especially if the controlling shareholder is another firm in the group' (Johnson et al., 2003: 618). The diverse patterns of finance–industry relations and corporate ownership evident across the EU are underpinned by a raft of corporate laws and regulatory practices, encompassing issues ranging from the protection of minority shareholders to the fiduciary duties of directors.

At the heart of these corporate laws and regulatory practices are the specific rules pertaining to the governance of corporations. These determine the legal structure of firms and the obligations and rights of the different actors within them. Across Europe, systems of corporate governance differ in fundamental ways that impact significantly on the capacity of socioeconomic actors to control or influence the behaviour of corporations. Most fundamentally, the nature of the company itself is differently conceived in EU member states. In the majority of countries, they are defined as private organizations owned by their shareholders. The duty of the company board and management is to protect and advance the interests of shareholders. All other considerations are deemed to be subservient to this core objective. In contrast, in a number of other states, the company is seen to be composed of a diversity of important actors, all with legitimate interests that should be safeguarded. In the Netherlands, for example, the governing board is legally obliged to protect the interests of the company as a whole and not just those of the shareholders (Moerland, 2002: 288). In France, while they are not formally members of the board, 'workers' representatives have the right to attend all board meetings as observers in all companies with more than fifty employees' (Allen and Gale, 2000: 86). This 'stakeholder' view finds its purest expression in Germany. There, the company is conceived to be a public entity, with substantial rights ascribed to management, employees, suppliers and other stakeholders as well as shareholders. There is also evidence that these differences impact upon corporate strategy and decision-making in very significant ways. In the mid-1990s, a survey of managers in the US, Britain, Germany and France enquired whether, in their view, the fundamental purpose of the company was to serve the interests of all stakeholders or simply those of the shareholders. In the US and Britain, 75.6 per cent and 70.5 per cent respectively plumped for shareholders, while in Germany and France the figures were, respectively, 82.7 per cent and 78 per cent for all stakeholders (ibid.: 113).

The basic structure of authority and control within firms also varies substantially. In most cases, there is a single-board structure (e.g., Britain, Ireland, Italy, Luxembourg, Spain, Sweden and France) (Adnett and Hardy, 2005: 179). The board of directors is charged with responsibility for guiding the company's operations and fulfilling its legal responsibilities to the shareholders, the tax authorities, etc. It is typically composed of senior management and outside 'non-executive' directors, though there are considerable differences in national rules concerning the origin of these non-executive directors and the nature of the links that they may have with the company. Thus, for example, in Britain, increasing emphasis has been placed in recent years on the independence of non-executive from executive directors. The former are presumed to be less likely to succumb to self-serving managerial perspectives and more likely to protect the interests of shareholders. However, the more substantial distinction among member states is between those with a single-board and a dual-board structure (e.g., Austria, Denmark, Germany, Greece, the Netherlands, Portugal) (ibid.). In both Germany and the Netherlands, for example, larger firms are subject to a dual-board structure that formally separates management and governance. The latter function is carried out by the supervisory board, which is composed entirely of non-executives. The management sits on the management board, which is answerable to the supervisory board.

To some extent, the single- and dual-board configurations are simply different ways to perform the key function of holding the management to account for its actions and performance. However, in both Germany and the Netherlands, related rules concerning the selection and composition of the supervisory board also reflect substantially different conceptions of the company and the nature of the interests that management should seek to further. In the Netherlands, for instance, places on the supervisory board are filled by a system of co-option. The existing board members choose the new members. While there is provision for shareholders and the employees' works council to recommend candidates for the board or object to those chosen, these opinions are not binding (Moerland, 2002: 288). The effect of this system is, on the one hand, to moderate greatly the capacity of both management and shareholders to influence the composition of the supervisory board and, on the other, to provide employees with some influence over its composition. The entrenchment of the supervisory board's ultimate right to determine its membership is justified thus: the lack of a representative-constituency relationship enables the board to pursue the interests of all the stakeholders in the company more effectively, rather than privileging one above the others (ibid.: 289). In Germany, the rules on supervisory board composition in large firms are much more favourable to employees. In this case, up to 50 per cent of the places on the supervisory board are reserved for employee representatives and the remainder for shareholders.[3] These differences in board structure and composition both reflect and substantiate contrasting views of the role and status of shareholders and other stakeholders in the firm, and significantly impact upon their respective capacity to influence the governance of the corporation and protect their own interests.

The links between corporate governance rules and forms of corporate ownership and control are close. Provisions concerning the types of shares that can be issued, the rights of minority shareholders, disclosure and accounting rules, etc. have major implications for how firms are held and by whom. Thus, the capacity of a dominant shareholder to retain control while raising additional finance is greatly facilitated by rules allowing multiple share classes.[4] Most commonly employed in Germany, Italy, Sweden and France, such practices have seen companies issue 'shares with no or low voting rights to allow a controlling shareholder to maintain control while issuing equity to which they did not subscribe' (Grant and Kirchmaier, 2004: 7). Similarly, the practice of 'pyramiding' discussed above requires a permissive set of corporate governance rules concerning the rights of minority shareholders (Becht and Böhmer, 2001: 148). In contrast, where ownership is widely dispersed, clear accounting rules and extensive requirements for public disclosure of financial information are crucial to the system's functioning. In practice, the precise legal form of these rules varies greatly from case to case. What is formally considered a matter of company law and what falls to separate laws on takeovers, bankruptcy, securities market rules, etc. is a product of local legal evolution. In Britain, important aspects of the rules concerning takeovers and minority-shareholder protection are the subject of voluntary 'City Codes', or stock listing rules. In Germany, these are typically a matter for state law. Yet, however they are formalized, their collective effect is to delimit a range of activities and shape a complex set of relationships with huge import for the conduct of corporations and the distribution of power among socioeconomic actors.

## The European Union and Reform

The EU has actively sought to reshape many of the regulatory arrangements that underpin these patterns of ownership, control and governance. Corporate law reform attracted the attention of the Commission from the earliest years of the Union's existence. Reform of the banking system became a growing concern from the 1980s, while in the first years of the twenty-first century, a sustained attempt to establish a European system of financial services regulation was launched. Gaining an understanding of the implications of these initiatives for the sustainability of national systems requires us to examine their content, purpose and impact.

### Company law reform

The legal basis of initiatives to harmonize company law in the EU was pro-vided by Article 54(3)(g) of the Treaty of Rome (now Article 44). This requires the union to coordinate 'to the necessary extent the safeguards which, for the protection of the interests of members and others, are required by Member States of companies or firms . . . with a view to making such safeguards equiva-lent throughout the Community'. For the treaty's authors, a degree of parity in the laws protecting shareholders and other stakeholders was necessary if disincentives to the movement of companies from one member state to another were to be removed (Deakin, 2006: 448). Initially, under the Hallstein Commission, this was interpreted as empowering the Community to institute an extensive harmonization of national company law systems in respect of the rules governing both public and private companies (Timmermans, 2003: 624; Johnson, 2009: 122). Subsequently, a growing appreciation of the scale of the task involved, its uncertain benefits and the level of political resistance that some early reform proposals provoked served to moderate the Commission's programme. Its initial intention to harmonize fully national systems of cor-porate law was substantially scaled back. Private company law reform was set aside and attention was fixed on public companies listed on stock exchanges, which typically encompassed many of the largest firms. In the 1980s, the approach shifted further towards the agreement of minimum harmonized standards in a broader context of mutual recognition.

Despite this diminution of ambition, there has been a considerable amount of EU activity in respect of public companies. Measures have been introduced on issues such as the formation of companies, distributions to shareholders, new issues of shares, mergers, accounting, auditing, mandatory disclosure of financial information, insider trading and takeovers (Enriques, 2005: 5). Among the most important of these was the adoption of the First Directive (1968), which harmonized national rules on disclosure of company documents and the legal validity of contracts entered into by the company. The Second Directive (1976) harmonized the rules for capital formation and protection with respect to the public limited liability company. Subsequent directives addressed mat-ters relating to domestic mergers, auditing and disclosure (see box 4.1). More recently, the Thirteenth Directive instituted a European takeover regime (Wouters, 2000: 259–60). In addition, after some 30 years of struggle, a legal framework for the creation of the European Company (*Societus Europea*, SE) was finally agreed. Under this regime, a company can incorporate as a European com-pany and operate without legal constraint across all member states, irrespective of the provisions of national law. It enables groups to merge their European sub-sidiaries with the SE, thereby avoiding the costs of maintaining separate boards of directors and auditors, of operating under a variety of accounting rules and of having to conform with a great diversity of corporate law requirements across the countries within which they operate (Pellé, 2008: 8).

## Box 4.1: Key EU company law initiatives

**Second Council Directive, 1976**
Sets down safeguards in respect of the formation of public limited liability companies and the maintenance and alteration of their capital, with a view to making such safeguards equivalent across the Community.

**Third Council Directive, 1978**
Sets down basic rules for the conduct of mergers of public limited liability companies.

**Fourth Council Directive, 1978**
Lays down rules concerning the presentation of the annual accounts of certain types of companies.

**Eleventh Council Directive 1989**
Establishes disclosure requirements in respect of branches opened in a member state by certain types of company governed by the law of another state.

**Thirteenth Directive 2004**
This establishes a European-wide regime for the regulation of takeover bids.

**European Company Statute (SE Regulation)**
Regulation (EC) no. 2157/2001, *OJ* L 294/1, 10.11.2001, established the framework for the European company. The SE Statute enables groups to merge their European subsidiaries with the SE. Companies can save on the costs related to running subsidiaries in different member states with different legal systems. There is no need for separate boards of directors, separate auditors or different accounting rules to follow. The entire company can operate according to a single set of corporate laws across the EU.

**Fifth Directive (withdrawn)**
This sought to coordinate the safeguards for the structure of public limited companies and the powers and obligations of their organs. This proposal engendered intense political conflict and was finally withdrawn in 2001 after almost three decades of debate.

**Fourteenth Directive (withdrawn)**
This sought to establish a European framework for the transfer of registered office from one member state to another. Depending on its precise terms it would have stimulated the development of inter-state regulatory competition in respect of firm incorporations. In 2007, the Commission decided not to proceed with the proposal.

*Sources:* The European Commission: The EU Single Market: Directives and Other Official Acts; Vossestein, 2008: 53; Johnson, 2009: 136; Pellé, 2008: 6.

It is evident, then, that a European web of rules and requirements has emerged that is designed to realize the freedom envisaged in the founding treaty, to trade and establish businesses across all member states. However, recognition of all of this activity cannot disguise the fact that many of the EU's more ambitious efforts at legal harmonization have met with failure. The proposed Fifth Directive on company law, which sought to lay down a European standard concerning the structure, powers and obligations of the organs of the public company, foundered on profound disagreements among member states over board structure, employee rights, etc. This directive was first proposed in 1971, amended on many subsequent occasions and finally withdrawn by the Commission in 2001 (Timmermans, 2003: 626). Different national practices in the treatment of groups and pyramids have also proved difficult to transcend. A Ninth Directive, covering the governance of corporate groups, never made it past the early drafting stages (Wouters, 2000: 262). In the Commission's 2003 Action Plan on Company Law and Corporate Governance, the need for action to be taken against abusive pyramids was asserted. Yet in its 2006 call to consultation, it was still 'wondering' whether there was any need for measures to be taken in this area.[5] In the course of 50 years, little has been achieved in relation to the protection of minority shareholders, even though this is widely perceived to be a weakness of many national systems (ibid.: 295). One observer has concluded that 'notwithstanding the steady stream of secondary EC corporate law rules over the last three decades, EC legislation is only marginally important for EU companies' (Enriques, 2005: 6). Moreover, despite all this activity, the Commission has fought shy of addressing some very important issues of company law, ranging from the fiduciary duties of directors, through the legal rights and remedies of shareholders against management of the company in the operation of the business, to the concept of limited liability itself. The coverage of harmonization directives in substantive areas of company law has been restricted and much of importance remains entirely a matter of national legal provision (Halbhuber, 2001: 1406).

### Corporate law and national capitalisms

The modesty of these achievements in corporate law reform is largely a consequence of the deep anxiety of member states to protect the essentials of their national institutional arrangements in this field. In its early reform programmes, the Commission was inspired by German practice. The first drafts of the Fifth Directive provided for a two-board structure and board-level representation for workers in firms with more than 500 employees (Johnson, 2009: 36) However, many member states baulked at the proposals on the grounds that they were far 'too German'. Enacting this directive would have transformed the nature of corporate governance and industrial relations in very significant ways in many member states and, unsurprisingly, it provoked intense opposition from many national business communities. Subsequently, the Commission reoriented itself in a markedly more liberal economic direction, adopting the conceptual framework of the shareholder-oriented model (agency theory) to develop reform proposals (ibid.: 302–3). The Commission's commitment to the virtues of a 'shareholder democracy', embodied in its 2003 Corporate Law Action Plan, illustrates this conversion. Now, however, it was Germany that baulked at key aspects of the proposals. It was as determined to protect its system of co-determination as other states had been to avoid having it foisted on them. These profound differences have resulted in the adoption of a piecemeal approach to company law reform, with doubts growing about the efficacy of harmonizing European company law through EU legal intervention (Wouters, 2000: 276).

Even when reform has been agreed, the obstacles to the effective Europeanization of national practice have proved difficult to surmount. Sometimes this has simply been a product of poor legislative design. Becht, for example, has found that the EU provisions on company disclosure are neither efficient nor flexible enough to adapt to changing circumstances, thereby inhibiting the very purpose for which they were promulgated (2003: 87). In the case of the SE, the high minimum capital requirement set out (some €120,000), the onerous demands concerning the negotiation of the terms of workers' participation, and the bar to the transformation of private companies into an SE have combined to limit greatly its appeal as a corporate form. As a result, by 2007, there were only 90 or so SEs in existence, rather than the hundreds of thousands that some had anticipated (Pellé, 2008: 8).

Most often, perhaps, European legal provisions have been deliberately subverted by national actors. Thus, a comprehensive corporate law reform introduced in Italy in 2003 blatantly violated the Second EU Corporate Law Directive in several important respects (Enriques, 2005: 12). In other instances, the actions of governments and the legal profession have combined to subvert the effect of European law through a mixture of intention and more inadvertent legal practice. Article 23 of the Second Directive, for example, offers a strong prohibition against firms providing finance to those acquiring their shares. This provision effectively renders leveraged buyouts illegal. Yet, in practice, such buyouts have become ubiquitous in EU member states. In some cases, such as Britain, this has been achieved by inserting exemptions in the process of national transposition of the directive. In other cases, national courts have been prepared to accept the inventive arguments of corporate lawyers as to why this prohibition does not apply to their case (ibid.: 31). Perhaps most tellingly, Halbhuber demonstrates the impact of 'national filters' in interpreting the meaning of EU law and its implications for national practice. He argues that German legal scholarship has systematically misinterpreted key ECJ judgments relating to the right of establishment provided for under the Treaty of Rome in order to protect established German legal practice. This may be partly a product of a desire by the German legal profession to protect their own expertise, relevance and, ultimately, economic position. Alternately, it may be an example of a wider phenomenon whereby 'the questions national lawyers ask when interpreting European legal materials determine the answers they get from these texts' (Halbhuber, 2001: 1410). Irrespective of the cause, however, the consequences are significant. In cases where national company laws conflict with an EU directive, they remain in effect as regards private parties until they are repealed by the national legislator, even if, in the meantime, the ECJ finds that they are in violation of the directive (Enriques, 2005: 13). National academic and judicial communities frequently either fail to recognize, or refuse to acknowledge, the potential clash of national and EU provisions and therefore neglect to make reference to the ECJ for interpretation and adjudication. As a consequence, the practical impact of EU law on national systems of corporate law is substantially contained.

The fate of efforts to establish a European takeover regime serves to demonstrate both the nature of the Commission's ambition from the 1990s onwards, and the degree of resistance offered by states to measures that risked undermining the structure of their national corporate systems. The Thirteenth Takeover Directive was agreed and passed into law in 2003. This was the outcome of 30 years of negotiation and conflict. Its stated purpose was to support the development in Europe of an active market for corporate control. The reference model that informed its development was that of Anglo-American securities markets. At the core of the conflict over its provisions lay the question of hostile takeovers. If a genuine European market were to emerge, cross-border bids would have to be facilitated by the removal of discriminatory national regulations. If such hostile bids were allowed in Britain but rendered prohibitively difficult in, say, Italy, British firms would be hindered from seeking to take over firms in Italy even while being themselves vulnerable to takeover bids by Italian firms. The encouragement of corporate restructuring through takeovers would require European restrictions on takeover defensives.

However, the introduction of measures to achieve this outcome threatened a wide variety of interests. National regimes that discouraged hostile bids would have to undergo fundamental change, and firms that had developed in these systems would have to adopt new strategies for corporate expansion and defence. Powerful corporate elites that had long exploited local regulation to control firms while only retaining minority stakes would face new challenges. Furthermore, the encouragement of corporate restructuring through hostile takeovers would place a far greater importance on the share price. A low share price would be likely to attract takeover bids. A higher share price would deter them. However, a greater concern with the share price is likely to shift the distribution of earnings within the firm towards profits and away from wages. A study of the 100 largest European companies demonstrated that in countries with an active market for corporate control, dividends are higher, while companies in countries where hostile takeovers are unknown pay a higher part of new value in wages (de Jong, 1997: 17). Firms may experience a profound change in the nature of corporate governance and employees in particular may be expected to suffer a loss of influence.

As Callaghan and Höpner establish in their close analysis of the takeover's fate, the radical thrust of European Commission proposals was well understood. In 2002, the Internal Market Commissioner, Fritz Bolkestein, stated bluntly:

[The trade unions] cling to traditional rights as though these were valid for ever, regardless of economic conditions. They want to remain within the comfortable and secure boundaries of what has been referred to as the Rhenish model of capitalism, where stakeholders are pampered instead of shareholders, and where consultations take place on numerous round tables. However, if Europe really wants to become the most competitive and most modern economic area, it must leave the comfortable setting of the Rhenish model and subject itself to the harsher conditions of the Anglo-Saxon form of capitalism, where the rewards, but also the risks, are higher. (Bolkestein, quoted in Callaghan and Höpner, 2005: 38)

Unsurprisingly, such ambition provoked considerable controversy and opposition. The measure's gestation had been long and painful. A first attempt to introduce reform in the 1970s only resulted in the issuing by the European Commission of a voluntary recommendation as member states were not prepared to address the question seriously (Johnson, 2009: 268). More determined efforts to introduce legal reforms followed the adoption of the single market project in the 1980s, but it was another decade and a half before a compromise agreement was finally reached. A draft directive produced by the Commission in 1989, focusing on market transparency and the avoidance of speculative abuses, drew heavy criticism from Britain for not addressing the problem of barriers to cross-border takeovers. A revised proposal sought to accommodate British criticisms and asserted the desirability of facilitating such activities, but it failed in the Council owing to insufficient support. In 1996, the Commission changed tactics, proposing a framework directive that established the general principles that member states would have to incorporate into national law without specifying detailed rules (ibid.: 270). This approach proved more successful and the Thirteenth Directive was endorsed by the Council of Ministers in 2000 and passed for final approval to the European Parliament.

A key element of its provisions concerned allowable forms of defence in the event of a hostile bid. In Britain, pre-bid defences are allowed in principle, but are rarely used while post-bid defences are subject to shareholder approval under the City Code. In many continental countries, in contrast, there are relatively high barriers to takeover and the laws regarding post-bid defensive action by firms vary greatly across states. Article 9 of the proposed directive committed the EU to a system very similar to Britain's City Code. The target company's board of directors were enjoined to 'abstain from any action which may result in the frustration of the offer' unless authorized by a shareholders' general meeting (Ferrarini, 2003: 246). This was unacceptable to many German MEPs in particular, who sought to extend the right to authorize defensive measures to the supervisory board (in effect, discriminating against companies with a single board structure). The central fear was that the EU proposal would open up German industry to hostile bids while leaving many other national corporate regimes secure behind other forms of defence, such as state-held golden shares or administrative protections that were largely absent in Germany (Gordon, 2002: 52). In a dramatic ballot on 4 July 2001, the proposed law fell on the casting vote of the European Parliament's chairman following a 274/274 tie. Tellingly, in many cases it was nationality rather than partisan affiliation that informed the voting pattern. More than 90 per cent of German MEPs voted against the proposed directive, while more than 90 per cent of British MEPs voted for it (Callaghan and Höpner, 2005: 308).

Attempts by the Commission to revive the measure by introducing a range of amendments generated more controversy. A so-called breakthrough rule, which would suspend voting caps and the restriction on the transfer of securities for the period of the bid, provoked opposition from France and the Scandinavian governments, which had supported the earlier proposal. In these states, the practice of attributing double or multiple voting rights for particular categories of shares was common. In the end, the directive agreed in 2003 allowed states to choose whether to incorporate the neutrality and/or the breakthrough rules into national legislation. Bolkestein viewed it as a catastrophic defeat. Member states were effectively allowed to retain their own rules on bid defences and the attempt to create a European market for corporate control was stymied (ibid.: 311).

## Regulatory competition and national capitalism

In the face of the immense political difficulties confronting it, the Commission has been forced to moderate substantially its reforming ambition in the field of European corporate law. However, a more indirect but potentially equally serious challenge to national systems has recently emerged in the form of ECJ judgments that serve to foster the development of regulatory competition between states. The most important example of this phenomenon came in the ECJ judgments in the *Centros, Überseering* and *Inspire Art* cases,[6] which together threatened the sustainability of crucial aspects of corporate law in a number of member states. The core issue revolved around the rules concerning incorporation. Within the EU there are two broad and distinct approaches to incorporation. In Britain, Ireland, the Netherlands and Denmark, the 'state of incorporation' rule lays down that the law to which corporations are subject is that law obtaining in the state of incorporation or registration (Johnson, 2009: 112). Under this principle, companies can choose where to incorporate and, therefore, the set of laws to which they must adhere. Moreover, it allows them to do all their business in one state while being incorporated in another. Under this principle, 'regime shopping' on the part of companies is entirely legitimate and practically feasible. In contrast, in Germany, Austria, Belgium, France, Luxembourg, Portugal and Spain, the so-called *siège réel* ('real seat' or 'seat of administration') rule obtains. Though subject to some variation across cases, the essential characteristic of such systems is that 'courts will regard the applicable law as that of the Member State in which the company has its main centre of operations – its head office or principal place of business' (Deakin, 2006: 448). This may be different from the country in which it is incorporated. Companies cannot escape the legal constraints of the state in which their activities are predominantly based, however onerous the conditions. To escape these restrictions would require uprooting the entire business and transferring it to another state. The effect of the *siège réel* principle is to secure the national character of firms, locking them into the 'organizational emphasis and stakeholder orientation of the company law system of those member states that had long recognized it' (ibid.: 451).

Nothing in the Commission's programme of corporate law harmonization since the 1980s had been designed to force member states to abandon this principle, if only because there was little likelihood of the Council of Ministers acceding to it. However, in its judgment in the *Centros* case in 1999, the ECJ's reasoning did challenge its legitimacy. Effectively, it appeared to maintain that *siège réel* was incompatible with the freedom of establishment enshrined in the Treaty of Rome. The case involved two Danish citizens incorporating a company called Centros in Britain. One of them subsequently applied to register a 'branch' of the company in Denmark in order to conduct business there. The Danish authorities refused the application on the grounds that the 'branch' would in reality be its principal business establishment and that the purpose of incorporation in Britain was simply to circumvent Danish rules on minimum capital requirements (Johnson, 2009: 154–5). The two Danes, strongly supported by the Commission, appealed this decision to the ECJ. The latter found in their favour on the grounds that the Danish authorities' ruling distorted competition in the internal market, a decision that placed the ECJ 'at the outer limits of free movement jurisprudence' (ibid.: 449).

The wider implications of this judgment were not entirely clear. After all, corporate law in Denmark was not based on the *siège réel* principle. However, two subsequent cases, building on the reasoning it contained, revealed its radical implications. In the *Überseering* case, the ECJ overturned a decision by a German court to dismiss a suit by a German-owned but Dutch-incorporated firm, Überseering, against a German subcontractor on the grounds that in its current legal form Überseering had no 'legal capacity' to take the action under German law. The effect of the judgment was to weaken the *siège réel* principle. Its implications were reinforced by the *Inspire Art* case, in which a firm sought to incorporate in Britain but effectively operate in the Netherlands (Johnson, 2009: 157–60). Once more, the Commission supported the case and the ECJ upheld the complainant, preventing the Dutch state from imposing its corporate legal requirements on Inspire Art even though it did not operate anywhere else but in the Netherlands (Höpner and Schäfer, 2007: 19).

The implications of these judgments are potentially dramatic. Where the place of incorporation and the effective place of business differ, it is the law of the former that takes precedence. This opens up the possibility that firms may regime shop, seeking to escape from the more onerous legal constraints of the country in which they conduct most of their business. In consequence, states may be constrained to alter their legal requirements in order to retain and attract incorporations. Thus, for example, the judgment appeared to open up the possibility that German firms might be able to incorporate in another country in order to escape the constraints of trade union representation on the supervisory board, a central plank of the co-determination system. To the extent that this occurred, a key building block of the German model of capitalism would be substantially weakened. Criticism by the German government of the *Centros* decision on these grounds was brushed aside by the ECJ, though in the *Überseering* decision the court did allow that, in exceptional circumstances, such as the protection of minority shareholder or employee interests, the application of the freedom of establishment principle may be restricted (Höpner and Schäfer, 2007: 20; Johnson, 2009: 155–6).

While the logic of these rulings clearly runs counter to the protection of national uniqueness and favours the growth of inter-state regulatory competition, their long-term impact on national systems of corporate law is difficult to predict. This partly stems from a lack of legal certainty about their meaning. It is not yet clear how far the ECJ will press the right of establishment and what national restrictions it will deem to be justified. However, there is also uncertainty about how they will affect corporate behaviour. Becht et al (2007) have identified a 'post-*Centros*' surge in incorporations by private limited companies from other EU member states in Britain. Between 2003 and 2006, there were some 67,000 of these, with the yearly average per EU country rising from 146 in the immediate pre-*Centros* period to 671 in the years after. These were firms that had no operational activity in Britain. Furthermore, these incorporations were overwhelmingly from countries that operated the *siège réel* system, with some 41,000 coming from Germany alone (ibid.: 2). Yet, while these figures are startlingly large, this incorporation migration does have some very specific characteristics that, in practice, limit the extent of the threat that it presents to national systems of corporate law and the socioeconomic compromises embedded within them. Firstly, public limited companies have not followed this path. The migration is confined to small, private operations, with entrepreneurs primarily motivated by the desire to escape high administrative costs and/or minimum capital requirement rules (designed to protect creditors) in their own country. In Britain, the costs of incorporation are low and minimum credit requirements entirely absent. Subsequent efforts by affected states to stem the outward flow of incorporations by reducing or eliminating minimum capital requirements and lowering administrative costs appear to have met with considerable success (ibid.: 2–4). Secondly, migration has been confined to new incorporations. Rules on mandatory dissolution and high legal costs make it extremely difficult for firms in any member state to reincorporate in another state. Attempts by the Commission to ease these constraints through the promulgation of a new corporate law directive (the Fourteenth Directive) were abandoned in 2007, at least partly owing to strong national political resistance to the proposals (Vossestein, 2008; 53).[7] Established firms remain 'trapped' within the national regime and the corrosive effect of incor-poration migration will take a very long time to alter this reality.

It may be that national systems of corporate law will be able to contain the implications of the *Centros* cases. In particular, whatever the attractions for German public companies of breaking free of the constraints of co-determination, the costs of so doing appear to be prohibitive in the short term at least. While the Court's decisions have weakened some key provisions of national corporate law, it has not 'forbidden Member States to impose restric-tions on the transfer of the real seat of a company incorporated under their law to another Member State' (Pellé, 2008: 10). However, the cases also clearly demonstrate the unpredictability and potentially radical nature of ECJ juris-prudence in this area and the deep liberal commitment of the Commission, which has consistently supported legal challenges to national authorities.[8] The transformational potential of the *Centros* and related cases may yet be realized through their combined efforts.

### The financial system

In addition to corporate law, the integrity of national systems of corporate ownership and governance is underpinned by the structure of the financial sector. As noted earlier in this chapter, the source of investment finance has a significant impact on the extent to which ownership is closely held or widely dispersed, readily contestable or insider-dominated. Thus, in systems endowed with large capital markets, it is possible to develop a broad-based ownership structure in a way that it is not where bank credit constitutes the principal source of external finance for firms. Similarly, different financial systems will affect the nature of relations between shareholders, managers and employees within the firm. Most basically, where firms are highly dependent on capital-market funding, the share price will exercise a powerful influence over man-agement behaviour. In contrast, where firms are closely held, it is the small number of dominant shareholders who will exercise a conditioning influence over managerial strategy. There is also evidence that the nature of control has an impact on the distribution of firm income between shareholders, manag-ers and employees (de Jong, 1997). Inevitably, then, major reform initiatives designed to integrate national financial systems into a European regime will challenge the sustainability of established patterns of ownership, control and governance in some member states. Where systems experience substantial restructuring, forms of ownership, contestability and governance are likely to alter.

In practice, in the first phase of integration EU policy offered little threat to national systems. The Treaty of Rome did include a commitment to the integration of financial markets. The right of firms established in one member state to operate in another and/or to supply services across national frontiers, embodied in Articles 52 to 66, encompassed financial as well as non-financial activities. Articles 66 to 73 provided for the abolition of restrictions on capital movements as they related to current payments. However, for the most part, the treaty also protected the freedom of the member states to control the extent and timing of any deeper form of integration. Thus, while Article 67.1 enjoined the member states to abolish progressively 'all restrictions on the movement of capital belonging to residents of the Community, and to eliminate any discrimination based on nationality, to the extent necessary to ensure the proper functioning of the common market', Article 68.1 encouraged them simply to 'endeavour to avoid' the introduction of new restrictions and to adopt a liberal stance on the granting of exchange permits. In short, the treaty's provisions amounted to an encouragement of liberalization rather than its command. Control over monetary, credit, insurance and exchange-rate policies remained firmly lodged within national finance ministries and central banks (Story and Walter, 1997: 7–8).

The legislative record of the Community in relation to bank regulation for the first three decades of its life was similarly cautious. The right of establishment was only implemented with the agreement of the Freedom of Establishment Directive in 1973. Fundamental regulatory questions concerning supervision, licensing, etc. were only systematically addressed with the agreement of the First Coordination Bank Directive in 1977, and its provisions were quite restrictive. Foreign banks that opened branches in other member states would be subject to the supervisory regime of the host country. This served to perpetuate quite prohibitive regulatory barriers to cross-border expansion. A decision to enter a foreign market meant adaptation to a different set of regulations, whether they concerned solvency rules, licensing arrangements, permissions for branch location, etc. Moreover, while laying down the ground rules, the First Bank Coordination Directive left much detail open to interpretation, and a more precise directive was necessary if cross-border provision of banking services was to be truly rendered practicable (Molyneux, 1996: 253).

As in so many areas of activity, it was only following the relaunch of the 1980s that the financial reform programme really began to gather momentum. The maintenance of distinct national financial systems was hardly compatible with the creation of a genuine common market. Thus, in the early 1990s, more far-reaching reforms of bank regulation were introduced with the specific purpose of breaking down the barriers that effectively protected national systems from substantial external competition. Moreover, as the 1990s progressed, EU policy came increasingly to favour a much-enhanced role for securities markets within the overall European financial structure. The Commission's submission to the important Lisbon summit in 2000 was strongly informed by its judgement that 'the bank-based systems of many EU countries were inferior to the more equity-based US system' (Grahl 2009b: 117). It urged the adoption of reforms designed to remove regulatory barriers and eliminate differences in financial practice that were perceived to have 'allowed inefficient financial systems to survive' (Block and Grahl, 2009: 141). More tellingly, the European Council statement issued on conclusion of the summit declared that 'it is essential to exploit the potential of the euro to push forward the integration of EU financial markets'.[9] The structural transformation of national financial systems has become a core objective of Union policy.

### Bank re-regulation

In respect of banking, the renewed impetus of European integration was manifested in two key areas. Firstly, it enabled the Union to agree new, common rules setting down what banks can and cannot do. Member states were distinguished by quite different regulatory traditions. In some countries, banks were allowed to offer a full range of services, from 'high-street' to investment banking. In others, this was illegal: different types of banks performed different functions. In some countries, banks were allowed to hold shares in non-financial firms; in others they were not. The range and diversity of prohibitions and allowances was complex and broad. The EU succeeded in sweeping aside most of these differences. The Commission won support for a broad and inclusive understanding of legitimate bank activity and the effect was to establish universal banking as the Union's preferred model.

The second innovation that proved pivotal to the realization of the project of bank integration was the application of the principle of mutual recognition to bank supervision. Many previous attempts to achieve a genuine integration of the European market had foundered on the need to harmonize the complex and extensive national regulations in order to establish a common European standard. This was a technically and politically demanding process that frequently ended in stalemate. The principle of mutual recognition offered a way around this impasse. The EU would only seek to agree a bare minimum of harmonized rules, such as the definition of legitimate banking activity. Beyond this, states would be constrained to accept the regulatory standards of other member states as a legally satisfactory basis for selling in their national market, even if these standards fell short of their own. Thus, while the goal of policy in the banking sector in the 1970s had been to substantiate the right of establishment subject to 'host' country supervision, in the mid-1980s the policy objective switched to the creation of a right of establishment subject to 'home' country supervision. This shift was embodied most significantly in the Second Banking Coordination Directive (now generally referred to as the Second Banking Directive). This was passed in 1989 and came into effect on 1 January 1993 (Frangakis, 2009b: 95). The directive created a 'single passport' system that enabled banks authorized to act as such in any single member state to set up branches or offer services in every other member state, without having to gain authorization from the host country. Under this system, the responsibility for supervising a bank wherever it operated in the EU fell to the banking authority that had first authorized its operation in one country.

The effect was to dramatically transform the economics of cross-border banking. Foreign expansion by banks no longer involved the assumption of a substantial additional regulatory cost and host country supervisors could no longer seek to protect domestic banks by imposing regulations that, for reasons of adaptive experience and familiarity, were less burdensome for them. The combination of a degree of harmonization with the application of the principle of mutual recognition facilitated a major integration of the banking industry.

### Financial markets

Until the 1980s, the EU's role in reshaping financial market regulation was minimal. Defenders of radically divergent national regulatory systems effectively prevented significant headway being made on cross-border integration. However, with the application of the principle of mutual recognition and the substantial advances in banking sector reform, a broader impetus for financial services integration developed. In 1985, a directive on the free marketing of units issued by so-called collective investment funds was passed. In 1987, a further directive laid down the requirements for the drawing up, scrutiny and distribution of the listings particulars to be published for the admission of securities to official stock exchanges (Molyneux, 1996: 257). The agreement of the Second Banking Directive also sharpened the reform imperative. From the perspective of non-bank investment firms, this directive threatened to weaken their position vis-à-vis a banking sector now operating according to a universal model of banking (Coleman and Underhill, 1998: 231). The Investment Services Directive (ISD) was introduced with the purpose of replicating in the securities sector the 'passport' model that promised so much in banking. In this case, however, the minimum level of harmonization required generated inter-state conflicts of interests that proved more difficult to reconcile. In those countries, such as Britain, where commercial banks and investment firms had been subject to different regulatory regimes, there was a determination that the universal banks would not be governed by what they considered a lighter regulatory burden than that faced by their own banks. In contrast, German universal banks saw the attempt to subject them to specifically investment-related regulation as an attack on the universal banking model (ibid.: 232). Ultimately, the universal bank model had to give ground and, in respect of their securities market activities, banks became subject to more demanding rules on capital adequacy and risk assessment.

Though these reforms were hard won, by the end of the 1990s there was considerable dissatisfaction with their impact. This stemmed from two factors. At a specific level, it became increasingly apparent that the 'passport system', based on a limited degree of regulatory harmonization and a substantial degree of mutual recognition, was less successful at furthering genuine integration in the securities industry than it had been in banking. The degree and diversity of securities market regulation was such that 'home' operators always enjoyed considerable competitive advantages. A very small difference in the nature of a financial instrument or transaction can have a major impact on the risks attached to it and how they are spread among the various parties involved (Grahl and Teague, 2005: 1012). Mutual recognition simply enabled national governments to maintain the home country regulatory bias in place. Moreover, the terms of the ISD still allowed 'host' country authorities to impose additional obligations on foreign entrants with regard to matters such as 'the constitution and administration of the firm, professional standards for staff, rules for clearing and settlements, and record keeping' (Thatcher, 2007c: 51). These were frequently exploited to protect established domestic firms from the threat of competition from new entrants. Even where there was no political motivation, differences in regulation tended to slow transactions and raise costs. Thus, in Europe, there was little agreement on which types of assets can be accepted as collateral against loans or the relative rights of counter-parties to the transaction if things go wrong. As a consequence, cross-border borrowing and lending against collateral was 'slower, more costly and much less developed' than the US (Grahl and Teague, 2005: 1013).

At a more general level, there had been a change of view within the EU and among a significant number of member states about the role of the financial sector. The contention that Europe must establish an integrated securities market system if it is to compete successfully on the world stage has gained many adherents within the Commission and among member states. The scale and flexibility of US financial markets is contrasted with the fragmented and comparatively 'shallow' resources of national systems in Europe. It is believed that bank finance is not capable of generating either the product innovation or the low costs of financial markets. Bank-based systems are not equipped to meet the competitive challenge from the US financial system (Block and Grahl, 2009: 143–4). The development of this perception reflected broad opinion in the financial industry itself. An ongoing process of financial 'dis-intermediation' has been taking place across the developed world for some time. Increasingly, corporations are coming to rely on the direct sale of securities to fund their activities. This trend has been favoured by a number of fundamental developments. Firstly, the long battle against inflation in the 1980s and 1990s, involving tight monetary policies and high interest rates, raised the cost of bank credit relative to share and bond issues (Grahl and Teague, 2005: 1007). Secondly, it is argued that the securities industries have proved more flexible and dynamic and have gained a competitive advantage over banks. The sheer scale of resources available in securities markets, partly as a consequence of global integration, greatly enhances their attractiveness to borrowers. The possibilities for 'securitization' that this facilitates offers greater liquidity to investors and a superior ability to manage interest rate risk exposures (Story and Walter: 1997: 122). Indeed, with the returns on deposit interests declining in the face of competition from new financial products, banks too have sought to 'dis-intermediate' some of their own activity

(Frangakis, 2009a: 67). However, whatever the precise cause, by the late 1990s the EU had concluded that a brighter future lay in the active encouragement of a European securities market system.

This widespread perception was manifested most clearly and significantly in the development and implementation of the Financial Services Action Plan (FSAP). Its purpose was to create a pan-European regulatory framework for an integrated European financial services industry (see box 4.2). Both the plan's content and the legislative strategy adopted to implement it reflected the general acceptance that mutual recognition could not provide an effective basis for genuine European financial market integration. A much more detailed set of harmonized regulations would have to be agreed, and a far greater degree of control exercised over how they were transposed into national systems. Such was the political commitment to FSAP that a new legislative procedure was agreed in order to realize these goals. Under the so-called 'Lamfalussy process', the standard legislative process was substantially amended (Hix, 2005: 248). In respect of FSAP-related lawmaking, the role of the Council of Ministers and the European Parliament would be to focus on the agreement of general framework directives setting out the general principles that should apply. The work of turning these frameworks into detailed legislation would then be undertaken by the European Commission, in cooperation with a committee composed of high-ranking officials drawn from the appropriate national ministries (the European Securities Committee). The conclusions of their discussions would be given legal force by means of secondary legislation, without the need for recourse to either the Council of Ministers or the European Parliament. The process of transposition and implementation of these provisions was also subject to special arrangements. Given the detailed nature of the regulations involved and the potentially significant impact of even quite limited variations in wording, a second committee of regulators was established and charged with ensuring a genuine and effective Europeanization of national regulatory arrangements (the Committee of European Securities Regulators). This remarkable departure from the standard legislative method demonstrated the depth of the EU's commitment to financial market integration. The purpose was both to speed up and improve the quality of legislation.

The specific objectives of this legislative activism were threefold. Firstly, it sought to create a single wholesale market to enable corporate issuers to raise finance on competitive terms on an EU-wide basis. In order to facilitate this, it allowed investors and intermediaries to access all markets from a single point of entry and enabled investment service providers to offer their services freely across borders (HM Treasury, 2004: 4). In practical terms, this involved standardizing the prospectus that accompanied a new security issue and adopting new European-wide reporting requirements that all companies listed on member-state stock markets had to fulfil. Secondly, the creation of an open and secure retail market for financial services was sought. Where the

## Box 4.2: Core objectives of the Financial Services Action Plan (FSAP)

**A Objective 1: To create a single EU wholesale market for securities and derivatives**

- enable corporate issuers to raise finance on competitive terms on an EU-wide basis;
- establish a common legal framework for integrated securities and derivatives markets;
- move towards a single set of financial statements for listed companies;
- contain systemic risk in securities settlement;
- encourage cross-border mergers and takeovers through the creation of a secure and transparent regulatory environment;
- establish a genuine single market for asset managers (pension funds, mutual funds, etc.).

**B Objective 2: To establish open and secure retail markets**

- equip consumers with the necessary information to permit their full participation in the single financial market;
- remove non-harmonized consumer-business rules;
- promote the development of effective instruments to resolve consumer disputes;
- establish a legal framework that facilitates the emergence of new payments and distribution systems on a pan-European basis.

**C Objective 3: To create a secure system of prudential rules and supervision**

- adjust national systems of prudential regulation to accommodate new international forms of business practice;
- contribute to the development of EU supervisory structures;
- establish the EU as a standard setter in global regulation and supervision.

**Concrete legislative proposals included (not all successfully achieved):**

- standardization of company prospectuses;
- improved company reporting;
- measures to safeguard against insider-trading and money laundering;
- more standardized forms of accounting practice;
- new measures to facilitate cross-border takeovers;
- new legislation clarifying the use of collateral to back cross-border securities transactions;
- agreement of a European Company Statute;
- legislation allowing the transfer of corporate seats to other member states;
- action plan to prevent fraud and counterfeiting in payments systems;
- measures to enhance disclosure of the activities of banks and other financial institutions.

*Source:* European Commission: Financial Services: Implementing the Framework for Financial Markets: Action Plan, 1999

wholesale market was designed for firms and financial market specialists, the retail market was designed to facilitate the integration of services such as pensions, insurance and collective savings instruments such as unit trusts, etc., which are primarily marketed to individuals and households that have no expertise in the functioning of such markets. Thus, legislation was designed to give retail customers the information and safeguards they needed to participate in a single financial market and reduce the charges on cross-border payments to render small value purchases feasible (ibid.). Thirdly, it sought to create an effective prudential and supervisory system to oversee and regulate these systems.

Though the legislative programme was extensive, perhaps the most significant single piece was the Markets in Financial Instruments Directive (MiFID), agreed in 2004. Its purpose was to advance integration by establishing a homogeneous set of rules for the sale of securities across all member states (Frangakis, 2009b: 99). It provided securities firms 'with an updated EU "passport", allowing them to offer a range of financial services across member states on the basis of home country control' (Haas, 2007: 56). It also incorporated a set of rules concerning the terms on which business must be conducted, sharply curtailing the latitude the ISD afforded national authorities to fill in the regulatory details of the passport system as they chose. Thus, it laid down the extent of protection to be given to investors when employing an investment firm and formulated a complex set of technical rules relating to order execution and transparency to ensure its effectiveness. The level of detail was substantial. The ISD had contained 32 articles and 14,381 words. The MiFID and its implementing measures contain 169 articles and 67,192 words (Frangakis, 2009b: 99). In addition, under the FSAP programme, individual directives covering the insurance market, transparency of financial information, money laundering, etc. were legislated, as well as a new Capital Requirements Directive that incorporated the provisions agreed for the global industry by the Basel II process. By the 2005 deadline set by the FSAP, 98 per cent of measures were completed and the emphasis was shifting to effective implementation at member-state level (European Commission, 2005a: 3). An ambitious regulatory framework designed to facilitate the emergence of a genuinely European financial services industry was put in place.

## Conclusion

In the early decades of its existence, the EU's role in relation to banking and financial market regulation was marginal. Initiatives were few and their scope limited. Where the Union did show more ambition, as in the case of corporate law reform, it had rapidly to curtail its programme in recognition of the unfeasibility of the task it had set itself. Indeed, in respect of key aspects of corporate law, Commission initiatives frequently continued to meet with disappointment into the twenty-first century. The rejection of the original version of the

Takeover Directive in 2001 was a major blow. Attempts to develop a harmonized set of legal protections for minority shareholders have borne little fruit. Proposals designed to facilitate incorporation transfers across member-state borders were abandoned in 2007. Notwithstanding these caveats, however, the weight and effectiveness of EU policy in respect of banking, financial markets and corporate law have grown very substantially since the late 1980s. National banking systems have been opened up to foreign competition. The basis for a truly integrated system of European securities markets has been agreed. Key provisions of national corporate law have been overturned by ECJ judgments. A European takeover regime has been established. Stronger rules protecting investors and prohibiting insider trading have been introduced. The quality of financial information that firms must publish has been improved. The EU is now a powerful presence in these key areas of national economic life.

In addition, it is apparent that EU reform has gained a new coherence of purpose that challenges the governing institutional structures extant in many member states. The early dalliance with the German model of corporate governance has been abandoned and the Commission's reform programme is now predicated on the general goal of reconstructing Europe's systems of corporate finance and governance along Anglo-American lines. Policies that support the development of a shareholder-oriented set of corporate practices are systematically favoured. Corporate law and securities market re-regulation are designed to facilitate the emergence of a market for corporate control and to prohibit the sort of 'insider-oriented' practices that have predominated in many of Europe's bank-based financial systems. The reforms pursued are hostile to the sorts of intimate, inter-corporate relationships that have been fundamental to the more coordinated forms of economic governance operating in many member states. In the next chapter, the success of this project of radical re-orientation will be assessed.

### FURTHER READING

Allen and Gale (2000) is an excellent introduction to the differences between financial systems and their implications. Grahl (2009) offers an up-to-date discussion of EU policy in this area. Johnson (2009) provides a very detailed and stimulating examination of corporate law developments in the EU.

5

# Finance, Corporate Ownership and Governance: National System Change

## Introduction

The liberal ambition of the EU's financial and corporate reform programme is clearly apparent. It has sought to reshape highly complex and deeply rooted socioeconomic structures of finance, corporate ownership and governance in ways that profoundly challenge the sustainability of key aspects of many national varieties of capitalism. What is much less evident, however, is whether the EU has the capacity either to enforce or to induce such radical changes in national practices. Its broader policy goals, such as those relating to the transparency of corporate ownership and its contestability, cannot be achieved through direct legislative *fiat*. National systems are highly diverse and, perforce, a liberal restructuring may require quite different forms of legal reform across member states. Effective change requires the alteration of complex, interrelated sets of rules and incentives that together sustain the traditionally highly localized, opaque and closed patterns of corporate ownership and control found in many European countries. While the EU can instigate a reform process, and has done so, significant change can only be achieved through multiple interventions by national authorities seeking to substantiate EU policy goals. However, this reliance on supportive national action inevitably subjects EU measures to the uncertain dynamics of Europeanization. Domestic policymaking pressures will exercise a major influence over the nature and extent of the change that is realized.

In order to assess the impact of the EU reform programme on national systems of corporate finance, ownership and governance, this chapter will firstly examine the evidence concerning the restructuring of banking and financial markets in response to EU policy change. Has a substantial pan-European integration of financial systems occurred? Has the relative importance of banking and securities markets in member states altered significantly? It will then seek to establish the cumulative effect of EU measures on national patterns of ownership and governance through two country studies. Is there evidence of a shift towards the precepts of the shareholder-oriented model in response to EU pressures? In what ways have domestic political factors mediated the impact of EU initiatives on national institutional arrangements, and what does this reveal about the capacity of national models to maintain themselves in the face of externally generated policy challenges?

The countries selected for closer examination are both 'hard cases': they embody principles and patterns of corporate ownership and governance that differ markedly from the prescriptions of the shareholder-oriented model. In Germany and Italy, EU reform presents a major challenge to key aspects of the established system. In both countries, banks rather than capital markets have played a predominant role in the financing of industry. In both countries, nationally focused financial systems have given rise to insider-oriented patterns of ownership involving high levels of blockholding. In both, the rules of corporate governance have served to sustain these patterns of ownership and control. In short, in their different ways they sit at odds with the essentially Anglo-American norms that have guided many of the EU's policy initiatives, particularly in more recent decades. The extent and the nature of restructuring in these patterns of finance and ownership offer a test of the impact of the EU's activities on the integrity of a key element of any national political economic model.

## Banking and Financial Services: The Impact of EU Re-regulation

In respect of the financial sector, EU policy has had two principal objectives. Firstly, the introduction of the principle of home-country supervision and the 'single passport' was designed to encourage the consolidation of the banking sector on a truly European basis. Domestic systems would be opened up to substantial external competition through mergers, acquisitions or direct entry by foreign banks. Secondly, it sought to enhance the role of securities markets within the European financial system. Changes in regulatory policy were designed to enlarge capital markets and increase the significance of financial market products such as asset management and investment banking. These objectives were pursued in the full understanding that they would damage the deposit and lending business of commercial banks (Barros et al., 2005: 15).

These innovations had enormous potential implications for the traditionally intimate linkages between national public authorities, industrial firms and the financial sector in member states. The creation of a larger more liquid capital market would contribute to the transformation of established patterns of corporate ownership. Larger markets would facilitate a wider dispersion of share ownership. More widely dispersed ownership would facilitate the emergence of a functioning market for corporate control. In conjunction with regulatory changes, these developments would render corporate ownership more contestable at a pan-European level. Deeply rooted patterns of ownership and governance that have prevailed in many states for decades could be transformed, with all that would entail for the distribution of economic power among socioeconomic groups.

Consolidating and integrating the banking sector threatened to have a similarly transformative impact on the nature of creditor–debtor relations in the corporate sector, especially among small and medium-sized enterprises

(SMEs). Analysts have drawn attention to the importance of the practice of 'relationship' banking in many European states. This can be said to occur when banks and firms develop a close and durable commercial relationship. Its existence sustains a practice whereby 'banks incur current losses on loans to companies in anticipation of compensating profits in the future', and firms are willing to 'incur relatively high costs in purchasing services from their relationship bank when they are doing well in return for assurance that they will receive support from the banks when they are doing badly' (ibid.: 6). In practice, such relationships typically have a strong territorial aspect and are underpinned by stable ownership patterns. They are deeply socially embedded. Reforms that substantially disturb these patterns may well destroy the social context within which they operate. Thus, if a regional bank is taken over by a foreign bank, with a corresponding shift in the locus of decision-making, the regional bank may no longer be free to adhere to the implicit relationship 'bargain'. The foreign bank is likely to be a larger and more complex organization. To ensure effective control, 'they may be obliged to operate with internal policies that are quite standard across countries and, thereby, lack the flexibility necessary to adapt to the specific needs of local borrowers' (ibid.: 8). As a consequence, particularly in a time of crisis, a foreign bank is unlikely to behave in a similar way to a local bank and a crucial instrument of economic management is lost to small and medium-sized firms. Critics perceive such practices to be potentially collusive and economically damaging, while many participants assess them more positively. What is evident, however, is that the logic of EU policy threatens their sustainability and, in the process, the sustainability of many of the linkages between the financial and corporate sectors that underpin established patterns of ownership and control.

### Banking

There is evidence that, in response to EU policy initiatives, the nature of banks and banking activity in the member states has indeed changed significantly. Walkner and Raes note that there has been a dramatic shift 'in the income profile of banks, with the proportion of interest income declining relative to income from more fee-based activities' while on the liability side 'a search for yield has prompted an outflow of depositor funds from banks to a range of competing financial products' (2005: 14). In response, banks have sought to diversify their activities, often moving into areas more typical of securities-market-based financial systems, such as insurance, mutual fund sales and asset management (Goddard et al., 2007: 1914). There is also evidence of substantial consolidation in the banking sector. Table 5.1 demonstrates a fairly general trend across EU15 states towards a reduction in the number of credit institutions. In countries characterized by a particularly fragmented credit sector, such as Germany, the trend has been especially marked with the number of institutions falling by approximately a third in just six years.

**Table 5.1** Number of credit institutions in EU15: percentage change

| Country/Year | 1997 | 2000 | 2003 | 1997–2003 % change |
|---|---|---|---|---|
| Belgium | 131 | 118 | 108 | −17.6 |
| Denmark | 213 | 210 | 203 | −4.7 |
| Germany | 3,420 | 2,742 | 2,225 | −34.9 |
| Greece | 55 | 57 | 59 | +7.3 |
| Spain | 416 | 386 | 348 | −16.3 |
| France | 1,258 | 1,099 | 939 | −16.3 |
| Ireland | 71 | 81 | 80 | +12.7 |
| Italy | 909 | 861 | 801 | −11.9 |
| Luxembourg | 215 | 202 | 172 | −20.0 |
| The Netherlands | 648 | 586 | 481 | −25.8 |
| Austria | 928 | 848 | 814 | −12.3 |
| Portugal | 238 | 218 | 200 | −16.0 |
| Finland | 348 | 341 | 366 | +5.2 |
| Sweden | 237 | 211 | 222 | −6.3 |
| Britain | 537 | 491 | 426 | −20.3 |
| EU 15 | 9,624 | 8,433 | 7,444 | −22.7 |

*Source:* European Central Bank, 2004 'Structural Analysis of the EU Banking Sector', Frankfurt

Crucially, however, this process of consolidation has occurred overwhelmingly within national systems. Mergers and acquisitions have largely been domestic in focus and arguably defensive in purpose, with cross-border activity accounting for 10 per cent or less of the total value of M&A in 13 of the 17 years up to 2004 (Walkner and Raes, 2005: 23). Thus, while the percentage of banking-sector assets held by foreign banks rose slightly in France and Germany between 1997 and 2003 (from 10.4 per cent to 11.15 per cent and 4.3 per cent to 5.95 per cent respectively), it fell in Italy and Spain (from 7 per cent to 5.8 per cent and 12.5 per cent to 11.04 per cent respectively) (Dermine, 2005: 55). From the late 1990s, there has been a trend towards mergers between banks and insurance companies but, again, the respective parties have almost invariably been co-nationals (Goddard et al., 2007: 1919). In 2004 and 2005, two major cross-border deals were agreed, with the Spanish bank Santander taking over the British bank Abbey and Italy's Unicredito purchasing the German bank HVB. However, the process of cross-border consolidation and restructuring in the banking sector that they appeared to presage has yet to occur. The one deal of similar magnitude that did subsequently take place, that between the British bank RBS and the Dutch bank ABN Amro, proved very damaging to both parties. The debt burden assumed by RBS in order to finance the takeover left it highly vulnerable when the financial crisis of 2008 struck, and it was among the first banks to turn to the state for recapitalization. The impact of the Second Banking Directive on the structure and operations of the banking sector has fallen significantly short of expectations.

A variety of explanations have been offered for this pattern of development. To some extent, it has been suggested, there was insufficient recognition of the importance of local knowledge in the conduct of banking activities (Grahl, 2009b: 204). As each 'loan applicant presents a specific adverse selection problem, banks already active in a specific market have an informational advantage over new entrants, not only in respect of potential clients but also in respect of local market characteristics' (Walkner and Raes, 2005: 22). Moreover, in many countries the local and regional banks that typically engage in 'relationship' banking with SMEs are savings, mutual or cooperative banks (Frangakis, 2009a: 65). The ownership characteristics of these institutions render them largely immune to efforts by foreign banks to buy their way into such markets. In this regard it is notable that, even at the end of the 1990s, the market share of cooperative and savings banks in France, Germany, Spain and Italy (as a percentage of total deposits) was 60.1, 50.2, 48.1 and 15.7 per cent respectively (Barros et al., 2005: 91–2). Both the activities and ownership of national banking systems are more deeply socially embedded than reformers recognized. Finally, persisting regulatory differences across states continue to inhibit the prospect of genuine cross-border banking activity. For example, different national rules on consumer protection render the provision of pan-European banking products difficult and relatively costlier. Different rules concerning double taxation, the treatment of losses and the management of mergers all complicate the process of cross-border consolidation (Walkner and Raes, 2005: 31–3). The myriad and complex variations across national economies present a continuing, substantial obstacle to integration.

These obstacles can only be overcome by a very significant political commitment by member states to push the process of integration further. However, there are serious reasons to doubt the support of many governments for a substantial reduction of national discretion in the regulation of their banking industry. Thus, while states have been forced to remove explicit barriers to foreign intervention, the use of more subtle instruments of protection has proliferated. Many have inserted 'public security' or 'general interest' provisions in national laws as part of the process of transposing European Directives. These have the effect of exempting state authorities from fully applying European law under certain circumstances. The EU has resisted such practices, but the challenge of effectively policing the behaviour of member states is enormous. Moreover, even when the ECJ has struck down such an arrangement, states continue to enjoy many opportunities either to evade or to delay effective implementation of European law and ECJ judgments. In 2002, the ECJ declared a Portuguese cap of 25 per cent on foreign ownership of a range of privatized banks to be illegal. Three years later, the Portuguese government had not yet changed the law (Walkner and Raes, 2005). In Italy, the central bank actively sought to protect Italian banks from foreign takeover (see below for details). The resistance of many national governments to the 'denationalization' of their system is evident.

### Financial markets

A similar pattern of significant change without transformation is evident in respect of financial markets. Important developments in relation to some aspects of corporate finance have taken place. In particular, the use of bonds to raise corporate finance has grown substantially in the last decade or so. By the end of 2006 the outstanding value of corporate bonds had risen to about €6 trillion from €2.1 trillion at the end of 1997 (Haas, 2007: 47). Greater reliance on bonds alters the relationship between corporations and banks in significant ways. Though banks play a role in the corporate bond market, they do so as fee-earning service providers helping to organize the bonds' issue rather than as providers of credit. A substantial degree of reform has also occurred in the regulation and ownership structure of stock markets in many member states. Regional exchanges have been integrated into national ones. Since the 1980s, many exchanges have been privatized. Under the EU's passport system, foreign operators have gained access to national exchanges. Most exchanges have become subject to stricter regulation. Moreover, the advent of the Euro has given greater impetus to cross-national integration. Thus, in September 2000, French, Dutch and Belgian exchanges merged to form Euronext (Faruqee, 2007: 87). Subsequently, the Milan market was taken over by the London Stock Exchange, while Scandinavian and Baltic exchanges have undergone a substantial process of consolidation. The structural basis for issuing and trading equities on a cross-national basis has begun to emerge.

However, it is not clear that the scale of change thus far, in respect of either corporate bond or equity markets, is sufficiently large to transform substantially the complex relationships between corporate finance, ownership, control and governance in member states. Thus, while the growth of the corporate bond market in Europe has been substantial, it still only amounted to some 8 per cent of GDP in the Eurozone by 2003, in comparison with 29 per cent in the USA and 25 per cent in Japan (Barros et al., 2005: 51). European firms continued to rely disproportionately on 'traditional' sources of external finance. Moreover, raising finance by issuing corporate bonds remains predominantly a practice of large firms. There is little evidence that SMEs have pursued this path to any substantial degree. In respect of equities, the extent of cross-national trading has been quite modest. Home bias, defined as 'the share of resident holdings of domestic stock in a country's overall portfolio of EU equities', remains very high at over 80 per cent (Faruqee, 2007: 103). While there is greater competition between national exchanges to attract listing business, the fact remains that the issuing and ownership of shares is still predominantly national in scope. Nor is there evidence that the changes that have occurred have generated a radical shift by European firms towards the use of capital markets to raise funding. Relative to their respective economies, EU capital markets in 2004 were 'much smaller and bank balance sheets much larger than those in the US' and even after recent developments they remain 'far smaller, less developed and more fragmented' than their US counterparts (Decressin and Kudela, 2007: 67, 85). Finally, though the size of financial markets grew fourfold in Eurozone countries between 2000 and 2006, the rate of growth has actually declined significantly since 2000 (Frangakis, 2009a: 58).

The key question is whether the mixed evidence of deepening integration evident thus far is simply a matter of 'early days', or whether fundamental obstacles to a deeper transformation of financial systems in Europe remain. The 'early days' thesis rests on the fact that much of the FSAP has yet to be implemented fully at national level. Transposition of the key MiFID Directive was only completed in November 2007 and its impact will take some time to unfold. Directives on Market Abuse and Transparency are even further from full implementation. With some justification, proponents of the FSAP can stress the need for patience before coming to any final judgement of the programme's impact. However, there are also grounds for scepticism about its longer-term transformational potential. Some argue that the scale of harmonization and liberalization embodied in the FSAP is insufficient to 'bring about full financial integration' (Block and Grahl, 2009: 148). More radical, but politically difficult, measures may be necessary if this goal is to be achieved. Considerable doubt also attaches to the EU's capacity to ensure the consistent application of the rules agreed under the Lamfalussy process, given the reliance on a country-based supervisory framework for implementation. Furthermore, it is questionable whether EU policymakers can react speedily enough to market innovations. Thus, for example, there has been an enormous growth of hedge funds, private equity, real estate and commodity funds in recent years, areas of activity that current EU provisions do not adequately cover. The response of national authorities to these developments has varied greatly, adding to the very fragmentation of the industry that the FSAP is striving to overcome (Haas, 2007: 48–9). Perhaps most fundamentally, it has been argued that 'financial products are essentially legally binding contracts that reflect the legal system under which they are executed, and these systems differ deeply across countries' (Fonteyne, 2007: 2). In this view, genuine financial market integration would require an almost inconceivable degree of legal integration across member states.

Clearly, the level of uncertainty concerning the consequences of recent EU initiatives in the financial sector is considerable. Moreover, the onset of a global financial crisis in 2008 has profoundly deepened this uncertainty. Many of the assumptions about the superiority of financial markets-based systems have been called into question. The disadvantages of their undoubted dynamism have become starkly apparent. Yet too much has changed to permit a return to the old order. Securities market trading is now central to the business strategies of many of the larger banks in Europe. European banks were very large holders of the CDOs (Collateralized Debt Obligations) that played such a central role in spreading financial turmoil in 2008 (Toporowski, 2009: 165). It is notable, for example, that highly globalized banks in bank-based Germany were among the hardest hit by the crisis. However, given that 'opportunities in domestic markets are limited and the lure of profits in risk-taking remains', a retreat to nationally oriented banking seems unlikely (Hardie and Howarth, 2009: 1034).

Another source of uncertainty stems from the political reaction to the crisis. The damage caused has led to the wholly unexpected return of the state as whole or part owner of significant segments of the banking sector in many countries. Banking regulation and remuneration has gained an enormous political salience, exposing it to the flux of party political and electoral dynamics to a degree that had not previously been the case. The effect of these developments on European policy remains to be seen. On one level, the depth of the crisis has demonstrated the limited capacity of national states to manage their own financial industries under conditions of extreme stress. The size of the financial sector and the extent of its regional and global integration render even the largest member state incapable of acting effectively alone. In particular, the feasibility of maintaining a nationally devolved system of prudential regulation under these conditions has been called into question and the crisis may serve to deepen the Europeanization of national systems of financial regulation. On another level, the Anglo-American financial system, as a guiding pole of attraction for the Commission and the European reform agenda in general, has been compromised. Whatever the ultimate cause of the crisis, it was precisely the more innovative financial instruments, developed in recent years by the financial markets, that contributed greatly both to its depth and the speed of contagion across the world. At the very least, it can be anticipated that the clear sense of direction that has informed Commission activity in recent decades will be subject to a greater level of critical scrutiny, if not resistance.

## Restructuring Corporate Finance, Ownership and Governance: Germany

German capitalism has long been characterized by a highly organized system of corporate ownership and governance that distributed power among a wide range of actors stretching beyond shareholders to encompass managers, employees, investors, regional authorities, suppliers, customers and cooperating companies (Beyer and Höpner, 2003: 179). This system was the product of dense, highly personalized business relationships underpinned by public policy. Firms traditionally have been closely held, with more than half of all listed companies controlled by a single majority block and only 17.4 per cent without a blockholder with at least a minority veto (Becht and Böhmer, 2001: 142). Cross-shareholding arrangements between firms have been ubiquitous. Interlocking directorates, whereby the governing boards of firms are well stocked with directors and managers from 'partner' firms, have been pervasive. Public policy was designed to support and sustain these networks, and the dispersion of power among national socioeconomic actors that they embodied. Thus, for example, to help firm management block unwanted takeover bids from actors, either domestic or foreign, outside the network, unequal voting rights for different types of shares was allowed. To support the economic integrity of inter-corporate cross-shareholding, profits earned from share ownership were taxed more favourably than profits from share sales (Beyer and Höpner, 2003: 190). To ensure the participation of employees and unions in the forming of company policy, a system of co-determination was established. This provided for a substantial representation of all sections of the firm on the governing supervisory board, with 50 per cent of seats allotted to workers in firms that employ more than 2,000 people.[1] In addition, firms were required to establish works councils within which management and representatives of the workforce would engage in sustained and detailed consultation about the running of the company. The corporate sector was owned and controlled by a broad-based but closed and highly personalized network of national actors, and the legal and regulatory system was shaped to facilitate and sustain these arrangements.

At the heart of this network lay the banks. Germany is widely viewed as the archetype of a 'bank-based' financial model. While stock markets have been marginal players in corporate finance – with the share of household savings held in equities never rising above 2 per cent throughout the 1950s (Thatcher, 2007c: 62) – relations between financial and non-financial companies have been extremely close. Industrial firms have traditionally raised the greater part of their external funding from banks. Banks have frequently bought substantial stakes in non-financial companies, taken seats on their supervisory boards and exercised voting proxy rights on behalf of the many shareholders who felt that their interests would be best protected by ceding these rights to the well-informed banks. In 1996, for example, some 29 of the supervisory board chairmen of the largest 100 industrial firms were representatives of Deutsche Bank alone (Lütz, 2005: 147). In a study of 372 industrial firms undertaken in the mid-1990s, it was found that banks held share blocks averaging some 24 per cent in 77 of them, while insurance companies held an average of 20 per cent of a further 34 firms (Becht and Böhmer, 2001: 140). In the case of 30 very large firms listed on the DAX share index, a survey of voting at the 1992 annual general meeting found that banks controlled more than 50 per cent of the voting rights in three-quarters of them (ibid.: 128–31).

One of the most important manifestations of these multiple ties of cross-shareholding, interlocking directorates and credit lending, was the *Hausbank* relationship between banks and industry (Lütz, 2005: 141). Firms tended to develop a close link with one or two banks and, in turn, these gained an intimate knowledge of, and became deeply entangled in, the vicissitudes of those firms' business. This intimacy and knowledge provided a basis for the development of 'patient capital', which involved a willingness on the part of bankers to finance investment with low short-term but potentially high long-term returns. Moreover, in the event that a company ran into trouble, these relationships often prompted banks to take the lead role in coordinating rescue operations. In short, banks played a central part both in financing and governing the firms with which they dealt. Together with insurance companies, industrial companies and families, they became deeply enmeshed in a complex network of 'insider' relations that controlled 'the strategies and decisions of large German firms (relatively free from the influence of stockmarkets or small shareholders)' (Deeg, 2001: 17).

Though pivotal to the system of industry financing and corporate control, the German banking sector was far from monolithic in structure. It was, in fact, exceptionally fragmented by European standards, with some 2,225 credit institutions in 2003 compared with France's 939, Italy's 801 and Britain's 426 (see table 5.1). The share of business held by the three biggest banks stood at 16 per cent in comparison to figures of 33 per cent for France, 47 per cent for Britain and 54 per cent for Spain (Grossman, 2006: 328). The substantial differences in historical origins, regional location and structure gave rise to a tripartite division of associational organization and governance that has given the political organization of German banking a very distinct profile. The first group, composed of the private commercial banks, includes the largest and most widely known German banks such as Deutsche Bank, Dresdner Bank and Commerzbank. Historically, these banks have had a close relationship with the largest industrial German companies, playing an important role both in their financing and in their governance. Consolidation among these private banks over the past decade or so has seen their number fall from a peak of 366 banks in 1990 to 261 by the end of 2003, with a combined market share of some 28 per cent (ibid.: 329). The second group is composed of publicly owned savings banks, which together serves approximately one-third of the overall banking market. Typically, these were initially founded to provide 'poor relief' but have gradually broadened their range of activities, moving into the provision of consumer-credit retailing, public infrastructure, communal finance, and mortgage finance (Deeg, 2001: 15; Lütz, 2005: 141). It is from the ranks of these banks that many small and medium-sized non-financial firms have found their *Hausbank*. Perhaps the most important of the publicly owned banks, however, were the 13 regional *Landesbanken*. Many of these are large banks owned by regional *Land* governments that require them to contribute to the achievement of local industrial policy objectives. Most importantly, the provision by the *Länder* of a public guarantee to the *Landesbanken* enabled them to raise capital cheaply on the money markets. With the benefit of such guarantees, risk for depositors or lenders was virtually eliminated and, unsurprisingly, of the 31 European banks awarded a 'triple A' standing by German credit-rating companies in 2000, 22 were German public banks with the remainder sprinkled thinly across the rest of the European Union (Smith, 2001: 127). In total, the savings bank and *Landesbanken* had a market share of approximately 36 per cent by the early twenty-first century (Grossman, 2006: 329). Finally, the third group is composed of mutually owned cooperative banks. Initially developed to meet the needs of craftsmen and local entrepreneurs, they now service much the same market as the savings banks, both in terms of the products offered and their focus on local communities. Though the number of cooperatives halved in the decade from 1992, there are still more than 1,600 in operation holding some 30 per cent of saving deposits and a total market share of 8.7 per cent (ibid.: 330).

### Change

The German system of finance and corporate governance has undergone major change and development in the last two decades. Policy has sought to enhance the role of securities markets and support the growth of more shareholder-oriented company behaviour. Moreover, important segments of the banking sector have chosen to alter their relationship with the non-financial sector. Though the breadth of reform was great, its key elements encompassed securities-markets re-regulation, tax reform and changes in corporate governance law.

In respect of the stock market, there has been a radical overhaul of its structure and regulation in the last two decades. In the mid-1980s, (West) Germany had eight regional stock exchanges that were owned by state governments and effectively operated as public utilities serving local needs (Thatcher, 2007c: 105). By the early twenty-first century, it had a single, privately owned exchange (*Deutsche Börse*) subject to a federal regulator. A host of new laws were introduced with the common purpose of stimulating the supply and demand for securities (Deeg, 2005a: 334). In particular, strenuous efforts were made to attract international investment. Policymakers sought to reassure new, foreign investors that their interests would not be sacrificed to benefit the traditional 'insiders' of corporate Germany. Illustrative of this new internationalism were the efforts of the *Deutsche Börse* to establish itself on the global stage, at various times pursuing mergers with the London Stock Exchange and the New York Stock Exchange (an initiative only abandoned at the end of 2008 in the context of dramatic financial and economic crisis).

These reform measures had a substantial impact. The number of IPOs (initial public offerings) soared in the 1990s. The market capitalization to GDP ratio rose significantly from 21.8 per cent to 43.7 per cent in the decade from 1996 (Franks et al., 2008: 41). The costs of raising finance fell, since, for large creditworthy firms in particular, it often proved 'cheaper to acquire

capital on international markets by issuing shares or bonds than to seek loans'
(Lütz, 2005: 144). As a consequence, 'the shareholder base of numerous large
German firms (and banks) has become more widely dispersed and internationalized' and German firms, of necessity, have become more responsive to their
preferences for corporate transparency (Deeg, 2005a: 337). Inevitably, such
developments had a profound impact on the integrity of the German bank-
based system as a whole. Just as the pursuit of cheaper finance induced firms
to look beyond their *Hausbanks*, the banks themselves had to look beyond a
credit business marked by declining profitability in order to boost earnings.
The effect was to weaken the ties between banks and industrial firms that
lay at the heart of the German system of corporate control. Since the 1990s,
the 'big three' private banks have decisively shifted their attention towards
investment-bank activities and sought to disentangle themselves from the
multiple networks of corporate control and the related burden of corporate
governance that accompanied membership of them. While Deutsche Bank
may have provided industrial companies with 29 supervisory board chairmen
in 1996, in 2001 it announced its intention to withdraw its personnel from
all such positions (Lütz, 2005: 147). Where the six biggest private sector banks
held stakes in 75 of the 100 largest companies in 1996, by 2002 the number
had declined to 30 (Grahl, 2009d: 227). Even in the savings bank and cooperative bank segments, securities market growth had an impact. As profits from
traditional credit activity declined in the face of new competition, many of the
larger *Landesbanken* have followed the private banks into investment banking.
In the cooperative sector, large-scale consolidation is under way as banks seek
to escape the squeeze on margins. The collective impact of these developments
has meant that, at least in the large-firm sector, the ties between banks and
non-financial firms have greatly loosened. Increasingly, firms borrow on securities markets and banks seek to provide the services required in these markets,
such as investment analysis, managing share issues, mergers and acquisitions,
etc. Contact may still be frequent and intense but it is also more fully mediated
by market mechanisms of competition and price. Finance–industry relations
are less opaque, less credit-based and less national. Firms are not as embedded in protective networks, while the logic of capital markets and the related
preoccupation with shareholder value holds increasing sway.

Reforms of corporate governance have been designed to bolster these
trends, introducing principles of regulation and governance that are compatible with and supportive of the operation of securities markets. Thus,
for example, the Control and Transparency Act 1998 (the KonTraG) partially
broke with the traditions of German corporate governance by emphasizing
the central importance of advancing shareholder interests, without making
any reference to the stakeholder model that had held sway for the previous
half-century or so (Beyer and Höpner, 2003: 191). The act also introduced
some significant specific rule changes. For example, it trimmed the power of
the banks by restricting the use of proxy votes, strengthened the role of the

supervisory board, introduced the 'one share, one vote' principle and allowed the use of share buy-backs and stock options. Tellingly, the only exemption from the 'one share, one vote' principle was designed to restrict the exercise of voting rights by inter-firm cross-shareholding networks. Moreover, these changes were reinforced by related reforms in takeover law and corporate taxation. In 2002, a new law was introduced to create a clear and coherent framework for conducting takeovers. In January 2002, capital gains tax rules were altered to facilitate the profitable unwinding of cross-shareholding networks. In short, as Cioffi has argued, the thrust of the legal changes was 'towards transparency, equal treatment of shareholders and curbing the rent seeking of corporate insiders' (Cioffi, 2002: 25).

It is undoubtedly the case that the German system of finance and corporate governance has undergone substantial change. The role of financial markets has been greatly enhanced. The large commercial banks have partially 'de-nationalized' themselves. The tax system no longer privileges the maintenance of cross-shareholding arrangements in the way that it used to do. Furthermore, there is evidence that these initiatives have had an impact on the structure of corporate ownership. Thus, between 1996 and 2006, the proportion of firms that can be described as widely held rose from 26 to 52 per cent (Franks et al., 2008: 5). Though still important, there is evidence that cross-shareholding arrangements are no longer quite as central to corporate strategy. Between 1996 and 2004, the total number of cross-shareholdings among the largest 100 companies fell from 51 to 28 and the 'number of enterprises (including banks) possessing such stakes from 39 to 17' (Grahl, 2009d: 227). Altogether, these developments represent 'a notable break from the old model in which banks and other large firms were long-term shareholders providing "patient" capital and protecting firm management from unwanted outside influences and takeovers' (Deeg, 2005a: 338).

However, the limits of change must also be recognized. Firstly, the role of the securities markets in comparison with its British or US counterpart remains considerably more modest. Germany's stock market capitalization rate of 43.1 still lags markedly behind Britain at 139.6 (Franks et al., 2008: 41). Secondly, the turn towards financial markets and the rapid erosion of *Hausbank* relationships were far more marked in the large-firm sector than among small and medium-sized firms. For the latter, banks continue to play a pivotal role in their financing and governance. Thirdly, in respect of corporate governance, important constraints on the embrace of a shareholder-oriented system remain. The institutions of co-determination, and the concomitant fiduciary duties of directors to protect the interests of employees as well as shareholders, are largely unaltered. Moreover, the evidence is that the social relations that the rules embody remain central to the productive strategies of even the largest German firms. It is notable, for example, that a study of corporate governance practice in Siemens during the early years of the twenty-first century concluded that its management strategy took into consideration more than the interests of shareholders and institutional investors and that 'in terms of consensual decision making the stakeholder model is alive' (Borsch, 2004: 381). German firms are still not private organizations owned by their shareholders, in the Anglo-American sense, and maximizing shareholder value is not their sole legal *raison d'être*. Fourthly, there is evidence that key aspects of the reforms introduced simply did not function as expected. Thus, Kirchmaier and Grant found that some recent takeovers excluded minority shareholders from reaping their proper share of the deal's benefits, despite the investor protection measures introduced by the KonTraG and the 2002 Takeover Act (2008: 11–12). Finally, attempts to facilitate the contestability of corporate ownership have largely proved unsuccessful. It is noteworthy that the controversial hostile takeover of the telecommunications firm Mannesmann in 2000 stands as an exceptional case, though at the time it was regarded as a harbinger of profound change

### The political dynamics of change

Notwithstanding the substantial continuities of practice, the changes introduced in Germany were both significant and broadly compatible with EU policy. The enhancement of the role of securities markets, the greater privileging of shareholder interests, the concern with improving the transparency of financial and ownership systems, the growing emphasis placed on ownership contestability, etc. have all served to shift the country markedly closer to liberal, Anglo-American practice, the reference point for all EU measures in this field. The role of the EU in initiating and shaping these changes, however, is considerably less clear. In relation to the source of reforming impetus, it is evident that it was not the only agent of change. The legal and regulatory reforms introduced were at least partly driven by the need to respond to the threats and opportunities stemming from the wider process of global financial market integration. The growth of international capital mobility presented new challenges that were impossible to ignore. Nor is it the case that the impetus for reform was entirely externally generated. In the German case, in particular, the impact of its specific historical experience in the late 1980s and 1990s must be recognized. Following unification in 1990, the country had been subject to enormous economic stresses that served to generate a pervasive sense of crisis. The perception that the *Modell Deutschland* was no longer working was widespread, as growth rates declined and unemployment rose. A corresponding sense of the necessity for fundamental reform developed and, by the mid-1990s, previously alien ideas had moved to the centre stage of the policy debate. Protecting 'shareholders and increasing the use of securitized finance had become important policy goals' (Cioffi, 2002: 8). Traditional mechanisms of corporate control such as interlocking directorates, insider-oriented accounting standards and limited minority shareholder protection were now deemed to be 'inconsistent with the political goals of an emerging "competitive state"' and German companies began to compete to establish a capital market orientation (Beyer and Höpner, 2003).

To a significant degree, the impact of EU initiatives derived from their compatibility with these other sources of reform pressure. Its policies tended to deepen the impact of globalization and legitimate the spread of new policy ideas. Most obviously, the single market and single currency projects served to intensify the impact of global financial market integration. Under the terms of the former, restrictions on the movement of capital were removed in all member states. As a consequence of the latter, the restrictive effects of prudential regulation related to exchange-rate fluctuation risks in insurance and pension investments were eroded. Fund managers were now free to look beyond the 'prison' of their national currency area. Equally, as many in Germany came to question the efficacy of established institutions, the importance of the EU in offering an alternative model of political economic organization should not be underestimated. The activism of the EU in this area fed the German debate. The need to transpose EU directives in the financial field and to apply competition policy weakened the position of those in Germany who sought to uphold the status quo. EU policy tended to work with the grain both of global economic change and domestic crisis. The conjunction and interaction of these factors greatly aided the project of liberal reform.

Similarly, in relation to the specific terms of the reforms introduced, the impact of the EU must be understood in its broader context. The legislative and regulatory interventions required of member states to substantiate the EU's liberal vision were many and complex. Inevitably, the success of its programme was dependent on the uncertain dynamics of domestic policy-making. This is illustrated by the experience of stock-exchange reform. The thrust of EU policy clearly favoured the development of the role of capital markets through their liberalization and integration and the enhancement of investor protection. However, for the most part, the degree of its legal imposition was low (Thatcher, 2007c: 112). Broad objectives were set out, but national authorities enjoyed a wide latitude over how to meet them. Thus, while the Investment Services Directive (1993) required member states to nominate a securities supervisory body that would undertake coordination with other member states, the structure and precise role of this body was left almost entirely to national policymakers to determine. Basic issues concerning its composition, its federal or regional structure, its powers, etc. were the focus of intensive lobbying in Germany from the late 1980s until the establishment in 2002 of the BaFin (*Bundesanstalt für Finanzdienstleitungsaufsicht*) (Thatcher, 2007c: 113). Change in response to EU initiatives was unavoidable, but the prescriptive content of EU measures was frequently quite modest.

In practice, the occurrence of EU-conformant change was greatly dependent on the development of a supportive and powerful coalition of domestic reformers. In respect of securities-market change in Germany, the process

began in the 1980s with the emergence of a reforming coalition compos-
ing large private German banks, the Frankfurt Stock Exchange, the Federal
Ministry of Finance and the *Bundesbank* (Deeg, 2005a: 334; Thatcher 2007c:
106). This so-called 'Frankfurt coalition' justified its project by reference to
the challenge presented by EU activity and the innovations of key competitor
states such as Britain. However, the extent to which the details of the changes
introduced were determined by domestic politics rather than EU prescriptions is striking. Ultimately, the terms of the new regulatory system were
shaped by the capacity of this coalition to overcome resistance to change and
drive through the reforms they sought. In many instances, national reforms
went well beyond what was necessary to satisfy the basic requirements of EU
legal transposition (Thatcher, 2007c: 112). While the EU's role as 'context' was
crucial, the precise nature of the changes introduced reflected the dynamics
of domestic coalition-building and policy conflict.

   Moreover, it is evident that national political and institutional factors play
an important role in facilitating or inhibiting the emergence of reforming
coalitions. This is exemplified by the response of business to the prospect of
substantial change in the system of corporate governance. While at a general
level there was widespread support for reform within the business community, there was little agreement about the precise nature of the changes that
should be introduced (Ziegler, 2001: 216). Differences of view reflected quite
different economic positions. Thus, while many large companies began to
espouse the importance of enhancing shareholder value as they invested
abroad, smaller firms were frequently alarmed by the prospect of unravelling
key relationships that underpin their productive strategies. While the large
banks became increasingly global in their thinking, even the largest manu-
facturing firms were cautious about undermining the general pattern of
cooperative relations with labour, of which the corporate governance system
formed an important part. Such differences of interest are unsurprising.
Substantial regulatory change is very likely to split any business community.
However, what is significant here is that the tradition of highly integrated
business representation in Germany inhibited the capacity of those who did
favour substantial reform to organize and press their case. On the one hand,
broad-based, peak business associations found it impossible to develop a
coherent position in relation to legislative reform in the face of significant
membership disagreement (Vogel, 2002: 1114). On the other, the organizational strength and representational legitimacy of these institutions made
them difficult to circumvent. In this instance, associational structures served
to mute the voice and disorganize the power of business, and the extent of
corporate governance reform was more modest than it might otherwise have
been.

   The interaction between EU policies and national institutions is very
sensitive to the specific character of each. As noted in chapter 1, institutions embody political compromises between conflicting actors. Inevitably,

therefore, they also contain points of tension and disagreement between those same actors. The success of EU initiatives in achieving effective implementation will be partly related to the degree to which its programme reinforces the logic of compromise or exploits the latent fissures within a particular institution. In the case of the Thirteenth Directive on Takeovers, for example, the EU's proposals succeeded in uniting many elements of business, most political parties and trade unions behind a policy of resistance. As noted in the previous chapter, this Directive was designed to create a European-wide takeover regime. After many years of negotiation, it looked set fair to pass into law in 2001 with the support of the Council of Ministers. By the spring of 2001, however, widespread opposition was growing in Germany. The major point of contention concerned its 'neutrality clause' (Callaghan and Höpner, 2005). This required management to remain neutral in the event of a bid but did not disbar the use of golden shares that were common in Italy and France but unknown in Germany. Under this provision, German firms would be defenceless in the face of bids from abroad, but would not gain a reciprocal advantage when seeking to buy firms in other countries. The Directive was attractive to shareholders who could expect to profit significantly in such a regime, but their lobbyists proved unable to resist the mobilization of a broad coalition of opposition to the measure in Germany. German management feared their vulnerability to takeover, especially from abroad. German labour feared the likely reordering of company priorities that would follow a successful bid. The CDU and the SPD united in defence of the national economy. A corporate governance reform designed to entrench key aspects of the shareholder-oriented model in European law provoked a powerful defensive reaction in Germany (Gordon, 2002: 52). The terms of the measure reinforced the socioeconomic compromises embodied in established institutional arrangements.

In contrast, where EU policy strikes at the fissures of conflicting interest that invariably exist within socioeconomic institutions, genuine Europeanization becomes much more feasible. This is perhaps best illustrated by the competition policy case taken by the Commission against the privileges enjoyed by the *Landesbanken*. The outcome of this action took two principal forms. Firstly, an agreement was reached in 2004, after 12 years of conflict, that six of these banks should repay some €4.3 billion of illegal subsidies to their respective regional governments. Secondly, in 2001, at the insistence of the Commission, it was agreed that the public guarantees provided by regional governments to public banks should end by July 2005 (Lütz, 2005: 143). This was a very significant policy shift that profoundly challenged the operation of these banks and their ability to perform the industrial policy and public service functions they had traditionally been charged with by their regional governments.

However, the course of this challenge illustrates the extent to which reform emerged from the complex interaction between EU policy and domestic institutions. As noted above, the banking sector was segmented into three distinct groups. The development and governance of German banking had been shaped by the relationship between them. Thus, rules governing the financial system had traditionally been developed consensually through a bargaining process involving the three associations representing the different sectors, each sharing a wholly national conception of themselves and the industry as a whole. Yet, at the same time, these groups were competitors, highly sensitive to transgressions by the others into 'their' area of activity. Governance of the banking sector rested on a complex equilibrium between cooperation and competition. EU intrusion destabilized this equilibrium. In particular, its competition policy rules offered an opportunity for some groups to 'renegotiate' the balance of advantage embodied in this institution.

Tellingly, the crucial first step along the path of reform came from the German private bank sector. Their initial concern that a loss of national policy cohesion might damage their interests gave way to a desire to realize the potential gains of a more European-oriented policy. Long resentful of the perceived competitive disadvantage that they had to endure vis-à-vis the public banks, and angered by the willingness of the *Landesbanken* to move into new business areas, it was they who initiated Commission action against regional subsidies and legal guarantees (Grossman, 2006: 333). The first breach came in 1993 when the private banks, following their failure to block the move at national level, complained to the Commission over the decision by the government of North Rhine-Westphalia to engineer a merger with a public housing company, the effect of which was to transfer approximately €3 billion to Germany's biggest public bank, WestLB (ibid.: 335). This move met with partial success, with the Commission obliging WestLB to repay some €870 million to the *Land* government. Emboldened by this success, and driven by the pressure to enhance their competitive position, the German private banks then plucked up the courage to challenge the public bank system more directly, instituting a formal complaint calling for the European Commission to investigate the competitive implications of the public banks' protected status in Germany.

The reaction to Commission involvement in this area from regional governments, a large part of the CDU and many segments of industry was extremely hostile. The conference of the heads of the *Länder*, under the leadership of the CDU/CSU future candidate for German Chancellor, threatened to block EU enlargement if the Commission did not desist from interfering with the *Landesbanken* (ibid.: 339). Ultimately, however, the Commission proved irresistible and a substantial regulatory change was forced upon Germany. The large private banks achieved reforms in regulation that they had long favoured by appealing to European agencies. If the conditions are right, national actors can leverage EU law and policy to strengthen their position within the institutional structures of the national political economy. Similarly, depending on the circumstances, the EU may be able to exploit existing intra-institutional tensions to Europeanize national institutions more effectively.

## Restructuring Corporate Finance, Ownership and Governance: Italy

In the area of corporate finance, ownership and governance, traditional Italian practice ran strongly counter to the liberal impulse of EU policy. As in Germany, banks have been the principal source of external funding for non-financial firms. Debt-to-equity ratios have been high and financial markets have played a relatively marginal role in providing investment finance to firms. Corporate ownership has been closely held, with opaque networks of families and financial firms dominating the corporate sector. However, its system differs from Germany's in important respects. In Italy, while most firms turned to banks rather than financial markets for outside capital, these banks were not universal in nature. They did not acquire ownership stakes in industrial firms nor did they play the active, directive role that German banks so frequently assumed. In this sense, they conformed neither to the securities market-based nor the standard bank-based ideal types.

The distinctive profile of the Italian system was largely a legacy of regulatory choices made in response to the profound economic crisis of the early 1930s. The Italian economy had been characterized by complex, large-scale cross-ownership links between banks and industrial firms. An effective run on the banks led to the collapse of the financial system and the near bankruptcy of the industrial sector. In the event, the state had to step in and nationalize most of the banking industry in order to prevent a total systemic failure. The Banking Act of 1936 established a new regulatory framework designed to prevent a repeat of this episode. A rigid separation between the banking and industrial sectors was introduced. Commercial banks were prohibited from taking ownership stakes in non-financial firms. Instead, they were confined to providing short-term credit, typically no longer than 18 months (Cobham et al., 1999: 328). More generally, intimate links between banks and industrial firms were effectively discouraged and the practice developed whereby firms tended to raise loans from a large number of different credit institutions rather than seeking to develop close and privileged connections with a few. Thus, relationships between banks and their debtors were not close and the former played little role in monitoring the latter's management or influencing the development of its ownership.

The 1936 Act also empowered the Bank of Italy to exercise a close supervisory role with a strong emphasis on maintaining system stability. In practice, this meant that the banks' competitive strategies were heavily constrained by public regulation. Banks were limited in the number of branches they could open and restricted in their ability to move beyond their geographical base. The provision of long-term credit to industrial firms was confined to a small number of state-owned Special Credit Institutions. Indeed, most banks remained within the ownership of the state or para-state institutions. As late as 1991, it was estimated that publicly owned banks collected some 80 per cent of all deposits and gave 90 per cent of all loans (Marrelli and Stroffolini, 1998: 152). The degree of control exercised by the state and public regulatory institutions over the functioning of the banking sector and its relationship with industry was enormous. One strand of court decisions even 'considered banking as objectively having some of the characteristics of a public service' (Ciocca, 2005: 7). Stability was heavily favoured over competition.

The specificity of the Italian system is also strongly evident in its pattern of corporate governance. Until recently, this has been characterized both by the extent of the state's role and the dominance of family capitalism in the private sector. In the early 1990s, a survey of companies listed on the stock exchange in Milan and those companies linked to them found that approximately 50 per cent were ultimately controlled by the state and 35 per cent by families or coalitions of family groups (Bianco et al., 1996: 8). No listed firm conformed to the Anglo-American public company model, with a widely dispersed pattern of share ownership. Furthermore, both the state and families exploited the weakness of investor-protection rules to develop extensive group pyramids. These enabled the ultimate entrepreneurs to maximize the reach of their corporate control at the lowest feasible cost. The pervasiveness of these techniques was such that in 1993 it was found that 55.4 per cent of Italian industrial firms belonged to pyramidal groups, including almost all firms with more than 1,000 employees (ibid.:11). Another survey established that, of some 9,500 firms examined, about 7,000 belonged to groups (Bianchi and Casavola, 1996: 6). Such pyramiding practices were favoured by a tax policy that ensured that dividends were taxed only once, no matter how many levels there were in the control chain. In addition, there were no legal provisions to prevent conflicts of interests between the controlling agent and minority shareholders in the subsidiaries (Bianchi et al., 2001: 161). The use of such techniques enables the Agnelli family, masters of FIAT, to gain control of up to eight times the amount of capital they themselves put into the group (ibid.: 182).

It is telling that the only Italian bank to play a significant role in the elaboration and functioning of these techniques of corporate governance, Mediobanca, exercised all its considerable might to sustain the power of the dominant families. It orchestrated a complex system of inter-corporate/inter-family alliances to maintain their respective empires even as the proportion of share capital each family owned dwindled. Equally tellingly, and somewhat ironically, its ability to develop this role derived from its state-protected position as the sole investment bank in the country. It exploited complex political and personal networks to gain access to cheap funds from cash-rich financial institutions such as Comit and Assicurazioni Generali (Tamburini, 1992: 126–8). These funds were then deployed to advance the interests and protect the patrimony of private family capitalism, which felt itself threatened by potential state encroachment and intervention by foreign or domestic outsiders. The system afforded little protection to minority shareholders. The market for corporate control was moribund, with privileged controlling shareholders well placed to command a *premio di maggioranza* (control benefit) in the event of a company being sold to other groups. A national system of ownership and control embodying a very particular distribution of economic power between public and private actors was facilitated and sustained by the systems of financial regulation and corporate governance.

### Change

There have been substantial changes in key elements of this system over the last two decades and many of them have been prompted by EU activity. Perhaps the most significant took place in the banking industry. Most directly, the Second Banking Directive effectively overturned many of the key provisions of the Italian system established in the 1930s. Legally sanctioned distinctions between savings banks and commercial banks were removed and broad-based integrated banking operations across a full range of financial services, including retail, investment, mortgage business, etc., emerged. Restrictions on bank holdings in non-financial companies were lifted. Regulatory support for the regional differentiation of the banking sector ended and, as a consequence, the national integration of the sector was greatly enhanced. More indirectly, the Maastricht criteria for EMU participation had a major impact. These laid down restrictions on the level of annual budget deficits and total public debt, setting them at 3 per cent and 60 per cent of GDP respectively. With deficits of up to 10 per cent and public debt of more than 100 per cent of GDP, Italian governments faced an enormous challenge if they were to realize their ambition of gaining early entry to the euro. In these circumstances, the attraction of raising finance by selling its enormous stock of banking and industrial assets proved irresistible and, by the early twenty-first century, the financial sector had been almost completely privatized. Finally, with the institution of a national competition policy in 1991 in response to EU demands, and the related enhancement of the Bank of Italy's powers to oversee the financial sector, the traditional emphasis on stability gave way to a greater concern with competition. Many of the restrictions on the conduct of bank business designed to restrict competition were substantially eased. Thus, Italian consumers saw a 70 per cent rise in the number of bank branches between 1990 and 2000, and the range, choice and price of banking services available to them improved significantly (Ciocca, 2005: 173). The structure and ownership of Italian banks was transformed, allowing them to develop new competitive strategies and enter new markets, in terms of both territory and product.

However, change in regulatory practice was not confined to banking. In an effort to align Italian practice more closely with EU norms, a substantial reform of key aspects of securities market regulation took place. *Il Testo Unico della Finanza* (Law 58/1998, generally known as the Draghi Law) represented an ambitious attempt to reorient financial sector regulation in a more liberal direction. In respect of corporate governance, the Draghi Law sought to substantially strengthen the capacity of shareholders outside the controlling group to influence the actions of management, by exercising an effective 'voice' within the company. Thus, Article 127 significantly simplified and eased the rules on correspondence voting, thereby reducing the cost to small shareholders of participating in company ballots. Article 125 lowered the threshold of shares required to convene a general shareholders' meeting from 20 to 10 per cent. New rules on the publication and dissemination of financial information, introduced as a direct response to EU measures, were designed to provide all shareholders and potential shareholders with a sound basis on which to make investment decisions (Belli et al., 1998: 173). Perhaps most importantly, Law 58/1998 sought to protect minority shareholder interests in the event of a takeover through the effective incorporation of large elements of the City of London's Takeover Code into Italian law. Thus, it introduced a new Mandatory Bid Rule (MBR) that required any shareholder – or group of shareholders acting in concert – gaining control of over 30 per cent of the voting stock to offer to purchase the remaining shares within 30 days of exceeding the threshold. The rule is designed to prevent the passing of control from one group of shareholders to another without benefit to minority shareholders.[2] Together with the greater resources that enhanced investor protection might stimulate, it was hoped that adopting the City Code would facilitate the development of a market for corporate control.

The scale of these reforms is undeniable. The banking sector became markedly more competitive. The regulatory system was reconfigured to mirror much more closely the practices of Anglo-American liberal capitalism. Moreover, changes in capital gains tax introduced in 2003 were designed to encourage the unwinding of pyramidal ownership structures. Together, the reforms represented a substantial break with the structures and practices that had dominated Italian capitalism since the late 1940s. However, their success in changing the dominant forms of governance is much more open to question. Central to a liberal market model of ownership are issues of transparency, contestability in the form of hostile takeovers, freedom from political intervention and openness to international capital. Privatization has, of course, changed the pattern of ownership and control in Italy considerably. A major process of consolidation has taken place, with a wave of mergers and acquisitions reducing the number of banks by approximately 400 to 778 between 1990 and the end of 2004 (Banca d'Italia, 2005: 414). There is evidence that the use of pyramids has lessened somewhat (Bianchi et al., 2001). Yet the manner of this process of consolidation and the ownership structures it has generated do not appear to adhere to liberal market norms. This is partly because efforts to exploit the privatization process to expand the size, liquidity and openness of the stock market have met with disappointment. This is particularly evident in the banking sector. In respect of the handful of sizeable, publicly owned commercial banks, the attempt to exploit the instrument of public share offerings to create a true 'public company' with a wide diffusion of shareholders has largely failed. In the case of Comit and Credit, for example, a process designed to ensure that they would not fall under the control of the dominant financial player, the merchant bank Mediobanca, completely backfired. Through determined, coordinated action with its allies, Mediobanca bought sufficient shares to ensure its domination of their strategic development and the appointment of a congenial management (Siglenti, 1996). The net effect was to buttress rather than transform the structure of ownership and control in the private sector.

In respect of the remainder of the banking sector, the Amato Law (1990) saw the large number of savings institutions split into public limited companies (banks) and private law 'not-for-profit' foundations, which were given ownership of the banks. This arrangement was intended to be transitional. Foundations were to sell 'their' bank to the public and use the funds to further their charitable mission. In practice, however, many foundations retained control, with the largest shaping a wave of cross-shareholding alliance building between banks from the second half of the 1990s onwards (Catelani 2005: 32). By 2004, foundations controlled just over 20 per cent of the shares of the 10 largest banking groups (Banca d'Italia 2005: 363). In a reflection of their power and ambivalent status, it has become common in Italy to distinguish between state ownership and public ownership. While by the end of the 1990s, the state had withdrawn from bank ownership, a large part of the banking sector was still partially protected from competitive pressures and still partially subject to the logic of power rather than profit. The principal author of the reform, Giuliano Amato, subsequently characterized his creation as a 'monster' and his own role as that of a 'Frankenstein' (Clarich and Pisaneschi, 2001: 43). Assessing the outcome, Inzerillo and Messori conclude that privatization and consolidation have failed to produce more transparency, contestability or efficiency in bank ownership (2000: 180).

The non-banking sector presents a similar picture of substantial continuity. As noted above, Italian private industry has long been marked by a tendency to construct cross-shareholding alliances designed to secure the economic and political power of key families and institutions, ranging from the Agnelli to the merchant bank Mediobanca. To date, the evidence is that privatization and regulatory reform have merely served to restructure these networks and alliances rather than supersede them as organizing mechanisms. A Bank of Italy survey of change in the pattern of ownership and control in the decade since 1993 concluded that ownership concentration continues to be high and direct family control remains as prevalent as ever. It is still the case that financial institutions rarely own capital stakes or play a role in controlling non-financial firms. Most firms continue to be owned by other firms and ultimate ownership is still generally in the hands of families. The market for corporate control remains underdeveloped, with 'insider', personal relations continuing to play a decisive role in determining the course of corporate restructuring (Giacomelli and Trento, 2005: 5). Foreign ownership of Italian industry has grown marginally but remains under 10 per cent (ibid.: 79). Furthermore, while new patterns of cross-shareholding alliances have emerged, the organization and management of these systems conform to traditional practice. Although the stock market capitalization to GDP ratio has risen from 18 to 63 per cent between 1996 and 2006, fewer than 25 per cent of the firms listed can be described as widely held (Franks et al., 2008: 5). The 'new' system of corporate ownership that had developed by the early twenty-first century can be described neither as transparent nor as open and contestable.

The durability of established patterns of corporate ownership and governance casts some doubt on the efficacy of legal and regulatory reform as an instrument of political economic transformation. In practice, the impact of any given reform is frequently highly dependent on developments in contiguous areas. Without related changes in these, the ambitions of reformers may well be confounded. Thus, for example, in an analysis of the 1998 Draghi reforms, Bianchi and Enriques conclude that even though the changes introduced did indeed strengthen the protection for small shareholders, the structural characteristics of the Italian financial sector restricted their impact on the conduct of corporate governance. In the ideal-typical Anglo-American model, such minority shareholder protection provisions enable a multitude of financial institutions holding relatively small individual stakes to exercise substantial influence over management behaviour. In Italy, by contrast, the absence of key public reforms in the pension sector means that the major financial institutions are insurance companies and mutual fund investors. The great majority of these are owned by banks anxious to maintain good relations with firms in order to protect their wider commercial relations (Bianchi and Enriques, 2001: 4). Consequently, financial institutions are reluctant to challenge practices that would be deemed unacceptable in London, irrespective of the formal regulatory rules. The dense networks of relations characterizing the Italian pattern of ownership and control prevent financial institutions from developing the sort of role that marks their behaviour in Britain.

The persistence of traditional, insider-oriented corporate practices, despite the introduction of stronger shareholder protection provisions, is perhaps best illustrated by the tortuous story of Italia Telecom, the large state-owned telecommunications provider. This company was privatized in 1997. Early fears that it would simply be incorporated into the opaque system of cross-shareholding alliances that had dominated Italian capitalism for decades were initially dispelled when, in a dramatic break with Italian tradition, Italia Telecom was the subject of a successful hostile takeover bid by the Italian firm, Olivetti. Exploiting the recent introduction of the euro to raise finance on a scale that would have been impossible in lira markets alone, Olivetti proclaimed its commitment to the advancement of shareholder interests and overcame the strong resistance of Italia Telecom's senior management to complete the bid. The international financial press hailed this as a triumph for liberal market capitalism and the promise of a bright, shareholder-friendly future. This judgement proved premature, however. Olivetti assumed a very large debt in order to finance the takeover. Subsequently, it repeatedly sought to reduce this burden by engineering complex share swaps between different elements of the Telecom group of companies (Kruse, 2005). However, the effect of these measures would have been to favour the interests of Olivetti over those of minority shareholders. Though the proposals were defeated by shareholder opposition, Olivetti's behaviour badly damaged its claim to be the outrider of a new, more shareholder-friendly Italian capitalism. One foreign investor remarked to the *Wall Street Journal* that 'when we met with Mr Colaninno [Olivetti's chief executive] during the takeover, he promised us to focus on shareholder value, this has all turned out to be a hoax' (quoted in ibid.: 17).

Subsequent events proved much more damaging to the proclamations of a new era. Unable to overcome its financial difficulties, in 2001 Olivetti sold its shares to Pirelli and Edizione Holdings, a Benetton family company, at an 80 per cent premium over the then current market price (Kruse, 2005: 34). The combined holding of 27 per cent of the shares allowed these two companies to enjoy effective control of Italia Telecom, while minority shareholders gained nothing from the transaction. Kirchmaier and Grant (2008) demonstrate that Pirelli was able 'to creatively comply with the law by acquiring control further up the control chain from a privately held company', thereby circumventing the Mandatory Bid Rule provisions of the 1998 Draghi reforms (which were not triggered until a holding exceeded 30 per cent). Moreover, while in Britain disadvantaged shareholders caught in such a situation could have realistic hopes of finding redress through the courts on the grounds that the company had breached its fiduciary duty to minority shareholders, no such option was feasible in Italy (ibid.: 19). Even though Pirelli's strategy damaged the interests of numerous Italian mutual funds that found themselves among the shareholders excluded from the deal's financial rewards, the fact that these funds were generally affiliated to the banks and insurance companies that held equity and/or debt in Pirelli meant that they were extremely reluctant to contest the issue (ibid.). Rules borrowed from the City of London Code find it difficult to gain traction amid the tangled web of relationships between banks, financial institutions and industrial firms that characterizes Italian capitalism.

The pattern of change in Italy is somewhat paradoxical. The occurrence of profound reform in the role of the state and in key aspects of the regulatory structure is undeniable. Moreover, it is clear that the EU exercised a substantial direct and indirect influence over these changes. Yet, thus far the impact of these measures on the structure of corporate finance, ownership and governance has been comparatively modest. The roots of established practices spread much more widely than reformers fully grasped. Without extensive reforms of social policy and/or judicial practice, the importation of Anglo-American regulatory standards may simply fail to have the anticipated effects.

At the very least, they cast some doubt on the efficacy of regulatory change to achieve substantial structural and behavioural transformations.

### The political dynamics of change

To a very great extent, capitalism in Italy has been national capitalism. Large parts of the financial and industrial system have been state-controlled. The level of foreign direct investment has been relatively low. Though Italy has had great success in exporting its goods, relatively few large Italian multinational companies have developed. Product, labour and financial markets have been restrictively regulated. The system has been overwhelmingly insider-oriented. The challenges presented to such a system by participating in the creation of a liberal European market are enormous. Effective integration into the European project requires the opening up of deeply rooted networks of economic and political power.

As noted above, Italy's response to this challenge has been complex and ambiguous. It has been marked both by significant regulatory reform and a substantial continuity of behaviour. The extent of reform largely reflects the success of a group of technocrats in exploiting the political turmoil of the 1990s, which followed the corruption scandals and the collapse of the dominant Christian Democratic Party, to push through major change. Led by the departmental head at the Treasury, Mario Draghi, the former Governor of the Bank of Italy, Carlo Azeglio Ciampi, and his successor, Antonio Fazio, this group played a leading role in driving through all the major reforms of the 1990s from privatization through corporate governance reform to monetary policy (Dyson and Featherstone, 1996: 278; Deeg, 2005b: 529; McCann, 2007: 105). However, the limited impact of these initiatives on the behaviour of economic actors reveals the powerful obstacles inhibiting the effective Europeanization of economic governance in Italy. One key barrier stems from the resistance to change manifested by large elements of the business community. In a comparative study of the extent to which liberal reforms have undermined the provision of 'patient capital' by the 'coordinated' financial systems of France, Germany and Italy, Culpepper concludes that in Italy 'there is no evidence that the provision of [such capital] to companies has changed at all since 1990', a factor he attributes to the attitudes of key business actors (2005: 188–9). In France, the AXA group had stood at the centre of cross-shareholding networks that bound the financial and industrial systems together. Following its decision to break from tradition and pursue profit maximization, even at the expense of its long-term relationships, the system quickly unravelled. In Italy no comparable transformative act has yet occurred.

A second major obstacle to reform stems from the administrative character of the Italian state. At a general level, its weak administrative capacity has meant that public regulation and surveillance have often been poorly executed (Ferrarini, 2005: 2). Even if willing, its capacity to implement effectively a liberal regulatory order has been doubted. At a more specific level, the application of EU legal norms has been greatly hindered by 'a judicial system ill-equipped to help enforce the new regulatory regime' (ibid.: 26). An empirical examination of the decisions of the Milan court, widely recognized as the most specialized and expert court in Italy in matters pertaining to corporate law, found it to be highly formalistic in its reasoning, reluctant to consider the substance of disagreements between parties, and extremely deferential to the decision-making of controlling shareholders (Enriques 2001: 86–98). None of these proclivities is appropriate to the role envisaged for the courts in a more liberal regime of corporate law and corporate governance. Many of the traditions and structures of the Italian state are inimical to the effective implementation of a liberal reform agenda. Effective Europeanization requires fundamental structural and normative changes in key national institutions that have eluded reformers for many decades.

The third key obstacle to effective Europeanization stems from the powerful influence of economic nationalist reasoning in Italy. Even among committed reformers there has been a persistent determination to retain in Italian hands as much control as possible of Italy's economic assets. This perspective was evident in the form of privatization adopted in the 1990s. In the case of Italia Telecom, the state retained a 'golden share' that would enable it to block unwanted takeovers. In addition, it sought to create a core shareholder group that would oversee the successful financing and management of the newly privatized company, while retaining it in national hands. Subsequently, when Olivetti launched its takeover, the Italian government supported it by effectively blocking a counter-bid by Deutsche Telekom on the grounds that such an important business asset should not fall into foreign hands (McCann, 2000: 57). When in early 2007 Pirelli sought to sell the company to foreign buyers, there was widespread political and public dismay. The centre-left government and business leaders quickly moved to establish an alternative consortium and the potential bidders from the US and Mexico were forced to withdraw.[3] Moreover, defensive nationalism was not confined to the centre-left. During the course of his successful general election campaign in the spring of 2008, Silvio Berlusconi denounced the prospect of a sale of the troubled airline, Alitalia, to Air France.[4] He called instead for an Italian solution and even hinted half seriously that his own family might participate in such a project. Subsequently, his new government successfully engineered a deal that kept the greater part of the airline in Italian hands. Repeatedly, governments of the left and right, in concert with leading financial and industrial business interests, have moved to protect the national control of large firms.

The depth and significance of this nationalist perspective is revealed by the actions of the Bank of Italy. Its reputation, both nationally and internationally, has been as a zealous agent of liberal, pro-competitive reform (Dyson and Featherstone, 1996; Deeg, 2005b). However, notwithstanding this record, the evidence of its economically nationalist behaviour is substantial. On the one hand, it exploited its considerable discretion in choosing the ownership of Italian banks to oversee the creation of complex new cross-shareholding arrangements between the newly privatized banks in order to protect national control (Catelani 2005: 140). On the other, it fought a determined campaign to restrict foreign investors in Italian banks to minority stakes. The depth of the Bank's determination to prevent foreigners from taking control became controversially apparent in 2005, following the launch of separate takeovers by a Dutch (ABN Amro) and a Spanish (BBVA) bank. In the case of ABN Amro's bid for Antonveneta, for example, its governor, Antonio Fazio, actively canvassed among Italian banks for a counter-bidder. He found a candidate in his close acquaintance Gianpiero Fiorani, who controlled the northern regional bank Popolare di Lodi, and gave every appearance of exploiting his regulatory powers in favour of the 'home' bid. The extraordinarily close nature of their relationship was revealed in July 2005 when verbatim reports from phone wiretaps were published in the national newspaper, *La Repubblica*. In these, Fazio expressed his deep gratitude to Fiorani for his (apparently) successful efforts to take over Antonveneta and block ABN Amro. The revelations caused a furore. By the high summer of 2005, Antonio Fazio was under judicial investigation regarding an alleged illegal conspiracy to block a foreign takeover of an Italian bank, and subject to ferocious condemnation for his actions both by the opposition and by some parts of the Cabinet, including the Finance Minister.[5] In November 2005, Italy found itself the subject of legal enforcement action by the European Commission for breach of European law in relation to the same events. By Christmas, Fiorani was in prison and Fazio had resigned (McCann, 2007: 113).

The logic of the Bank's behaviour is revealing. Fundamentally, its function is to protect the integrity of the Italian financial system and of the Italian economic system in general. A central feature of this system is its localism and the intimate links that exist between regional banks and industry. The Bank had long recognized the importance of these relationships and deployed its regulatory authority to foster their development. Its influential post-war governor, Donato Menichella, believed that the role of local banks in funding the small firm sector was crucial to the economy's growth and deserved protection.[6] Such territorially and socially rooted networks, already under pressure from regulatory changes, would be threatened by the intrusion of foreign owners employing different metrics of business success (Conti and Ferri 1997: 459). Even in the changed context of the twenty-first century, the Bank of Italy could not be indifferent to the fate of these relationships. Cesare Geronzi, a long-time ally of Antonio Fazio and the influential chairman of Capitalia, one of the five largest Italian banks, clearly expressed this concern about the loss of economic control: '[W]e must recognize our weakness, that our system is the most open to attack in Europe . . . if one loses control over bank decision-making, we could find ourselves in a position where we aren't able to contribute to decisions that govern our country's economy.'[7] Carlo Giovanardi, a minister in Berlusconi's government, publicly expressed his belief that 'if anyone thinks that Italian banks, bought by foreign banks, would still help our small and medium-sized businesses on the ground, they are greatly mistaken'.[8] Though less stark in its declarations, it is evident that the Bank of Italy shared many of these anxieties. In his annual statement in May 2005, Governor Fazio noted the importance of Italian banks in financing Italian industry, with over 70 per cent of small and medium-sized firms relying on them for external funding. Given this importance, he argued that it was vital in this transitional phase 'that the support of the credit system remains strong'.[9] The Bank's ambition was to combine liberalization, privatization and the protection of the integrity of these crucial bank–industry relationships. This required the maintenance of a substantial degree of decision-making power in Italian hands, even if such a strategy risked a clash with the European Commission. To achieve this end, the Bank had to pursue the restructuring and consolidation of the sector while relying on Italian agents. However, with pension funds little more than embryonic and the financial markets still underdeveloped, its overriding difficulty was to find private Italian investors capable of securing national control while achieving the necessary consolidation and enhancement of efficiency. To overcome these problems, it chose to exploit rather than transcend the traditional mechanisms of Italian inter-corporate alliance building. Such alliances facilitated consolidation and the creation of stable ownership structures without the need for vast sums of capital on the part of the constituent members. For the same reason, the Bank allowed the foundations to play a pivotal role in effecting consolidation, praising them for their contribution to ownership stability.[10] It could not afford the luxury of marginalizing such well-resourced actors on the basis of their peculiar legal status. A project that sought to integrate the Italian into the European financial system on the best terms possible required the exploitation of many traditional mechanisms that would be anathema to Anglo-American capitalism and, perforce, the European Commission.

## Conclusion

The European Union has launched an ambitious programme of banking and securities market reform since the 1980s. Its twin purpose was to integrate and reorient the financial systems of member states. More integrated markets would offer greater scale and flexibility to both creditors and debtors. The reorientation of European finance towards the Anglo-American securities market-based model, it was argued, would enable investors to benefit from the perceived superior innovative capacity and enormous resources of such systems. Ultimately, the availability of more flexible and cheaper finance would raise investment and growth levels in Europe. In addition, such a reorientation would support the emergence of a market for corporate control. This, in turn, would facilitate necessary acts of corporate restructuring and constrain managements to be more efficient and less self-serving in their actions. Given the scale of this project, it is perhaps unsurprising if it remains far from fully realized. Consolidation of the banking industry has taken place. However, this has occurred overwhelmingly within rather than across national borders. Securities markets have expanded. Yet banks continue to play the central role in corporate finance, especially outside the large-firm sector. Moreover, the financial crisis of 2008–9 has added a great deal of uncertainty to the exercise. The weaknesses of securities-based systems have become starkly apparent and regulatory authorities and policymakers are likely to be more concerned with stability than innovation for some considerable time to come.

However, evidence from the two case studies does indicate that while change has fallen far short of transformation, EU initiatives have had a major impact on the structure and governance of national financial systems. In Germany, for example, securities markets have undergone substantial re-regulation, at least partly in response to EU measures. The application of European competition policy has transformed the status and role of Germany's publicly owned regional banks within the national financial system. Though not directly mandated by EU policy, important regulatory changes have been introduced, which strengthen minority shareholder protection and render networks of ownership more transparent. Large banks in particular have embraced the language and practice of 'shareholder value' and withdrawn from the role of 'inter-corporate network manager' that they had traditionally played. In Italy, the Second Banking Directive necessitated a fundamental transformation in the regulation of Italian banks. A major reform of corporate governance designed to enhance shareholder protection and facilitate the development of a market for corporate control was introduced, largely in response to EU activity. More indirectly, the fiscal pressures unleashed by the single currency project prompted an enormous wave of bank privatization in Italy. In short, the EU has played a central, though not exclusive, role in promoting the fundamental restructuring of regulation in the financial and corporate sectors in both countries.

Yet it is equally evident that, in relation to corporate ownership and governance, practices persist in both countries that are anathema to the norms of the Anglo-American, shareholder-oriented model. In Germany, the key institutions of co-determination remain largely unaltered. Companies are governed by a form of power-sharing between shareholders, managers and employees. Insider networks built around corporate cross-shareholding arrangements and/or interlocking directorates are still common. Hostile takeovers remain very uncommon. In Italy, corporate control continues to be dominated by families and complex inter-firm alliance structures. Hostile takeovers are rare and can only succeed if there is powerful political backing. The terms of corporate restructuring deals still tend to favour privileged 'insiders' over other shareholders. More problematically, the case studies also suggest that the capacity of the EU to enforce a radical reform of these practices is quite limited. In Germany, for example, the degree of its influence was greatly dependent on domestic developments. The real political impetus for change arose from a general sense of economic crisis and the particular proposals of powerful actors, such as the large private banks. It was the compatibility of the EU's proposals with these domestic developments that afforded it some influence. In the absence of such a congenial political context, it is doubtful that the EU would have been capable of enforcing significant change in Germany. The Italian case casts an even greater degree of doubt on the transformative power of the EU. In many respects, the regulatory reforms of investor protection and takeover law were more extensive than those introduced in Germany. Yet, despite these changes, the mechanisms of corporate ownership and control continue to exhibit their traditional characteristics. Though many of the reforms were modelled on City of London practices, the broader legal and judicial context was very different and this greatly diminished their impact. A genuine liberal transformation of the Italian system would require legal, administrative and institutional changes of enormous breadth and depth. It is inconceivable that the EU could ever gain the political and legal capacity to enforce them. Radical liberal reform must await domestic political developments.

### FURTHER READING

Frangakis (2009a, 2009b) and Grahl (2009a, 2009b, 2009c, 2009d) give detailed information concerning the progress of EU financial reforms. Deeg (2005a/b) examines the extent of reform in Germany and Italy. Thatcher (2007c) offers a very detailed accounted of securities-market reform in a number of EU member states.

6

# Work and Welfare: National Capitalism and Social Europe

## Introduction: Labour Markets and Social Models

The nature of the relationship between employers and workers in the labour market is of central importance to the functioning of economic systems. A poorly performing labour market will inhibit efficiency and growth. Firms will not find appropriately skilled labour at an affordable price and/or workers will not find employment at acceptable wages (Adnett and Hardy, 2005: 45). The particular institutional structure of a labour market will also strongly affect the distribution of power among socioeconomic actors, and the form of their interaction. Different sets of laws and associational structures inhibit or facilitate quite distinct forms of behaviour, whether of a cooperative or a conflictual nature. In turn, the properties of a given labour market are closely linked to the wider structures of the welfare state. The specific provisions of welfare policies acutely affect a range of labour market issues. Thus, the terms of social security programmes have major implications for the cost of hiring labour and the willingness of workers to strike. Pension rules have major consequences for the costs to employers of shedding older workers (Pierson, 2001: 5). Conversely, the model of employment relations, the structure of bargaining systems, rules of employment protection, etc. fundamentally influence welfare state institutions and policies (Wood, 2001: 368). Thus, for example, there is a close relationship between the development of employment-protection regulations and systems of financial provision for the unemployed.

Collectively, the complex mix of welfare and labour market arrangements found in individual states is characterized as a 'social model'. Such models 'structure individuals' access to resources through income from work and its alternatives, such as transfers and public provision, . . . before, during, and after the stages in life when they participate in the labor market' (Martin and Ross, 2004a: 11). They are composed of a specific mix of institutions that 'govern market-society relations in a particular national-specific combination' (Ebbinghaus, 1999: 3). Much of the recent discussion of social policy reform in the EU has been conducted in terms of the existence and malfunctioning of a 'European Social Model' (ESM). This ESM stands in counterpoint to the 'Anglo-American' model, exemplified by the USA, Britain, Australia and New Zealand. ESM states are said to rely more on public institutions and collective choice than on markets and individual choice. Taxes tend to be higher to sustain more generous transfer payments to cover loss of earnings from unemployment, ill-health or old age. Protection against arbitrary management power in areas such as hiring and firing and the control of the workplace is more highly developed. The substantial earnings inequality and job insecurity that typically characterize the operation of markets are significantly curtailed (Martin and Ross, 2004b: 24; Adnett and Hardy, 2005: 78–9). Employment relations are typically much more highly organized and corporatist (Grahl and Teague, 2003: 397).

Of course, this broad characterization of the ESM needs some qualification. Comparative analysts of 'welfare capitalism' in Europe have identified three distinct types of system, in addition to the Anglo-Saxon/Anglo-American variant (Ebbinghaus, 1999; Amable, 2003; Sapir, 2006; also see table 6.1). All differ substantially in relation to the rules covering employment protection, the arrangements for collective bargaining over wages and conditions of work, provisions for the representation of employee interests within the company, the terms of social security support for the unemployed, the nature of public employment policies, etc. Thus, while sharing a commitment to high levels of social protection, *Nordic* countries (Sweden, Finland, Denmark and honorary member, the Netherlands) place a far greater emphasis on 'active labour market policies' that seek to re-skill the unemployed and render them fit for the jobs that are actually available than do *Continental* countries (Austria, Germany, France and Belgium). In contrast to both these types of system, *Mediterranean* countries (Italy, Spain, Portugal and Greece) tend to impose strong employment protection mechanisms that make it difficult to fire workers rather than rely on unemployment benefit or retraining to facilitate the operation of labour markets (Amable, 2003: 106–7; Sapir, 2006: 376). Similarly, there are marked differences between these models in relation to the extent and nature both of centralized bargaining and workplace employee representation. Yet the general point remains valid. In comparison with the USA, most EU15 states exhibit a strong tendency to mitigate the impact of market forces on the material wellbeing of their citizens.

In recent years, the effectiveness and sustainability of the ESM has been the subject of growing scepticism. It has been argued, for example, that the highly interventionist and protectionist approach to labour market regulation that typically characterizes EU15 states has been partly responsible for Europe's relatively poor record in employment creation since the 1980s. The perceived inferiority of its performance in comparison with the USA has been attributed to the generally far more highly regulated character of national labour markets, the strength of trade unions and the propensity to centralize collective bargaining. Rules protecting employed workers from dismissal are said to increase the adjustment costs of firms, thereby weakening their capacity to respond quickly to competitive challenges. Centralized forms of collective wage bargaining are similarly criticized for inhibiting necessary flexibility in the face of economic change. The insensitivity of such institutions to the specific conditions of individual firms and industries is said to produce competitively inappropriate wage levels, hindering economic efficiency. The most notable proponent of this analysis is the OECD, which has argued that wage-setting arrangements in 'continental Europe' were much more detrimental to employment growth than those in the USA (Casey, 2004: 335). Recommendation five of its influential jobs study urged European governments to 'make wage and labour costs more flexible by removing restrictions that prevent wages from reflecting local conditions and individual skill levels' (OECD, 1994: 35). This criticism was extended to what are perceived to be overly generous unemployment benefits that inhibit the development of necessary wage flexibility by allowing the unemployed to hold out for better job offers than the labour market is actually generating. It argued that such 'temporary income support systems . . . have drifted towards quasi-permanent income support in many countries, lowering work incentives' (ibid.: 48). The general contention is that such 'rigidities' play a pivotal role in shaping the functioning of labour markets, the strategies and opportunities of different actors and, more critically, the relatively disappointing economic performance of many states over the last two decades or so. The implication is that labour market regulations, collective-bargaining institutions and social policies that distort the interaction of labour supply and demand should be reformed, if not eliminated.

Further doubts about the sustainability of the European social model have been raised following the establishment of a European monetary union. It is argued that membership of the Eurozone removes the national sovereign control necessary for the effective functioning of welfare systems. With fiscal policies significantly constrained by the Stability and Growth Pact and the option of currency re- or devaluation removed, the solution to problems of competitiveness and employment creation at national level must now be sought by governments 'within the heart of European social models' (Hemerijck and Ferrara, 2004: 248). Without national governmental control over the macroeconomy, 'labour market institutions and social protection arrangements' can no longer be shielded from 'the need to adjust to international competition' (ibid.). As a consequence of monetary union, welfare states are now much more fully exposed to the competitive pressures generated by the single European market. Some critics regard the enforcement of a neo-liberal reconstruction of the ESM now to be a real possibility (McNamara, 1998).

The EU's response to these criticisms and challenges is the subject of considerable dispute. Judgements concerning the nature of its ambition and effectiveness as an agent of substantial reform of national welfare systems vary greatly. Sapir, for example, laments the EU's failure to reform 'outdated labour market and social policies' at the national level despite deepening integration (2006: 373). He perceives the development of a dangerous disjunction between integrated European product and financial markets and enduring national labour market regimes. In contrast, Raveaud believes that the EU is

**Table 6.1** Varieties of 'social model' in EU15: some key features

| Type | Nordic | Continental | Mediterranean | Anglo-Saxon |
|---|---|---|---|---|
| Labour Markets | Regulated labour markets<br>Active labour market policies | Coordinated labour markets<br>Varying levels of employment protection | Regulated labour markets<br>High levels of employment protection | Flexible labour markets<br>Limited employment protection |
| Industrial Relations | Centralized trade unions' and employers' associations with high rates of membership<br>Coordinated bargaining<br>Highly compressed wage structures | Centralized trade unions' and employers' associations<br>Coordinated bargaining<br>Works councils | Fragmented trade unions<br>Decentralized bargaining with ad hoc state interventions<br>Legal extension occurs State–union crisis pacts | Fragmented unions<br>Decentralized bargaining<br>Voluntarism<br>Wide and increasing wage dispersion |
| Welfare support | Universalist model Social service orientation | Mostly employment-based benefits | Limited support with patchy coverage | Large reliance on 'last resort' social assistance<br>Increasing activation orientation. |

*Sources:* Ebbinghaus, 1999: 15; Amable, 2003: 174-5; Sapir, 2006: 376–7.

imbued with a reforming zeal that is infused with a monetarist, neo-liberal agenda that amounts 'to an attack on the European social model' (2007: 430). Finally, Hemerijck and Ferrara argue that the advent of EMU has actually triggered a 'building and deepening of social Europe' (2004: 251). Important initiatives pursued at the European level have sought to buttress the ESM in the face of new economic challenges. Basic questions concerning the coverage, logical (and ideological) thrust and effectiveness of the EU policy are the subject of dispute.

It is not the intention to examine here the course of national welfare reform in EU15 states over the past two decades. Rather, the focus of attention will be on EU efforts to develop an effective social policy role for itself. How important an actor is it in the field of social and labour-market policy? Has it developed a coherent programme of reform? Is it seeking to advance the restructuring of national systems along substantially more liberal lines, as advocated by the OECD? Can its efforts be more accurately characterized as a threat to the ESM or as an aid to its survival? This chapter will examine the developing remit, objectives and methods of the EU's social policy since its creation. The following chapter will then focus on the specific issue of industrial relations and collective bargaining. Are these fundamental systems changing in response to EU policy? The central concern of both chapters will be to establish the extent to which the actions of the EU are serving to undermine and transform the integrity of national systems of labour-market governance.

## Social Policy and the European Union

The full flowering of Europe's welfare regimes occurred between the 1950s and the 1980s. The systems that developed were state-based and exclusive. Membership and entitlement were rooted in national citizenship. While the markets of member states integrated, the thrust of social policy was in a decidedly less open direction. This disjunction reflected the nature of the political deal embodied in the Treaty of Rome. Economic integration and social protection were effectively decoupled. Integration was framed exclusively in terms of market integration and liberalization (Scharpf, 2002: 646–7). This was deemed to be both desirable and feasible. The Paris Treaty, which set up the European Coal and Steel Community, clearly stated that social policy competency would remain with national states. For the signatories of the Treaty of Rome, there appeared to be no incompatibility between open economies and closed welfare states. Indeed, Alan Milward has argued that European integration in the economic sphere helped provide the economic resources necessary for the full development of systems of national welfare. Rather than a threat, the creation of the European Community should be seen as 'an external buttress to the welfare state' (Milward, 2000: 216).

For these reasons, the social policy activity of the early EU was extremely modest. Commission efforts to develop a substantial European role in the regulation of labour markets were hamstrung by the fact that treaty provisions concerning social and employment policy were vague and afforded the EEC few concrete powers. Article 118 of the Treaty of Rome, for example, provided for the Commission to promote cooperation through studies, opinions and consultations. Though the general liberal market orientation of the treaty suggested that these should be supportive of competition, the direction and purpose of cooperation and consultations were not laid out with any clarity. One of the few concrete provisions concerned equal pay for men and women undertaking the same jobs. This was the result of a French effort to ensure that its somewhat higher standards would be exported to other member states rather than undermined by regulatory competition. More generally, however, Commission proposals in the social and employment area were predicated on more generic treaty articles that provided for the approximation of national regulatory systems when necessary for establishing a common market, such as Article 100 (now 94). Under such legal cover, directives on dismissals (1974) and workers' rights in the event of a merger (1975) were introduced. However, they could not provide a legal basis for a more ambitious social and employment policy agenda. While the ECJ provided legal backing for these measures, it refrained 'from over-zealous judgements where the treaty basis was unclear' (Rhodes, 2005: 285).

The one exception to this modest social policy agenda concerned the free movement of labour. In this area, the treaty provided a solid basis for action. Article 48 (now 39) prohibited all forms of discrimination by member states regarding employment, including nationality. The practical implementation of this basic right took approximately a decade and a half. By 1961, all intra-European visa requirements had been eliminated while in 1970, all remaining obstacles were removed (Ferrara, 2005: 100). Passed in 1970, regulation 1251 introduced the right of workers to remain in the member state in which they worked after retirement. Simultaneously, measures were introduced to protect the social rights of mobile workers. Regulation 3/1958 established the principles that should govern their treatment by host states, which included non-discrimination and equality of treatment, eligibility of all periods of insurance in whatever country, benefit exportability from one member state to another and the principle that laws of the country in which the work took place should apply in determining rights (ibid.: 101–2). Collectively, these directives and regulations were not insignificant. However, with the exception of equal pay, their applicability was quite narrow and in relation to the general areas of welfare and labour market regulation, the EU was a marginal actor.

The relaunch of European integration in the 1980s began to undermine the neat and politically convenient division of labour between European and national authorities in the field of social policy. In the context of a genuine single market, the distinction between economic and social regulation became increasingly unsustainable. A truly integrated European market for product and services inevitably had substantial implications for labour markets. The rights and status of workers posted to other countries as part of the supply of goods or the provision of services assumed a much greater significance as more and more companies began to operate on a European scale. Intensifying capital mobility and the growing multinationalization of production opened up the spectre of 'social dumping', whereby states with the lowest and least costly social standards are rewarded by higher levels of investment. The rise in the number of multinational firms also threatened the power and influence of national systems of worker representation. Frequently, works councils were confronted by the fact that the location of ultimate managerial control had migrated to another jurisdiction where they struggled to exercise influence. Moreover, the advent of monetary union served to transform what had previously been largely national matters, such as wage-setting, into issues of general European concern. Employment and unemployment developments were increasingly, if indirectly, affected by European decision-making. Though the general architecture of national welfare systems was not directly challenged, those aspects most closely linked to the operation of labour markets came under great strain. The new phase of European integration threatened to 'dis-organize' and undermine the functioning of national labour-market systems.

In these circumstances, the EU and its member states faced a choice between substantially enhancing the EU's role in relation to these matters, leaving any process of adjustment to the discretion of each individual member state, or pursuing a mix of the two. A few modest efforts were made to adopt the first option. The terms of the SEA provided some additional powers to the EU in relation to workplace health and safety matters. A process of social dialogue between the Commission, employers and trade unions, designed to broaden the EU's social function, was initiated in 1985 (see next chapter). Yet the development of a broad-based European social policy would require much more substantial treaty changes than those included in the SEA, and the political conditions for such an ambitious project were far from propitious. A broad range of forces consistently resisted the EU's acquisition of new legal powers over social policy on principle. Unsurprisingly, proposals for such a major enhancement of EU prerogatives have been strongly resisted by those who oppose welfare development at any level of government. Anti-federalists, hostile to the EU role in public policy per se, naturally resisted its development of a social policy role. Both groups tended to view the market-integration project as deregulatory in nature. Certainly, this was a view prominently supported by Britain, many elements of business and parts of the European Commission, most notably in the single market directorate. While many social democratic governments, trade unions and elements within the Commission saw the need to create a substantial social policy at the European level, the constitutional architecture of the Union presented an enormous obstacle to any such project (Larsen and Taylor-Gooby, 2004: 184; Scharpf, 1999).

These tensions were evidenced in the debates of the Convention on the Future of Europe, from which emerged the proposed EU Constitutional Treaty. The right sought to keep the question of social Europe off the agenda altogether. In contrast, a substantial part of the left pressed for the initiation of a fully fledged social policy based on parity with economic objectives, and the creation of a policymaking system based on the extension of Union competence and qualified majority voting in the Council of Ministers. Yet the ultimate success of the right in blocking radical initiatives also revealed the complexity of the political calculations of actors. It benefited greatly from the decision of the Nordic Social Democrats and the British Labour Party to break ranks and join with Conservatives and the Christian Democrats to oppose granting new competences to the EU because they feared that it might affect and damage the core functions of national welfare states (Zeitlin, 2005: 237). Even among those who were more supportive of European integration, there were some who doubted the EU's fitness as a social policy actor, given its weak democratic credentials and the absence of the necessary bonds of social solidarity among its peoples (de Búrca, 2005: 4). 'More Europe' could not be simply equated with the defence of social Europe for a substantial segment of opinion on the centre-left.

However, while the obstacles to building a fully fledged EU 'welfare state' proved insurmountable, the alternative strategy of doing nothing also proved problematic. Preparation for membership of the single currency was a painful process for many member states. Unemployment rose, and social democratic parties, many of which were ascending to national power in the mid- to late 1990s, were particularly concerned that the Union take action to ameliorate the problem. More broadly, the growing perception that the EU was falling adrift of international competition – most particularly the USA – led to the initiation of the Lisbon process. At the core of this programme lay the premise that many aspects of national labour market and social policies were obstacles to economic growth and job creation. Lisbon's stated goal of making the EU 'the world's most dynamic and competitive economic area' could only be realized if major liberalizing reform took place. Social and employment policy would now be much more concerned with protecting and enhancing competitiveness than with equality (Adnett and Hardy, 2005: 93). The programme sought to modernize social protection, the subtext being that established national systems were 'old fashioned, their view of social protection an artefact of a pre-modern age' (Daly, 2006: 466).

### New aims, new instruments

By the end of the twentieth century, the broad outline of a new EU social policy remit was discernible. It was predicated on an acceptance that the attempt to foster substantial EU-wide social policies or to harmonize national systems must be abandoned as unfeasible (Larsen and Taylor-Gooby, 2004: 182). Article 137 of the EU Treaty provides for the development of a European social policy, but it also boldly states that the provisions adopted pursuant to this article 'shall not affect the right of Member States to define the fundamental principles of their security systems and must not significantly affect the financial equilibrium thereof'.[1] It would remain the case for the foreseeable future that EU social policy 'is most hollow in the domains that are considered the core of social policy at national level, that is social protection and income redistribution' (Daly, 2006: 463). Instead, a new, narrower agenda has been adopted that emphasizes employment and labour market issues, namely 'jobs, skills and mobility' (Larsen and Taylor-Gooby, 2004: 186). This was clearly articulated first in the Commission's Fourth Action programme in 1998, but it was subsequently confirmed and generalized at the Lisbon summit in 2000, where member states agreed to broaden the social policy agenda to include combating poverty and reducing social exclusion. However, these goals were to be achieved by improving the functioning of the labour market and by job creation. Labour markets and employment policy became the core focus of European social policy.

The formulation of a new strategic approach to social policy did not, however, resolve the problem of implementation. Under any circumstances, the diversity, complexity and political entrenchment of national systems of labour market and employment regulation would make them difficult targets for liberal reform and Europeanization. Without the acquisition of new powers and/or the development of new policy instruments, the EU risked developing a reform agenda without possessing the capacity to act upon it. Acutely aware of the dilemma, the Commission's response has been highly innovative. Beginning in the mid-1990s, it has developed a new method of policymaking that, following its adoption as a core element of the Lisbon process, has become central to many areas of EU activity. This approach seeks to overcome the EU's 'hard' power deficit by developing new, so-called 'soft' instruments. Developed piecemeal in the context of an evolving European strategy on employment, this 'new mode of governance' was formalized and generalized by the Lisbon process. Now commonly referred to as the Open Method of Coordination (OMC), it involves:

- fixing guidelines for the Union combined with specific timetables for achieving the goals which they set in the short, medium and long terms;
- establishing, where appropriate, quantitative and qualitative indicators and benchmarks against the best in the world and tailored to the needs of different Member States and sectors as a means of comparing best practice;
- translating these European guidelines into national and regional policies by setting specific targets and adopting measures, taking into account national and regional differences;
- periodic monitoring, evaluation and peer review organized as mutual learning processes.[2]

Such an approach is designed 'to permit exploratory learning within and among Member States by contrasting different problem-solving strategies, each informed by a particular idea of the good, with the aim of both improving local performance and creating frameworks for joint action at the Union level' (Zeitlin, 2005: 214). The emphasis is placed on deliberation, policy learning and peer evaluation rather than on forging and implementing Council directives. The objective is to encourage 'social learning' and, ultimately, to create an epistemic community that will drive forward European policy and national adjustment (Trubek and Mosher, 2003: 39). Its supporters argue that the OMC can be an effective mechanism for pursuing common European concerns while respecting legitimate national diversity. It 'commits Member States to work together in reaching joint goals and performance targets without seeking to homogenize their inherited policy regimes and institutional arrangements' (Zeitlin, 2005: 218). Moreover, the open and deliberative quality of the process offers a means to depoliticize the issues (Goetschy, 2003: 73). The language of policy debate shifts from relative advantage and national interests to efficiency-oriented and technocratic concepts of 'benchmarking' and 'best practice'. Through such mechanisms, it is hoped that a substantial Europeanization of labour-market policy can be achieved.

The advent of the OMC partly represents an attempt to reconcile the perceived need to address Europe's labour market-related problems at the European level with member states' determination to retain sovereign control over these areas of policy. It also partly reflects the distinct character of many such policy areas where, in all jurisdictions, 'law, classically understood, has a less direct role' (Chalmers and Lodge, 2003: 1). Devising a new, all-encompassing policy at the European level would be unrealizable in practical terms even if it were politically feasible. Ultimately, however, this leaves the EU's effectiveness as a social policy actor very dependent upon the success of the OMC as a mode of governance.

## The European Employment Strategy

The European Employment Strategy (EES) lies at the heart of the EU's social policy as it has evolved from the mid-1990s. It was launched in December 1997 at a special heads of government 'jobs summit' in Luxembourg. Its formulation had been stimulated by the publication of the Commission's White Paper, *Growth, Competition and Employment*, in 1993. It was prefigured by the agreement of a series of employment recommendations at the Essen summit in December 1994 and finally crystallized in the Amsterdam Treaty of 1997. This empowered the Council of Ministers to set out recommendations on employment, to which member states had to respond (European Employment Guidelines – EGLs). The objective was to initiate a process of dynamic interaction between the European institutions and the member states that would lead to the restructuring of national labour market policies and a return to employment growth.

The strategy's vision was, and remains, essentially technocratic. It seeks to involve a broad range of national and European actors in a collective search for solutions to Europe's employment problem. The method of policy formulation devised reflects this approach. The Commission's initial policy ideas develop in the context of wide-ranging discussions with the Council of Ministers, member state governments, trade unions and employers' associations, etc. It then formalizes these into annual guidelines following further discussion with, and endorsement by, the Council of Ministers. On the basis of these guidelines, member states are required to draft a 'National Action Plan' (NAP). These plans are then subject to extensive scrutiny. Thus, in the first stage, the Commission and the Council of Ministers assess their merits, make new recommendations and issue new guidelines to individual states. In the second stage, a process of peer review is undertaken by the Employment Committee (EMCO), which is composed of two representatives from each state and two from the Commission. On the basis of EMCO assessments and follow-up discussions with the Commission, national policymakers are pressed to make further adjustments where necessary. Through participation in these processes, member states are drawn into a complex, iterative Euro-discourse that is focused on problem-solving. By adopting this approach, the strategy seeks to circumvent potentially damaging debates between member states about fundamental matters of policy principle or institutional design.

The strategy was developed within the context of the commitment to establishing a monetary union. The Maastricht Treaty laid down a set of fiscal criteria for membership of the single currency that necessitated the adoption of deflationary policies by many member states. Inevitably, these measures had the effect of driving up unemployment rates. Social Democratic governments in particular demanded that the EU take some positive, countervailing measures to improve the situation (Rhodes, 2005: 291). More fundamentally, however, the strategy's adoption reflected a general recognition of the fact that, in a single currency system, many traditional policies of economic adjustment can no longer work and that, in consequence, new instruments need to be developed. One alarming scenario that attracted considerable attention concerned what would happen if the monetary union were struck by an asymmetric shock, i.e. a powerfully disturbing economic event that strikes some states much more forcefully than others. If a state controls its own currency in such a situation, an act of devaluation can absorb some of the adjustment costs. International competitiveness can be partially regained by allowing the value of the national currency to sink. In a single currency zone, however, this option is closed off and the costs of adjustment have to be borne by fiscal policy and wage and price developments. Higher unemployment is likely to be one major consequence of this. Moreover, in a single currency zone, the political and economic fallout from such a development can quickly spill over into other member states (Hodson and Maher, 2001: 733). It was clear that some alternative mechanism was needed to ameliorate these effects. In relation to fiscal policy, the response to these new interdependencies was institutionalized in the Stability and Growth Pact. In the case of labour markets, the response was the creation of the EES.

Yet however great the perceived need, the obstacles to the establishment of an effective employment strategy are formidable. Most problematically, the diversity in regulatory practices across member states is enormous. This is exemplified by the different approaches taken by countries to employment protection (see table 6.2). Such systems encompass a range of issues the most important of which pertain to the rules for hiring and firing workers and regulating fixed-term contracts. In some states, workers can be fired readily and cheaply. In other, more heavily regulated states, the procedures for dismissal of full-time contracted workers are complex and slow; the severance pay that must be offered for 'no-fault' dismissal is substantial; the definition of 'unfair' dismissal is broad; and the notice periods required before 'fair' dismissals can take effect are lengthy. Thus, in Germany, for example, workers employed for 20 years must be given seven months notice, and pay-offs are substantial (Pontusson, 2005: 120). In Britain, in contrast, both the period of notice and the statutory minimum redundancy payment are considerably less generous to workers. Moreover, attempts to reform such provisions are greatly complicated by the highly diverse functions that they perform within the overall mix of labour market regulation and welfare provision. Thus, for example, by comparison with most OECD countries, EU15 members have relatively generous unemployment benefit systems with high replacement rates and relatively long duration periods. However, the Mediterranean states have quite a distinct profile. In these countries, the level and coverage of unemployment benefits are relatively restricted and employment-protection legislation has provided the principal form of security for workers (Lodovici, 2000: 42). Consequently, any liberalization of employment protection across Europe would present a far greater threat to workers in Italy than, say, in the Netherlands. Similarly, the implications of moves to limit the duration of unemployment benefit will differ greatly between states. Some states, such as Sweden, have successfully established so-called 'active labour market policies' (ALMP) designed to re-skill workers and equip them to find new jobs. In such cases, unemployed workers are much less threatened by policies that force them back into the labour market (ibid.: 36). By contrast, in states where ALMPs are less developed or entirely absent, early curtailment of unemployment benefits would present a much greater threat to workers. Developing a single European policy that can encompass and reconcile such complexity and diversity is virtually impossible.

Both the content and method of the EU's employment policy reflected the recognition of the scale of these difficulties. Afforded limited powers by the terms of the Amsterdam Treaty, the EES has made a virtue of necessity and focused on supply-side reforms to remove structural impediments to employment, developing policies on quality and productivity at work, and social cohesion and inclusion (Trubek and Mosher, 2003: 41; Rhodes, 2005: 295). Moreover, in developing these policies, it has sought to push beyond existing national practices rather than challenge them or seek to harmonize them. By identifying new issues, it sought to find policy space that had not already been fully colonized by national actors. Thus, for example, demographic trends that threaten to reduce the working population dramatically in future decades have been used to justify focusing on policies to drive up labour-force participation rates to 70 per cent. Such a policy focus was wholly new to policymakers in many member states (Raveaud, 2007: 414). Similarly, the increasingly rapid rate of economic change has been harnessed to support a shift towards more active labour employment policies that seek to match job-seekers with the skills for which there is a demand. In the name of both labour-force participation and flexibility, considerable attention has been paid to the development of 'lifelong learning' policies. In short, the EES has sought to carve out space for a European policy by identifying new problems and/or new linkages between old problems. Its *modus operandi* has been to develop and propagate new ideas. The central thrust of policy has been to build a common discourse concerning the nature of the problems faced, a common knowledge

**Table 6.2** Employment protection and labour market expenditure: EU15

| Country | Employment protection Summary indicators Point scale From least to most protective[a] | Active labour market policy expenditure as % of GDP[b] | Out-of-work income maintenance and support as % of GDP[b] |
|---|---|---|---|
| Britain (L) | 0.5 | 0.116 | 0.187 |
| Ireland (L) | 1.0 | 0.481 | 0.769 |
| Denmark (N) | 1.5 | 1.433 | 1.833 |
| Finland (N) | 2.1 | 0.711 | 1.466 |
| Belgium (C) | 2.1 | 0.852 | 1.940 |
| Sweden (N) | 2.4 | 1.097 | 1.198 |
| The Netherlands (N) | 2.4 | 0.582 | 2.021 |
| Austria (C) | 2.4 | 0.458 | 1.232 |
| Germany (C) | 2.8 | 0.616 | 2.297 |
| France (C) | 3.1 | 0.664 | 1.567 |
| Spain (M) | 3.2 | 0.583 | 1.424 |
| Italy (M) | 3.3 | 0.461 | 0.719 |
| Greece (M) | 3.5 | 0.061 | 0.438 |
| Portugal (M) | 3.7 | 0.517 | 1.194 |
| Luxembourg (C) | NA | – | 0.475 |

L = liberal welfare state; N = Nordic; C = continental; M = Mediterranean
[a] Nicoletti et al, 2000, p. 84, table A.3.11.
[b] Table B1.3, Eurostat, Labour Market Policy – Expenditure and Recipients 2007 (2005 data) Luxembourg.

base encompassing descriptive statistics and a mechanism to disseminate knowledge (Jacobsson, 2004: 361–3). It is believed that such systems will provide a basis on which member states can, or can be persuaded to, develop shared interpretations of the problems to be addressed and common views of the most effective way to do so. It is anticipated that the 'soft law' character of the EES will facilitate the emergence of a political consensus on employment policy (Rhodes, 2005: 298).

### Neo-liberal reform?

Some critics have characterized the EES as a neo-liberal assault on the ESM (Raveaud, 2007: 430). Its thrust represents a transformation in the politics of the welfare state, 'whereby it becomes less centred around a discourse of social citizenship and more around economic growth and competitiveness'

(Chalmers and Lodge, 2003:10). This reading is not without validity. Much of the economic analysis that informed the EES derived from the OECD Jobs Survey published in 1994, reflecting a market-oriented, deregulatory agenda in respect of labour market issues. Both the OECD and the ESS identified the inability of European states to adapt to change as a major contributing factor to Europe's high level of unemployment and, particularly, structural unemployment (Casey, 2004: 333). Both the 1993 Delors White Paper which initiated the development of the EES, and the OECD study place great emphasis on the need to 'make work pay'. If work does not pay, people will be reluctant to do it. Yet for work to pay, greater flexibility in labour markets was needed. Economic growth alone could not solve the jobs crisis.

Notwithstanding these important commonalities, however, there were also certain significant differences between the analyses and policy prescriptions of the OECD and EES that cast some doubt on the neo-liberal characterization of the latter. Most crucially, while the OECD sees no genuine merit in the functioning and maintenance of the welfare state, the EES does. For the OECD, the influence of trade unions in the workplace, income maintenance policies and collective bargaining are structural obstacles to the proper functioning of the labour market. They cause unemployment. In contrast, the EES regards the security these measures can provide to workers as beneficial, at least potentially. In addition to OECD analysis, a study of the origins of the EES has identified the significant role of 'the conventional centre-left ideas of a network of Commission officials who worked on these issues' (Johnson, 2005: 106). Chief among those officials was Allan Larsson, who declared that the objective of policy is 'to develop labour markets that are adaptable to change, offering flexibility for enterprises and security for workers' (Larsson, 1998: 399). Reflecting a strong Scandinavian influence, the EES embodied a belief that employees are willing to accept change if society provides a sufficient safety net. People are 'willing to participate towards full employment if you only give them half a chance' (Noaksson and Jacobsson, 2003: 39). Furthermore, it maintained that substantial employment protection, retraining schemes, supportive childcare arrangements, etc. can be economically beneficial. It is telling that Larsson directly attacked the validity of the concept of NAIRU (the non-accelerating inflation rate of unemployment) that underpinned much of the OECD's analysis. He argued that the claim that full employment could only be bought at the price of an unsustainable level of inflation was false. The objective of full employment was feasible and should lie at the centre of the EES. Rather than seeking to roll back the welfare state, one of the justifications offered for raising labour-force participation rates was that this would help to generate the additional social insurance contributions necessary to sustain benefits at existing levels (Casey, 2004: 340). Rather than encouraging 'regime competition', the Commission has sought to enact directives that would curtail the practice of social dumping (Adnett and Hardy, 2005: 39). More recently, it has explicitly encouraged EU states to emulate the Nordic model of 'flexicurity', a 'combination of flexible employment rules, solid social safety nets and active support for those who become unemployed' (Barysch et al., 2008: 82). Clearly, in its own eyes, the Social Affairs Directorate General of the Commission is engaged in saving the ESM by modernizing it.

What is more debateable, however, is whether the context within which the EES operates has enabled it to perform the rehabilitative role that it has set itself. One important constraint on its effectiveness has been its subordinate place within the Union's macroeconomic framework. The EES is subject to the constraints of monetary policy, the overwhelming concern of which is to contain inflation. Additionally, until 2005 it has had to conform to the Broad Economic Policy Guidelines (BEPGs), set out annually by the EU. These guidelines were formulated by the Commission's DG EcFin (Economics and Finance Directorate General). In terms of its economic orientation, DG EcFin is much closer to the OECD's liberal economic orthodoxy. As a result, the BEPGs typically embodied a strict monetarist agenda of reduced public deficits and taxes and the intensification of market competition (Raveaud, 2007: 428). Indeed, it has been suggested that, over time, the BEPGs tended to intervene in labour market policy with increasing frequency, 'making recommendations often substantively different from those in the EGLs, and circumventing the discussion processes with the social partners and the central role of DG Employment and Social Affairs that had helped to make the employment guidelines comparatively "progressive" in the first place' (Watt, 2004: 13). Though the EES is not intrinsically a neo-liberal policy, in practice it has been 'subservient to the ideologies, path dependencies and structures of Economic and Monetary Union, as institutionalized in the Broad Economic Policy Guidelines' (Chalmers and Lodge, 2003: 2). Though the BEPGs and the EGLs were merged into a single set of Integrated Guidelines in 2005, there is little evidence to suggest that this reformulation of process has reversed these underlying policy principles and priorities (Armstrong et al., 2008).

### EES and OMC: evaluation

Given the very different starting points of the EU15 states, a simple comparison of the degree to which national labour market arrangements conform to the prescriptions of the EES would tell us very little about its impact. As Scandinavian ideas strongly informed its development, it is hardly surprising that Sweden exhibits EES-conformant traits to a far greater degree than any Mediterranean state. A more frequently adopted method of evaluation is the 'scorecard'. This ranks states on the basis of the reform measures they have introduced and the extent to which they contribute to realizing the broad EES goals of bringing people into the workforce, upgrading skills and modernizing social protection in ways that encourage and equip workers to return to work. To date, such scoreboards do not make particularly impressive reading. In one authoritative evaluation of recent developments, for example, of the five best performing countries, four were Nordic welfare systems that already embodied many of the approaches favoured by the EES (Finland, Sweden, Denmark and the Netherlands), while the fifth was a continental system (Austria). The laggards were three Mediterranean systems that started from a very different position (Italy, Greece and Portugal) (Barysch et al., 2008: 123). An analysis of the Greek case acknowledges that the EES has succeeded in forcing the introduction of policies in areas that the Greek government had traditionally ignored. However, it also noted the existence of both a widespread feeling among Greek policymakers that these policies would not be effective and a degree of resentment at the fact that Greece so frequently ranks towards the bottom of EES league tables. Peer review and benchmarking tend to alienate and demotivate rather than galvanize Greek policymakers (Johnson, 2005: 135–6). There is little here to suggest any substantial transformation in national practice.

Defenders of the EES suggest, however, that such assessments are premature and fail to understand the fundamental nature of the OMC as a mechanism of policy formulation and implementation. It is contended that its impact is achieved through its capacity to alter 'the beliefs and expectations of domestic actors' (Hodson and Maher, 2001: 740). It seeks to create a 'Eurodiscourse' that establishes common problem definitions and views on causal relationships. The development of such a language 'is important because it steers thought and focuses attention, that is, it frames conceptions of reality' (Jacobsson, 2004: 361). If the hearts and minds of national policymakers can be Europeanized, their institutions and policies will follow. Both the existence and effective impact of such a discourse have been discerned by a number of analysts. Goetschy argues that the EES is contributing to the 'emergence of an "epistemic community" at the EU level, where experts and social and political actors share similar cognitive and normative orientations towards the key objectives and issues for employment reforms' (2003: 72). Jacobsson has found evidence that the language and outlook developed in the EES colours national policy discourse, especially as practised at elite political and civil service level (2004: 366). Specifically, as a consequence of the EES, issues such as labour market 'activation',[3] gender mainstreaming, lifelong learning, etc. have gained much greater prominence in many member states. Similarly, because of EES initiatives, across the Union attention has shifted from combating unemployment to raising employment levels and labour-force participation rates. In a study of German labour market policy reform, Fleckenstein found evidence of social learning from European initiatives in the area of activation, active ageing and gender mainstreaming (2006: 295). A study by Zeitlin found evidence that OMC processes raised the political profile of employment and social inclusion issues at both national and EU levels. These measures contributed to general shifts in national policy orientation and thinking, with EU concepts increasingly coming to inform national debates (Zeitlin, 2005: 232).

Such claims of success for the EES and the OMC have been strongly contested. Critics argue that there is little to suggest that the EES has succeeded in transcending intergovernmental bargaining or in depoliticizing potentially contentious issues. At the European level, rather than being a deliberative chamber contributing to the development of a positive-sum consensus on desirable employment policies, policymaking has become increasingly politicized as member states have sought to use the EES as a mechanism to favourably shape the policy agenda (Rhodes, 2005: 298). While in the early years of the strategy's operation the Commission directed the review process and publicized the results as a means to encourage states to implement its recommendations, member state representatives have more recently wrested back control, pursuing traditional self-interested strategies. As a result, policy outcomes often owe more to old-fashioned intergovernmental bargaining than to deliberation (ibid.). Claims that the OMC represents a more inclusive form of policymaking have also been contested. Participation in the EES by non-governmental actors has been very uneven and in all but one member state (Luxembourg), the national action plans were governmental rather than jointly produced documents (de la Porte and Pochet, 2004: 74). In practice, the EES has reduced social partnership to a 'managerialist façade', with both employers and trade unions co-opted into a process beyond their influence (Gold et al., 2007: 20).

Perhaps most damaging of all is the claim that even when national policy does follow the lines recommended by the EES, it does not do so because of the EES. A number of studies suggest that the strategy's impact is dependent on the prior existence of domestic support for such measures. Thus, in respect of active labour-market measures, it was found that their success was 'conditional on domestic politics, institutions and extant policies' (Armingeon, 2007: 906). They were widely adopted because many European states were already well disposed to such initiatives. Indeed, in Germany, it was found that the introduction of 'labour market activation' measures by the Red-Green government in the early 2000s 'would have occurred without the Luxembourg process' (Fleckenstein, 2006: 29). In contrast, where proposals were not already on the domestic agenda, or faced very active political resistance, they go unimplemented. Thus, for example, EES proposals on tax reform have generally been completely disregarded (Trubek and Mosher, 2003: 45).

It appears that the impact of the EES on national labour market reform is little more than a matter of domestic convenience. Where its proposals run with the grain of national debate and are compatible with the structure of established systems, the EES may contribute to change. Where these conditions are absent, member states can and do ignore it without any fear of adverse consequences (Gold et al., 2007: 21). In this sense, critics argue that the consensus on labour market reform that European policy seeks to generate is in fact a precondition of its effectiveness, raising the question of whether it has any significant independent impact at all (Fleckenstein, 2006: 29). It may well be that the opportunities for genuine policy transfer will be rare given the diversity of national systems (de la Porte and Pochet, 2004: 72).

## Conclusion

The EU has struggled to establish itself as a significant social policy actor. In the first 30 years of the Union's existence, member states effectively refused to allow it to intrude into what they considered to be their domain. Even with the 'relaunch' of the 1980s, it failed to establish a significant role for itself in relation to the core activities of the European welfare states – i.e., social protection and income redistribution. However, since the mid-1990s, the Union has succeeded in carving out a significant niche for itself in relation to labour market and related social policy reform. Responding to the particular challenges generated by the transition to EMU, it has devised a complex, institutionally innovative employment strategy with an ambitious agenda to encourage/induce member states to restructure key aspects of the welfare state policy as it affects employment. In the process, new policy objectives and policymaking techniques have been developed. Furthermore, these policies and methods have gained greater prominence since the Lisbon summit in 2000. The policy priorities and policymaking techniques developed in the EES are the core around which the Lisbon programme of economic modernization has been built.

The central objectives of the strategy reflect a widespread perception that unless EU product and financial market reforms are matched by corresponding changes in the structure and governance of labour markets, Europe will be condemned to a future of low labour-force participation, high unemployment and low growth. Its central goal has been to improve labour market flexibility, eliminate disincentives to work and increase employment. In many respects, its rationale reflects the liberal reform programme long advocated by the OECD. However, the influence of Scandinavian social democratic ideas in the strategy's design is also apparent. Most basically, it has sought to modernize rather than destroy the European social model. Thus, for example, its justification for striving to raise employment levels is that this will help to generate the resources required to maintain generous welfare state provision. It is telling that 'flexicurity' rather than 'flexibility' has become one of the strategy's key buzzwords. Indeed, in key respects, the EU's social and employment policy can be regarded as an attempt to extend Scandinavian best practice throughout the Union.

The implementation of this reform programme has faced, and continues to face, many obstacles. Even within the Commission, the perspectives and priorities that the strategy embodies are strongly contested by powerful actors in other directorates who generally favour more robust liberal reforms. In key instances, employment guidelines have been overridden by the liberal economic priorities of more influential officials. Most fundamentally, however, its success as a policy greatly depends on the OMC's effectiveness as a mode of policymaking. Though it is too early in the OMC's life to come to a definitive judgement about its merits, there is reason for scepticism. The weight of current research suggests that participation in the EES has only marginally influenced the substance of national employment policy or the mindset of policymakers. While concerns about the economic sustainability of existing national labour market and social policies in Europe deepen, the EU continues to struggle to develop a significant and effective role in directing the process of change.

### FURTHER READING

Hantrais (2007) provides a good comprehensive introduction. For a more detailed discussion of the fate of recent reforms of the EES and the operation of the OMC, see Armstrong et al (2008). De Búrca (2005) includes some very informative chapters on the operation of the OMC.

7

# Social Europe and Industrial Relations

## Introduction: Social Models and Industrial Relations

Industrial relations systems form a central component of social models. They encompass the interaction of labour, business and government, which engage in a complex and often conflictual process of strategic choice affecting the content and regulation of employment relations (Visser, 1996: 2). At the heart of these systems lie the institutions and conduct of collective bargaining between employers and employees over wages and conditions and the provisions made for employee representation within the firm. As is the case for political economic institutions more generally, the particular character of industrial relations systems is predominantly shaped by national traditions, laws and power relations, and they vary considerably across the EU. Thus, the conduct and legal status of bargaining take radically different forms in different states. The organizational character of employers' and employees' representative associations varies greatly. Employee works councils assume quite contrasting forms and perform different functions from country to country. The degree of state involvement in collective bargaining differs markedly.

Table 7.1 illustrates the nature and extent of this diversity. Trade union membership density rates vary from a low of 9 per cent in France to 78 per cent in Sweden. There are wide divergences in the coverage of collective bargaining, with agreements in Austria encompassing some 91–100 per cent of the labour force, while in Ireland the corresponding figures are 51–60 per cent.[1] The level of bargaining that predominates in EU15 national systems also differs substantially. Thus, in Belgium, Finland and Ireland, national bargaining plays a dominant role in collective bargaining. In another set of countries, stretching from Germany, Italy and the Netherlands through to Denmark, Portugal, Austria, Sweden and Cyprus, collective bargaining is principally conducted at the sectoral level. Uniquely among EU15 states, bargaining in Britain is generally conducted at the level of the individual enterprise. More broadly, there are very marked differences across members in respect of the regulatory function of the state. Thus, where in some countries it plays a central role in industrial relations, both through the constitutional provision of workers' rights and through comprehensive labour market legislation (e.g. Belgium, France, Germany, the Netherlands, Luxembourg, Italy and Greece), in others it has traditionally abstained from regulating such matters extensively either

**Table 7.1** Key features of national industrial relations systems in the EU

| Country | Trade union membership density (%) 2001 (a) | Employers' associations organization rate (%) (a) | Dominant level of collective bargaining (b) | Extension provisions in operation? (legal or administrative) (a) | Collective bargaining, % of wage and salary-earners covered (a) |
|---|---|---|---|---|---|
| Sweden | 78 | 55 | Sectoral | No | 91–100 |
| Denmark | 73.8 | 52 | Sectoral | No | 81–90 |
| Finland | 71.2 | 60 | Inter–sectoral | Yes | 81–90 |
| Belgium | 55.8 | 72 | Sectoral | Yes | 91–100 |
| Ireland | 35.9 | 60 | Inter–sectoral | No | 51–60 |
| Austria | 35.7 | 100 | Sectoral | Yes | 91–100 |
| Italy | 34.8 | 51 | Sectoral | Yes | 61–70 |
| Greece | 26.7 | 70 | Sectoral | Yes | 61–70 |
| Portugal | 24.3 | 58 | Sectoral | Yes | 71–80 |
| Germany | 23.5 | 63 | Sectoral | Yes | 61–70 |
| The Netherlands | 22.5 | 85 | Sectoral | Yes | 81–90 |
| Spain | 14.9 | 70 | Sectoral | Yes | 81–90 |
| France | 9.7 | 74 | Sectoral/ enterprise | Yes | 91–100 |
| Luxembourg | 33.7 | 80 | Enterprise | Yes | 71–80 |
| Britain | 30.7 | 40 | Enterprise | No | 31–40 |
| *2004 entry states* | | | | | |
| Cyprus | 70 | 60 | Enterprise | NA | 61–70 |
| Malta | 63 | NA | Enterprise | NA | 51–60 |
| Slovenia | 41 | 100 | Sectoral | Yes | 91–100 |
| Slovakia | 35.4 | 65 | Sectoral | Yes | 41–50 |
| Latvia | 20 | 30 | Enterprise | NA | 11–20 |
| Czech Republic | 27 | 35 | Enterprise | NA | 21–30 |
| Hungary | 19.9 | NA | Enterprise | Yes | 31–40 |
| Estonia | 16.6 | 35 | Enterprise | NA | 21–30 |
| Lithuania | 16 | NA | Enterprise | NA | 11–20 |
| Poland | 14.7 | NA | Enterprise | Yes | 41–50 |

*Sources:* European Commission, 2004: 23–35; European Commission, 2006a: 47.

by codes or legislation (e.g. UK and Ireland) (Rhodes, 2005: 282). In yet a third group, a functional equivalent to legal and legislative frameworks is provided by corporatist-type agreements between employers and unions (e.g. Denmark and Sweden) (ibid.).

Despite this diversity, the existence of fundamental, shared orientations and characteristics across the industrial relations systems of many of the EU15 states must also be acknowledged. Most basically, the interactions of labour, business and government are invariably conducted in a highly regulated and organizationally dense environment. Actors are numerous, relationships are complex and choice is subject to considerable regulatory constraint. More specifically, the interaction of employers and employees is typically heavily collectivized and multi-employer bargaining at the sectoral or inter-sectoral level is exceptionally well developed. Indeed, not only is bargaining rarely conducted at an individual level between employer and employee, in many countries there is provision for extending the terms of agreements reached between employers' associations and trade unions to firms and workers that are not members of any organization. Thus, in France, despite a trade union membership density rate of only 9 per cent, some 91–100 per cent of workers are covered by collective agreements as a consequence of state-enforced extension. Moreover, when account is taken of the nature and degree of state support for labour in the form of rights to representation, information consultation and collective bargaining, the extent of the commitment to sustaining highly institutionalized forms of industrial relations is apparent (Marginson and Sisson, 2004: 41). With the notable exception of Britain, associations are generally strong, bargaining is highly collectivized and states are strongly supportive of highly 'organized' forms of industrial relations practice (European Commission, 2004: 33).

On initial examination, the role of the EU in relation to the operation and development of these systems appears marginal. The Amsterdam Treaty explicitly denied it any function in respect of pay determination, the right of association or the right to strike and impose lockouts.[2] These matters remain subject to national regulation. Yet more careful attention suggests that, despite these prohibitions, the impact of EU activity on established systems of industrial relations is both substantial and deepening. Indeed, by 2007, many national trade unions across Europe expressed fears that the EU was actively facilitating the practice of social dumping, whereby countries with lower social protection standards exploit the cost advantage this gives them to gain a competitive advantage over those countries with higher standards. The established highly organized institutions of industrial relations in Europe were perceived to be under threat from the application of EU laws that are essentially liberal economic in nature.

The EU's threat to established industrial relations practices takes three distinct forms. Firstly, notwithstanding the prohibitions of the Amsterdam Treaty in relation to pay, EU policies do impact substantially on the economic environment within which national industrial systems must operate. In a context of 'opened' national product markets and a Europeanized monetary system, the retention of formal authority over collective bargaining at the national level may not obviate the need for major structural change in response to EU initiatives. Secondly, the apparent clarity of the Amsterdam Treaty in relation to protecting the national character of industrial relations and collective bargaining has been challenged by developments in ECJ case law. In particular, judgments concerning the implications of treaty rules on freedom of establishment and the provision of services appear to undermine significantly the demarcation enshrined in Amsterdam between national and European competence with regard to industrial relations. Thirdly, the 'Amsterdam exclusion' does not preclude the EU from addressing non-pay industrial relations issues that emerge at the European level. The potential importance of such activity is perhaps best illustrated by the issue of employee representation rights within the large emerging group of 'Euro-companies'. What arrangements, if any, should be instituted to ensure that companies operating across a number of member states do not escape the requirements for effective workplace representation and consultation imposed at national level? How should European management be forced to engage in meaningful exchanges about the running of the company with essentially national workforces? These issues have been the focus of considerable EU activity and controversy.

In this chapter the extent and nature of the EU's role in relation to industrial relations will be examined. Firstly, is there evidence of substantial changes in national systems of collective bargaining and, to the extent that there are, can they be attributed to the EU? Secondly, is it correct to characterize recent ECJ judgments as representing a fundamental attack on the balance between liberal economic principles and the values of the European social model that many thought had been struck in the Amsterdam Treaty? Thirdly, to what extent has the EU developed a substantial industrial relations function at the European level? At the root of these questions lies the broader issue of whether it is correct to characterize the EU as a threat to the integrity of national industrial relations institutions and the balance of socioeconomic power they embody.

## European Markets, European Money and National Industrial Relations

Europe's industrial relations systems developed within the framework of nationally regulated economies. Nationally organized employers' associations and trade unions have engaged in collective bargaining within a context of national economic management and a national currency. Consequently, the processes and outcomes of collective bargaining were to a significant extent protected from the impact of the wider international environment. However, with gathering pace, European integration has stripped away much of this insulation. Economic regulation and management are increasingly constrained by EU rules. The level of trade and investment across member states has grown hugely. In many cases, a national currency no longer mediates the relationship between the national and international economies. The implications of these changes for the conduct of industrial relations at the national level are considerable. As product-market and monetary integration deepens, the degree of shelter from international market developments afforded to governments, employers and workers has diminished. The advent of the euro in particular has greatly intensified this process of change. If a given national economy becomes uncompetitive relative to its trading partner or undergoes an economic shock, exchange-rate movements can no longer act as a mechanism of adjustment. The use of fiscal policy by national governments to ease economic adaptation is heavily constrained by the terms of the Stability and Growth Pact. Potentially compensating policy mechanisms at the European level have not been developed. There are virtually no Eurozone fiscal stabilizers, while cross-national labour mobility is very limited (Dølvik, 2004: 281). In consequence, much of the burden of adjustment to exchange-rate movements or the impact of economic shocks now falls much more directly on labour market actors; the pressure on employers and trade unions to negotiate a reduction in real wages in response becomes much more intense (Marginson and Sisson, 2004: 6). More broadly, as integration deepens, 'regime competition' between states becomes more likely. Holders of mobile capital gain increasing leverage over national governments, forcing them to create a more congenial regulatory environment if they do not want to see investment go elsewhere (Adnett and Hardy, 2005: 67–8). In respect of industrial relations, such competition manifests itself in demands for less restrictive regulation on hiring and firing, greater pressure on trade unions to consider productivity issues in setting wage rates, etc. There is evidence that pressure for wage-rate convergence across states is growing (Dølvik, 2004: 281). In some states, public authorities have made adjustments to render their system more compatible with the perceived preferences of investors (Traxler and Woitech, 2000: 155). The deepening of European integration witnessed over the last two decades presents a major challenge to the integrity of national industrial relations institutions.

These complex developments have generated a contrasting range of expectations concerning the impact of European integration on national industrial relations. Some analysts anticipate that market and monetary integration will ultimately serve to 'dis-organize' and liberalize national systems, initiating a general turn towards highly fragmented, company-based bargaining systems. It is argued that the emergence of a genuinely integrated market with a single, and generally restrictive, monetary policy will greatly intensify the level of market competition. In such an environment, firms will need to restrain costs and enhance the flexibility of work organization (Traxler, 2003: 86). Over time, the attraction to employers of individually tailored agreements will grow and, in consequence, multi-employer bargaining will fade from use and trade unions will be severely weakened. An alternative scenario predicts a rather different outcome. Accepting the unsustainability of the status quo, it anticipates the development of an industrial relations system at the European level in response to economic and monetary integration. Social policy will follow the market in a process of 'spillover' (Marginson and Sisson, 2004: 6). In particular, trade unions and sympathetic governments will seek to replenish labour's diminished bargaining strength through European-level re-regulation. A third perspective contests the premise that the EU will necessarily transform the institutional structure of national systems of industrial relations that lies at the core of both of these scenarios. Rather, it anticipates the defensive 're-nationalization' of industrial relations in the face of the new competitive challenge (Dølvik, 2004: 279). States, employers and trade unions will exploit the established mechanisms of industrial relations to strengthen their relative competitive position vis-à-vis other member states. Such nationalistic 'competitive corporatism' may involve a 'beggar-thy-neighbour' policy of wage restraint and work intensification that embodies a major shift in the balance of power within the institutions of collective bargaining in favour of employers. It does not, however, necessarily transform the essential institutional structure of the national system.

## European Market Integration and National Industrial Relations

There is clear evidence of substantial change in the organization and conduct of national collective bargaining across EU15 states in the past two decades or so. The highly developed associational structures that sustain sectoral and/or national forms of collective bargaining are coming under increasing strain. Trade union membership densities in EU15 states have declined significantly, falling from an average of 27.8 per cent in the period 1995–2003 to just 24.4 per cent in the period 2004–6 (European Commission, 2008: 22). An ever-increasing proportion of the labour force is unorganized. Though employers' associations have fared better, there is evidence in many countries of growing disagreement within associations concerning bargaining priorities. In particular, small firms have grown more hostile to sectoral agreements, the costs of which they find difficult to absorb, while larger firms continue to appreciate the price stability and industrial peace that they deliver. One consequence of these tensions has been a significant growth in the number of small firms defecting from employers' associations and/or seeking to escape from the full application of agreements entered into by sectoral associations. This problem has been particularly evident in Germany, where the membership coverage of Gesamtmetall, the metalworking industry's employers' association, fell from 58 per cent of all firms in the sector in 1980 to 34 per cent in 1998 (Hassel, 2002: 312).

The stresses revealed by these organizational developments have also found reflection in bargaining processes and outcomes. A tendency to decentralize collective bargaining to the company or enterprise level is evident across the member states of the EU (European Commission, 2006c: 46). Where bargaining remains sectoral, 'inability to pay' clauses have been incorporated into agreements in recognition of the very diverse positions of firms operating in the same industry. So-called 'opening' clauses that allow exemption by individual firms from the general provisions of an agreement under specified conditions have become common. In some countries, a practice of setting minimum wage levels and then allowing firms to adjust upwards if necessary has emerged. In others, wage ceilings have been agreed, with individual firms allowed to agree lower pay rates with unions locally. Simultaneously, the formation of company-level 'pacts for employment and competitiveness' (PECs) has spread widely across almost all member states (Marginson and Sisson, 2004: 155). Though diverse in form, typically these pacts are agreed between the management and workers of a given company with the purpose of preserving employment, reducing costs and enhancing flexibility. By their nature they ensure that the content of employment relations in a given firm is much more closely linked with its specific competitive circumstance.

The challenge to established collective bargaining institutions from decentralization is compounded by the growing sensitivity of national labour markets to external wage developments. Agreements reached in other countries may substantially influence the course of negotiations between employers and labour. In response to such effects, some trade unions have sought to develop mechanisms to coordinate pay negotiations across national borders (European Commission, 2004: 55). Perhaps most significantly, since 1998, the European Metalworkers' Federation (EMF) has tried to develop a common negotiation formula, based on productivity increases plus inflation, which would serve to ameliorate the danger that competition between national bargaining rounds would depress wage levels (European Commission, 2004: 55). In practice, these efforts have encountered major obstacles. The absence of significant sanctions has made it difficult to punish defectors from this formula. IG Metall, the powerful German union that played a central role in initiating the process of coordination, has concluded that there was virtually no awareness of these coordination problems at national level (Visser, 2005: 290). In addition, the coverage of these efforts tends to be geographically limited. To date, they have been confined to Germany and its immediate neighbours, on the one side, and the Nordic countries on the other. Moreover, even where there is evidence of significant cross-border interaction in bargaining outcomes, as is the case in the German and Austrian metals industries, this tends to reflect the depth of economic interdependence between the countries rather than explicit acts of coordination (Traxler et al., 2008: 232). Indeed, it is frequently the case that efforts at cross-border coordination fall foul of differences in national structures and traditions. In the case of working time, for example, there were heated debates among national representatives over whether working hours should be expressed in terms of a yearly or a weekly figure, with each trade union concerned to uphold the integrity of existing national arrangements. Furthermore, beyond the metalworking industry, the capacity of European trade union sector associations to coordinate such policies appears to be even less developed (Marginson and Sisson, 2004: 109–11). Yet, the very existence of these initiatives reveals the depth of anxiety felt by trade unionists. National systems of collective bargaining that for decades had largely satisfied the aspirations of organized labour are no longer perceived to be capable of performing this function effectively.

Clearly, the evidence of change in national industrial relations systems is substantial. A generalized process is under way whereby collective bargaining is significantly decentralized. However, whether this process can legitimately be characterized as transformational in nature is much more contestable. Notwithstanding these developments, multi-employer bargaining at the sectoral level remains the dominant type of wage-setting in EU15. Bargaining coverage has proved to be stable overall, with only Britain (49 per cent to 36 per cent) and Germany (72 per cent to 63 per cent) witnessing marked falls in the 1990s (European Commission, 2004: 31). In the period 2000–6, only Britain and the Netherlands among EU15 states witnessed further reductions, while some, such as Spain, Finland and Sweden, saw rises (European Commission, 2008: 78). While the practice of extension has also been the subject of 'opening' clause exemption in some cases, there has been no general move to end it in EU member states (Visser, 2005: 301). If market pressures for the devolution of bargaining are strong, the existence of powerful structural factors serving to sustain traditional practices also need to be recognized. As Marginson and Sisson point out, apart from Britain and Ireland, multi-employer agreements are not simply legally enforceable contracts between the parties, but also compulsory codes. They have effectively become systems of private law the termination of which would necessitate more rather than less government intervention in the bargaining process (2004: 169). Yet, ultimately, the persisting importance of traditional structures of collective bargaining reflects the fact that, aside from Britain, neither the majority of firms nor employers' associations in most EU member states are keen to embrace a wholesale shift to company-level bargaining. It is noteworthy that while PECs may have proliferated, these are typically designed not to contravene the terms of sectoral or inter-sectoral agreements. The clear trend has been for the employers to seek a greater degree of flexibility within traditional bargaining systems. Thus, it has been concluded that notwithstanding striking recent developments, most EU15 countries have shown remarkable stability in their wage-bargaining structure, the same stability observed in bargaining coverage (European Commission, 2004: 4; 2008: 77).

## Monetary Union and Social Pacts

The complex dynamic of continuity and innovation in national collective bargaining systems, and the central role of EU policy in driving this process, are perhaps best exemplified by the proliferation of so-called 'national social pacts' across member states from the 1990s. Such pacts have met with greatest success in the Netherlands, Ireland, Italy, Denmark and Finland, but among EU15 states only Britain failed even to countenance their negotiation (Hassel, 2003: 709). Though diverse in their structure and content, most pacts share a number of fundamental characteristics. Firstly, they take the form of national agreements between employers, trade unions and the government that cover a wide range of industrial relations and related social policy issues. Secondly, the goal of moderating wage rises in order to protect competitiveness lies at their heart. Often, the principal mechanism of restraint takes the form of guidelines setting the parameters within which sectoral or company-level bargains can be struck. These guidelines frequently emerge from some sort of external benchmarking process. In smaller countries in particular, they are often set in reference to wage developments in other European states. They are explicitly related to competitiveness concerns and have contributed to the emergence of a 'European going rate' (Marginson and Sisson, 2004: 121). Thirdly, such pacts encompass a much wider range of issues than is normally the case in collective bargaining. In contrast to the redistributive focus of the 'incomes policy' agreements of the 1970s and 1980s, social pacts link supply-side reform with overall wage formation in order to buttress the credibility of macroeconomic policy (Dølvik, 2004: 293). Most frequently, the agenda encompasses social protection reform, including issues such as pension and unemployment benefits; employment policy reforms, involving the development of active labour markets; the re-regulation of employment protection; and the reform of collective bargaining structures themselves (European Commission, 2008: 53). The terms of agreements between employers and trade unions are tightly coordinated with government social, taxation and employment policies. The central objective has been to contain and reduce non-wage costs and improve the flexibility of labour markets.

The development of the social pact phenomenon can be directly linked to EU initiatives (Natali and Pochet, 2009: 147). Frequently, they have been formulated and justified explicitly by reference to monetary union. Across member states, it was widely believed that in order to meet the financial criteria for membership of the single currency, a coordinated adjustment strategy by trade unions, employers and governments was required. As the external constraints on national fiscal and monetary policies tightened, the cross-linking of wage policies, social reforms and labour-market practices was deemed to be an urgent necessity if inflation, loss of competitiveness and rising unemployment were not to result (Hassel, 2003: 710). It is notable that the greatest innovations were evident in states that had a propensity to high inflation. Italy, Spain, Portugal, Greece and Ireland underwent a recentralization of wage bargaining and the development of social pacts as they sought to adjust to the anticipated constraints of monetary union. In several instances, the revival of tripartite bargaining between employers, trade unions and the state 'occurred in response to failed attempts to curb inflation through monetary policies in fragmented bargaining systems' (Dølvik, 2004: 287). Where states already possessed highly coordinated bargaining institutions, these have been adapted to serve the goal of protecting national competitiveness. Perhaps most famously, the Dutch 'Polder' model has combined its 'Rhenish' institutional inheritance with a substantial degree of liberal reform to lower its relative wage costs and enhance the country's ability to compete within the Eurozone (de Beus, 2004: 195).

These strategies have been criticized as a form of 'beggar-my-neighbour' politics. Through the agreement of a substantial package of wage moderation and labour-market reform, a country may gain a substantial competitive advantage vis-à-vis other member states, thereby driving out their products and services and gaining a greater 'share' for itself. From this perspective, European integration has unleashed a destabilizing 'arms race' of competitive reductions in wage rates and worker-protection measures. It is also suggested that they reflect a shift in bargaining power from labour to employers. In many instances, unions have had to make very substantial wage concessions in return for social policy reforms that they favour. Moreover, doubt has been cast on the sustainability of social pacts as an industrial relations practice. Visser argues, for example, that labour's weakening bargaining position will ultimately obviate the need for them. As integration deepens, neither employers nor states will have any need to 'buy' the acquiescence of trade unions to pay moderation through social policy reforms (2005: 293). The intensity of market pressures will achieve the same end. However, in a number of cases, such as Ireland and Spain, 'the progressive stabilisation of the pacts has been witnessed despite changing economic and political conditions' (Natali and Pochet, 2009: 148). At least in some instances, they have proved to be more than a transitional strategy in the adaptation of industrial relations in Europe to the euro.[3]

The pact phenomenon demonstrates the powerful impact of the EU on national industrial relations. The problems addressed, the processes of formulation and agreement, and the substantive outcomes of bargaining have all been strongly affected by European developments. Indeed, it has been argued that the similarity in the structure of pacts represents an important example of 'Europe learning from Europe' (Marginson and Sisson, 2004). Faced by a common challenge, states have borrowed from each other in the search for viable solutions, and countries such as Portugal, Spain, Italy and Ireland have demonstrated substantial innovation in managing industrial relations. However, it is also apparent that the general pattern of innovation in response to EU development cannot properly be characterized as an 'Americanization' of European practice. Industrial relations in EU states remain 'embedded in fairly coherent national polities where social institutions, legislation, and state support facilitate multi-employer bargaining and cross-sectoral coordination' (Dølvik, 2004: 294). The precise structure and content of pacts has been strongly conditioned by the established organizational forms and rules of national industrial relations systems (Hassel, 2009: 13). Rather than simply being the product of relative bargaining strength between employers and workers within labour markets, the pacts embody 'the persistence of the politics of exchange' (Rhodes, 2003: 143).

## European Law and National Industrial Relations

In recent years, a more direct challenge to the sustainability of national industrial relations institutions has come from decisions taken by the ECJ. In a series of politically controversial judgments, the court has effectively restricted the strong defence afforded by Article 137 of the Amsterdam Treaty to the institutions of national industrial relations. These protections were widely understood to exempt collective bargaining from the application of EU law on competition, freedom of establishment and the free movement of labour. Supporting evidence for this interpretation was provided by the ECJ judgment in the Albany case in 1999. This stated that 'agreements concluded in the context of collective negotiation between management and labour in pursuit of [social] objectives must, by virtue of their nature and purpose, be regarded as falling outside the scope of Art 81', the legal basis of competition policy (Reich, 2008: 129). Social rights were held to have primacy over competition rules. It was not unreasonable to anticipate that a similar privileged status would be accorded in respect of other fundamental economic freedoms. However, in its findings in the Laval (2007), Viking (2008) and Rüffert (2008) cases, the ECJ effectively set aside this exemption. Though the details of the cases vary, they all revolved around the use of collective action to prevent foreign firms from undercutting the costs of local labour by failing to adhere to terms of local collective agreements. Though the court's judgments were complex and their full implications uncertain, their combined and clear consequence has been to limit the special protection afforded to collective bargaining and its outcomes by the Amsterdam Treaty. In future, in cases where the right to take collective action by trade unions conflicts with the economic freedoms guaranteed by the treaty, national courts will have to adjudicate between them on the basis of principles of 'balance of interests' and/or the 'proportionality' of the actions taken in relation to the scale of the threat posed to established social arrangements.

It is no accident that these cases emerged following enlargement of the EU in 2004, which saw the accession of 10 new member states. Both social protection standards and wage rates in these states were substantially inferior to those obtaining in the great majority of existing members. In consequence, there was a sharp clash of interests between the two groups. Older member states sought to protect established social institutions and resist what they perceived to be social dumping. By contrast, new members sought to exploit one of the few competitive advantages they enjoyed, namely low-cost labour.

Bercusson has demonstrated the fundamental significance of this division for the legal arguments presented to the ECJ by the member states. New members consistently advocated the application of the principles of economic freedom enshrined in EU law, older states (frequently supported by the Commission) sought to protect the integrity of established collective bargaining regimes and the social settlement that they embodied (2007: 292–300). Of the established members, only Britain tended to side with the advocates of market freedom. The clash between the liberal economic principles informing European integration and the purposes of national social models was stark.

### Viking and the right of establishment

The core issue raised by the Viking case concerned the right of establishment and its applicability in respect of collective action by labour.[4] The case revolved around the attempt by a Finnish shipping company to re-flag a ferry in Estonia, thereby allowing it to replace its predominantly Finnish crew with Estonians, who would be employed on inferior terms and conditions (Reich, 2008: 136–7). This action was resisted by the Finnish Seamen's Union (FSU) and, following the failure to negotiate a deal with Viking, it gave notice of industrial action. Its stance was supported by the International Transport Workers' Federation (ITF), whose 'flag of convenience' rules stipulated that the wages and conditions of employed seafarers should be negotiated by the union 'in the country where the ship is ultimately beneficially owned' (Bercusson, 2007: 281). Following Estonia's accession to the EU, Viking applied for an order in the High Court of Justice (England and Wales) to prevent any action being taken by the FSU and the ITF to prevent the re-flagging. Though successful in this action, the unions appealed the decision and, in the course of hearing the case, the Court of Appeal sought clarification from the ECJ in respect of a number of key aspects of European law.

In its determination, the ECJ first rejected the analogy made by the FSU and the ITF between the Viking and Albany cases. It reasoned that such collective actions did indeed fall under the scope of Article 43 of the treaty, which protects the right to establishment. Moreover, while accepting the fundamental right under European law to take collective action, it also held that this right might be curtailed in certain circumstances (Zahn, 2008: 4). In this instance, it concluded that the actions of both the FSU and the ITF amounted to a restriction on Viking's right to freedom of establishment. It then outlined the criteria that should be applied in the adjudication of such clashes of freedoms. Paragraph 77 of the ruling stated that 'the right to collective action for the protection of workers is a legitimate interest which, in principle, justifies a restriction of one of the fundamental principles guaranteed by the Treaty'. However, the action must be proportionate to the level of threat posed to those workers. Factors to be considered include 'the seriousness of the threat to jobs or conditions of employment' and the 'exhaustion of other possible means before the initiation of collective action' (ibid.: 6). The court made it clear that, in the case of Viking, the actions of the FSU and ITF were disproportionate and unjustifiable.

### Laval, Rüffert and the right to provide services

The Laval and Rüffert cases concerned the principle of free service provision and the status and treatment of so-called 'posted workers' – that is, workers 'who for a limited period carry out their work in the territory of a Member State other than the State in which they normally work' (Adnett and Hardy, 2005: 20). A framework for the treatment of these workers had been established prior to the accession of new members in 2004. The *Rush Portuguesa* decision of the ECJ in 1990[5] had determined that a Portuguese company had the right – based on the freedom to supply services provided for in the Treaty of Rome – to carry out a contract using its own workforce. However, at the same time the ruling allowed that France had the right to force the company to comply with French social and labour legislation during the period of the contract (EIROnline, 1999). Essentially, member states were free to regulate the conditions that should apply to posted workers in their jurisdiction as they saw fit. In practice, the terms adopted by states tended to reflect the preferences of trade unions and employers' associations, the degree of their relative organizational strength and the quality of their respective access to government (Menz, 2003). Subsequently, the Posted Workers Directive,[6] agreed in 1996, confirmed the general determination to prevent the right to provide services from becoming a mechanism to facilitate the practice of social dumping. It embodied the basic objective 'that working conditions and pay in effect in a Member State should be applicable both to workers from that State, and those from other EU countries posted to work there' (EIROnline, 1999). Specifically, the directive required member states 'to determine the terms and conditions of employment, including minimum rates of pay of posted workers either by law, regulation or administrative provision, or by collective agreements which have been declared universally applicable' (Zahn, 2008: 7).

Following the 2004 accession of poor, low-wage countries, this legal equilibrium came under increasing pressure, as demonstrated in the Laval case. This involved a dispute between a Latvian construction company, Laval un Partneri Ltd, and the Swedish Building Workers' Union (Svenska Byggnadsarbetareförbundet). At issue was the question of social dumping. The Latvian firm won a contract to renovate a school near Stockholm. In order to fulfil the contract, the Riga-based firm posted 14 Latvian workers to undertake the task, paying them some 40 per cent less than their Swedish counterparts. Concerned that this practice would threaten the position of Swedish construction workers, the trade union requested Laval to pay their Latvian workers the standard Swedish rate of pay as laid down in the collective agreement for the sector. Following the company's refusal to do so, the Swedish union, supported by the Swedish Electricians' Union, instituted a picket on the building site. Laval requested that the Swedish Labour Court declare the picket unlawful. The unions contended that Swedish legislation relating to collective agreements stipulates that organized labour can resort to industrial action to force an employer to sign a collective agreement, irrespective of where it is based (EIROnline, 2008). Uncertain of the situation, the Swedish Labour Court sought guidance from the ECJ on whether the actions of the trade union breached EU law and, more specifically, the provisions of the Posted Workers Directive.

The opinion offered by the Advocate-General, one of eight legal advisers to the ECJ, essentially upheld the trade unions' position. While adjudging that the issues raised did fall within the scope of European law, he rejected the contention that the negotiation of employment terms and conditions by Sweden's social partners prevented the satisfactory implementation of Directive 96/71/EC. Rather, Mr Mengozzi concluded that the construction site picket was acceptable as it was motivated 'by public interest objectives, such as the protection of workers and the fight against social dumping, and is not carried out in a manner that is disproportionate to the attainment of these objectives'.[7] However, crucially and unusually, the ECJ's final judgment did not confirm Mr Mengozzi's conclusions. While recognizing the right of the trade unions to take action, it stated that this action did represent a restriction on the freedom to provide services, making their provision less attractive. Where there was a legitimate issue of public interest, this restriction could be tolerated. In this case, however, the court found that the trade unions' action did not promote public interest even though it was designed to prevent social dumping in the Swedish labour market. Such action would be permissible only where an undertaking fails to comply with the minimum protection standards applicable within the host country. In the case of Sweden no such minimal standards were deemed to exist. Such a conclusion was based on the fact that, in Sweden, minimum rates of pay are agreed between management and labour and embodied in collective agreements that are not declared universally applicable by legislation. Consequently, none of the methods for establishing a minimum level of pay provided for in the Posted Workers Directive was used (Zahn, 2008: 7). As the Swedish system of industrial relations is built on cooperative, voluntary arrangements between employers and trade unions, the court's judgment represented a profound challenge to the essential institutional character of Swedish collective bargaining. These institutions may now need to be buttressed by legal interventions at odds with the logic and traditions of Sweden's 'flexicurity' model. Introducing a national minimum wage is one possible remedial response. More generally, the ECJ's judgment in Laval served to establish that the Posted Workers Directive effectively set a minimum floor of rights that cannot be improved upon by trade union collective action (Zahn, 2008: 16).

The implications of this judgment were confirmed, if not deepened, by the ECJ decision, issued on 3 April 2008 in the Rüffert case.[8] In this instance, subcontractors, based in Poland, but operating in Germany, were fined for failing to pay their posted workers at the rate of pay of the applicable German collective agreement. They were employed as subcontractors on a public contract in Niedersachsen and the state law provided that such work could only be awarded to undertakings that committed in writing to pay their employees at least the level of pay prescribed in the applicable collective agreement. This commitment also required the contractor to ensure that all subcontractors complied with this requirement. In this case, however, the Polish contractor only paid its 53 workers 46.57 per cent of the prescribed minimum wage. Ultimately, as part of the legal proceedings, the ECJ was asked to rule on whether the freedom to provide services precluded a statutory obligation requiring a contractor on a public works contract to undertake to pay its employees at least the remuneration laid down in the applicable collective agreement. In its judgment, the ECJ determined that the Niedersachsen state law, which does not itself fix any minimum rates of pay, cannot be considered a law, within the meaning of Article (1) of Directive 96/71, which fixed a minimum rate of pay. As in the Laval judgment, the ECJ's restrictive interpretation represented a fundamental challenge to the institutions of collective bargaining and agreement. Long-established institutional arrangements have to be reconfigured in order to conform to EU law as interpreted by the ECJ.

### Implications

The net effect of these cases is to subject the operation of national industrial relations systems to the application of European law. The purely national character of established systems of collective bargaining and enforcement has been substantially circumscribed. In the case of the Posted Workers Directive, fundamental institutional change may be necessary if states are to conform to the court's interpretation of its meaning. More broadly, while the right to collective action has been deemed fundamental to European law, it is not unrestricted. Where there is conflict with equally fundamental commitments to free movement, principles of 'balance' and 'proportionality' must be applied. While the objective of combating social dumping has been deemed to be legitimate in the court's judgments, the protection of firms' economic freedoms is considered to be equally important. Thus, the absolute right to use established collective bargaining systems to resist the threat presented by low-cost competition to the integrity of national labour markets, which many trade unions thought they had won at Amsterdam, has been substantially curtailed. Furthermore, the introduction of concepts of 'balance' and 'proportionality' will create great uncertainty with regard to the practices of collective negotiation and agreement, inevitably involving national courts in the adjudication of matters that would traditionally have been beyond their remit. Indeed, it has been argued that the reliance on judges to apply these concepts inevitably 'leaves a lot of room for interpretations by national courts and influence by national political sentiments' potentially creating 'wide disparities in the protection of collective action across the Member States of the European Union' (Zahn, 2008: 11). In this respect, Europeanization may serve both to destabilize established systems of collective bargaining and to accentuate, rather than moderate, the degree of divergence in the protection afforded workers across member states.

## Industrial Relations at the European Level

Though the core collective bargaining issues concerning pay, the right of association and the right to strike and impose lockouts have been explicitly excluded from the EU's competence, the ongoing integration of Europe's markets and the growing multinationalization of its firms inevitably generate problems and conflicts that require European-level action. Certainly, the European Commission has sought to develop a significant industrial relations role for the EU in managing the emerging European market. Two initiatives in particular have been significant. The first concerns the sustained attempt to foster a process of 'European social dialogue' (ESD) between the European representative associations of the 'social partners', employers and labour. The second concerns the attempt, in response to the growing number of Euro-companies, to establish a legal framework for representing worker interests within their managerial structures. An analysis of the evolution and impact of these initiatives can offer insight into the extent to which the EU should be regarded as an agent of liberal transformation in the institutional character of industrial relations in Europe.

### European social dialogue

In 1985, a process of European social dialogue was instituted at a meeting between the representative associations of labour and business under the auspices of the European Commission. The Commission President, Jacques Delors, declared his intention that the ESD should, in the future, produce collective European agreements between the 'social partners' that would complement national industrial relations activities. Such ambitions were given a more secure legal foundation with the agreement of a Social Protocol appended to the Maastricht Treaty. Subsequently, in the Treaty of Amsterdam, the protocol was incorporated into the body of treaty law. Under Article 136, the Community and the member states committed themselves to promoting social dialogue between management and labour at the European level. To facilitate this dialogue, the social partners were accorded a privileged position within the policymaking process. Thus, on the one hand, the Commission was required to consult the partners on any matter of social policy. This encompassed a large range of issues, including matters relating to the working environment, health and safety, social security and social protection, gender equality of opportunities and treatment at work, employment protection, representation of and collective defence of the interests of workers and employers, and financial contributions for promoting employment and job creation. On the other hand, where the social partners reached an agreement on a matter of policy, they had the right to request the Commission to submit their proposals to the Council of Ministers as a proposed directive. Taken together, it was hoped that these provisions would encourage the emergence of substantive forms of interaction between the associational representatives of employers and employees over many other aspects of industrial relations.

Some headway has been made towards establishing the necessary organizational preconditions for such a dialogue. At the peak level, the European Trade Union Confederation (ETUC) brings together all major national confederations, largely managing to escape the political and confessional divisions that fragment trade union movements in many member states. Almost 90 per cent of all union members in Europe are indirect members of ETUC, totalling approximately 60 million people in some 35 countries (European Commission, 2004:17). On the employers' side, the representation of employers' interests is similarly united and comprehensive. BusinessEurope (formerly UNICE) has successfully established itself as the recognized representative of business in the dialogue with organized labour at the EU level. Its membership encompasses almost all the main national cross-industry confederations of private sector employers. A separate organization, Centre Européen des Entreprises Publiques (CEEP), was founded in 1961 to represent firms with some element of public ownership and/or publicly oriented function. A distinct European-level body representing smaller firms, the Association of Craft and Small and Medium-sized Enterprises (UEAPME) has also emerged. Since 1968 UNICE (now BusinessEurope) and UEAPME have worked effectively together in EU-level social dialogue and in negotiations with trade unions (European Commission, 2004: 27). Despite this impressive façade, however, the actual representative effectiveness of these organizations is quite restricted. In practice, the national federations comprising BusinessEurope exercise very tight control over its policy, with each retaining the right to block any measures regarded as undesirable. As a consequence, BusinessEurope's capacity to govern and lead its members is very limited. When members are divided over an issue of strategy or policy, its propensity is to remain inactive in order to avoid a damaging internal conflict. In effect, its capacity to engage with trade unions is largely determined by the most recalcitrant among its members. Moreover, when the analysis is extended beyond the peak employers' associations to the sectoral level, the picture is even less impressive. Thus, the European Industry Associations that represent the interests of national sectoral trade unions at the European level frequently lack employer counterparts (Keller and Platzer, 2003: 3).

The pattern of organizational development among employers reflects their general reluctance to engage with the process of ESD. This reluctance is manifest in the record of legislative initiatives taken under the special procedures agreed at Maastricht and strengthened in the Amsterdam Treaty. Thus, while social framework agreements concerning parental leave, part-time work and fixed-term work have been reached under this procedure, and subsequently given legal form through council directives, it is apparent that employers only engaged in serious negotiations when there was a possibility that the Commission would initiate its own proposals. Their objective is generally to prevent rather than facilitate the agreement of European legislation (Falkner, 2003: 22). Indeed, the evidence is that even where there is a credible threat of Commission action, the energies of employers' associations will be directed towards obstruction. Given the need of the Commission to find agreement across the full range of social partners, both European and national, such resistance has every chance of success. For these reasons, expectations of the evolution of a substantial role for the social partners in shaping the emergence of European labour markets and industrial relations regulation have largely been disappointed. With few exceptions, employers see no merit in the development of a European role.

On initial examination, the picture looks somewhat rosier at the sectoral level. It is estimated that, since the 1980s, such dialogue has generated some 300 agreed texts. These encompass a wide range of issues, including health and safety, vocational training, equal opportunities and the working environment (European Commission, 2004: 71–3). However, on closer scrutiny, the situation is considerably less impressive. Most activity is heavily dependent on the substantial support that the Commission provides. Not only do many of the topics discussed reflect the Commission's agenda, but without its financial support for translation, travel, accommodation, secretarial services, etc., the organizational apparatus necessary for the dialogue to continue might well collapse (Keller, 2003: 35). Indeed, even with this support there is often difficulty in finding representative employers' associations willing to participate in the process and with the capacity to do so. In practice, genuine engagement by employers' associations as well as trade unions has largely been confined to sectors where the Commission is a major regulatory actor. Thus, by far the greatest activity has been in industries undergoing a process of liberalization that was at least partly a consequence of EU policy. Of the top four sectors of ESD activity, three were the liberalizing industries of telecoms, postal services and railways, and the fourth was agriculture, always the most Europeanized of industries (de Boer et al., 2005: 60). Moreover, much of this activity amounted to little more than lobbying for policy amendments with little or no industrial relations content. It has been estimated that 'three quarters of all joint statements are targeted exclusively at EU politics, which means that these results are in no way intended to commit the national affiliates to anything, but are targeted purely at influencing European policy in some way' (ibid.: 61).

Given this motivation, it is unsurprising that the value of the ESD's output has been heavily criticized. The great majority of the documents produced embody agreed statements of view and take the form of non-binding guidelines, codes of conduct and policy orientations. They lack 'hard', legal force; even as 'soft' forms of regulation they are often very soft indeed. In most cases, the minimum provisions these agreements lay down are far below those already obtaining in individual countries (Visser, 2001). When the social partners came to review the process in 2001, the vision they offered in the Laeken Declaration was one of autonomous, bipartite dialogue designed to conclude voluntary, non-legally binding agreements (de Boer et al., 2005: 64). Some have suggested that ESD has been unfairly criticized for failing to produce outcomes it was never designed to achieve (Marginson and Sisson, 2004: 103–4). However, the increasing tendency for the practice of social dialogue to be conducted within the framework of the EES bodes ill for its future (Gold et al., 2007: 20). There seems little reason to challenge Keller's assessment that ESD is unlikely to contribute significantly to closing the gap between economic and social integration at the European level (Keller, 2003: 53).

### European integration and works councils

A central feature of industrial relations in many European countries is the provision for employee representation in firms, typically known as works councils. Their character differs substantially across national systems. In many states, their function is to facilitate information sharing and consultation between management and employees. In a minority of cases, there is provision for co-decision-making, with employees enjoying substantial rights to participate in developing company policy in respect of personnel and even investment matters. Irrespective of these differences, however, works councils share some features common to all those states that have them. Most fundamentally, they are institutions of public governance with employers unable to evade or buy out their obligations to participate and practically to support their operation. Councils embody a substantial public commitment to rebalance employment relations in the employee's favour. In order to substantiate this right in the face of market pressures, workplace participation in post-war Europe has been institutionalized in legal statute. In effect, this served to insert them 'as compulsory elements in any individual employment contract regardless of the will of the contracting parties, and if necessary against their will' (Streeck, 1997: 644). The form of this statutory provision has varied. Where there is provision for a degree of co-decision-making, thereby curtailing the rights of private property, the purpose and remit has generally been embodied in company law. In contrast, where the business of councils was confined to modifying 'management's prerogatives in the day-to-day governance of the employment contract', they were more usually a matter of labour law (ibid.). However, irrespective of the formal legal mechanisms, these arrangements shared 'the promise, and in most instances also the reality, of constructive, forward-looking interaction between labour and management' (Hancké, 2000, 37).

There are substantial differences in the status and design of these arrangements across countries. Thus, while in most states they are composed of employee representatives elected by their peers, management also enjoys membership rights in Belgium, Luxembourg and France. More significantly, the relationship between councils and trade unions varies greatly across states. In so-called 'single channel systems', the right to workplace representation for the purposes of information is expressed through workplace unions. In effect, union and council functions are merged (European Commission, 2004: 21). Such systems obtain in Finland, Sweden, Denmark, Poland, Lithuania, Cyprus and Malta. In dual channel systems, in contrast, the works council system operates separately from the trade unions. In this model, the rights to representation, information and consultation are conferred on individual workers, independently of trade union representation (European Commission, 2004: 21). Such a separation holds in many member states, including Germany, Austria, France, Belgium, the Netherlands, Luxembourg, Spain, Slovenia and Slovakia. In a third group, the single and dual channel models are blended. In Italy, for example, works councils do not distinguish between union and non-union members, and the unions voluntarily extend union rights and benefits to non-union members (Regalia, 1995).

Councils also differ in their remit. In all cases, their primary function is to facilitate communication and consultation between management and employees, especially in relation to social and personnel policies. Many works councils also have a monitoring function with regard to collective agreements or statutory rights. In general, however, the rights of councils in the Rhineland and Nordic states are considerably more developed in comparison with the Latin states of the Mediterranean (Marginson and Sisson, 2004: 47). It is in the former states that works councils typically enjoy co-determination privileges, which affords them a significant influence over company decision-making regarding social and human resource management policies. In some cases, these rights even extend to economic policy matters including mergers and takeovers, work organization and investment. Finally, in most of the systems where co-determination rights exist, works councils must be consulted over the implementation of pay systems and working-time schedules, even if they are barred from participating in the collective bargaining process itself (European Commission, 2004: 23).

It must also be recognized that there are significant limits to the coverage of works councils, both across and within member states. Neither Britain nor Ireland has any national legal provision for such employee representation. To the very limited extent that workplace representation exists in these two countries, it is entirely voluntary. Many of the post-2004 entrants operate less developed and less encompassing systems, while employers frequently evade the responsibilities to which they have been legally subjected (ibid.). Moreover, even within those states with strong provision, coverage is not total. Thus, though the size threshold varies across states, works councils are generally a phenomenon of larger companies. This is partly a matter of law. In almost all countries, the smallest firms are exempt from the requirement to establish a council. In the Netherlands, for example, only firms with 50 or more employees need establish one, while in Germany the figure is 5 workers. In many instances, however, it is evasion rather than exemption that limits coverage. Even in Germany, where in many respects the system has reached its purest, most developed form, it is estimated that a third of the workforce is not covered by a council, far more than can be justified by exemption provisions. In France, it is estimated that of small firms (1–19 employees), fewer than 20 per cent have a form of workplace representation, while in firms with more than 50 employees, that figure rises to over 90 per cent (ibid.: 22).

Notwithstanding these caveats and qualifications, however, among the continental member states of the European Union, works councils do constitute significant institutions that shape the interaction between management and workers and, in particular, serve to bolster the position of labour in the employment relation. It is also apparent that the deepening of European market integration presents a considerable challenge to the sustainability of these national systems. In a context of free capital mobility and the increasing multinationalization of firms, national systems are unavoidably drawn into competition with each other. More onerous systems of industrial citizenship may deter foreign investors and/or encourage outward investment. Multinational companies operating across a range of member states may be able to leverage inter-plant rivalries to test the solidarity of workers. Moreover, with more and more plants ultimately subject to decisions made by management based in other countries, works councils outside the 'home' country may find it difficult to exercise their rights if the company chooses to make key decisions at headquarters level and marginalizes local management. In such instances, foreign firms escape controls to which domestic firms are subject, while the workforce of domestically controlled firms retain rights which are effectively denied to those employed by foreign multinationals.

The implications of these developments for works councils are a contested issue. Some anticipate that, as the process of market integration deepens, there will be a steady erosion of national systems. Employers will exploit the new competitive environment to free themselves from the constraints of consultation with their workforces. From the 'varieties of capitalism' perspective, such a liberal market response is far from preordained. Thelen and Kume (1999), for example, suggest that in coordinated market economies, employers may in fact respond to globalization by strengthening their works council institutions in order to secure labour cooperation and boost productivity. To date, the empirical evidence does not definitively point in either direction. In respect of foreign investment and 'regime shopping', Traxler and Woitech have suggested that there is little evidence that the character of particular labour-market regimes weighs heavily in determining the location of multinational corporation investment (2000: 155). However, a study of the impact of foreign direct investment on works councils in Germany found that employers were able to exploit the threat to direct investment elsewhere to win substantial concessions from works councils in respect of work practices, often to the fury of trade unions, which found that the hard-won fruits of collective bargaining were effectively undermined (Raess and Burgoon, 2006: 296). While national systems of works councils still exercise considerable influence over develop-ments, the integration of European markets does appear to strengthen the negotiating position of employers.

### The European response

The corrosive potential of market integration for national systems of work-place employee representation was recognized early by the European Commission. Proposals were formulated to address the issue and these were characterized by a marked bias towards the introduction of a common system modelled on German practice. As noted in chapter 4, in the early 1970s the Fifth Directive in Company Law proposed the introduction of a full-blown system of co-determination across all member states. At the same time, pro-posals were presented for a European Company Statute, again modelled on German corporate law. If enacted, together these directives would have simul-taneously harmonized and substantially Germanized corporate law across Europe, largely eliminating the possibility of regime competition between states and entrenching a very substantive form of industrial citizenship rights in the European economy as a whole.

The strength of these provisions, the depth of opposition from business and the fact that they were extremely alien to traditional practice in a number of member states ensured that the directives were never passed. Though the Commission did not abandon its ambition to build a European regime of employee representation rights, its proposals became progressively more modest as successive rounds were rejected by the Council of Ministers. Thus, in 1980, the draft Vredeling Directive set down a wide-ranging list of information and consultation rights to which employees were entitled, but it abandoned the attempt to enshrine strong co-decision-making rights. It also left the pre-cise composition and operational rules of works councils to be determined at national level, in accordance with established law and practices. In regard to multinational companies, its provisions were somewhat more demanding. It would have empowered workers at plant level to bypass local management and deal directly with central management when necessary, even if the latter were based in a different national jurisdiction (Streeck, 1997: 650). However, partly because of this aspect, the directive drew strong criticism from business across Europe and fell before the certainty of a veto by Britain, for whom such proposals were particularly alien.

Over the following decade, the Commission's strategy and objectives altered considerably. Discussions of employee representation schemes were referred for consideration to the 'social dialogue' process. Although the Commission and the European Parliament created a budget line to promote and finance transnational social partnership arrangements, the voluntaristic nature of these initiatives revealed the increasingly restricted range of ambition in comparison with the 1970s (Müller and Platzer, 2003: 62). The terms of the European Works Council Directive, finally agreed in 1994, reflect the growing liberal orientation of the EU generally. While its agreement was facilitated by the adoption of QMV and the British opt-out for social policy matters agreed at Maastricht, even in comparison with Vredeling its provisions were very modest. It did establish a set of procedural rules for the creation of works councils and laid down a set of statutory minimum provisions that would apply to all firms with more than 1,000 employees in a member state and at least 150 employees in two other member states (Adnett and Hardy, 2005: 184). Yet it also provided ample space for the accommodation of different national and corporate traditions, and for the individual enterprises to negotiate their own distinctive terms. The directive simply obligates member states to require 'nationally based firms with significant employment in other European Union countries to negotiate, with a body representing their entire European workforce, on a European-wide workplace information arrangement' (Streeck, 1997: 651). A wide range of areas are deemed suitable for such cooperation, stretching from the introduction of new working methods through employment, investment and organization changes to questions of transfers of production, mergers, cutbacks and closures. However, this represented a set of options and there was no compulsion to incorporate any of them into the terms of reference of a European Works Council (EWC). Moreover, not only was there no provision for co-decision-making in the directive, but, even where consultation rights are agreed, their effectiveness may be marginal. Management is not required to await a considered response from the employee representative body before moving to action. In fact, if management and workforce are in agreement, there is no obligation to establish an EWC at all. The directive turns 'industrial citizenship, from an institutional condition of negotiations between employers and workforces, into their result' (ibid.: 653).

The relatively undemanding terms of the directive are also reflected in the mode of its implementation. Most particularly, two distinct regimes are provided for. Firms that established their EWC by September 1996 were subject to Article 13, which set a quite undemanding set of minimum requirements for the functioning of the council. More laggardly firms were, instead, subject to Article 6, which laid down somewhat more rigorous demands in relation to the nature of the information that management had to disseminate and the depth of the communication between management and employee representatives that had to take place. By 2002, some 639 EWCs representing around 11 million employees had been set up in major European companies, creating an institutional basis for transnational social dialogue (European Commission, 2004: 144). Of these agreements, some 72 per cent were set up under Article 13 of the directive, while the remainder were subject to Article 6.

The EWC Directive is viewed by some as offering the basis for developing a European system of industrial relations. Marginson and Sisson suggest that EWCs are incrementally opening the door to forms of European collective bargaining, contributing to the emergence of a 'Euro-company dimension to industrial relations' (2004: 242–3). Arrowsmith and Marginson perceive them as offering 'an institutional framework which can potentially underpin cross-border bargaining' (2006: 255). In support of such optimism, the Commission itself has cited evidence that, on expiry of the initial agreement to establish an EWC, the growth of trust and experience between the parties has frequently facilitated the agreement of a stronger form of council (European Commission, 2004: 144). The processes that 'are triggered by the EWC Directive's mode of regulation develop their own, and often unpredictable, dynamics, potentially generating surprising developments' (Müller and Platzer, 2003: 80). In the case of General Motors, the EWC succeeded in generating effective cross-border trade union cooperation (Fetzer, 2008: 304). Moreover, the optimistic view has been bolstered by the agreement of Directive 2002/17 that creates 'a framework of minimum standards for informing and consulting employees at company level in all member states', thus forcing Britain and Ireland to introduce a statutory provision for works councils at the national level for the first time (European Commission, 2006c: 59). The base upon which EWCs can be built has been broadened. Yet if this optimism is to be justified, an enormous amount of development must occur. It is notable that in one recent study, it was found that only one in ten councils makes provision for consultation beyond 'dialogue' or 'exchange of views', including the right of employees to give considered comments or make recommendations. Only 3 per cent of agreements afford the EWC a negotiating role (Marginson and Sisson, 2004: 232). Another detailed study of 23 EWCs demonstrated that approximately half were purely 'symbolic' in nature, formally constituted but effectively inoperative. The remainder had developed a role in relation to providing information but only one-sixth were engaged in negotiating substantive agreements and joint initiatives with management (Müller and Platzer, 2003: 81). EWCs need to undergo major development if a substantial European dimension to industrial relations is to emerge.

Furthermore, based on the balance of evidence to date, it would appear that whatever does emerge in the future will more closely reflect the ambitions of management than those of employees. Analyses of EWCs reveal that it is company management that tends to determine their terms of reference. They drive forward the cross-border articulation of local bargaining agendas and outcomes within multinational corporations (MNCs) 'often through 'coercive comparisons' of labour costs, working practices and performance' (Arrowsmith and Marginson, 2006: 246). In a study of the chemicals sector, Waddington found that management had effectively prevented EWCs from impinging on their decision-making (2006: 348). In contrast, employee representatives had failed to force the issues that most concerned trade unions onto the agenda (Waddington, 2006: 337). In the motor industry, Hancké found a marked lack of inter-plant solidarity. The acquisition of information about plant performance was not used by trade union representatives to build a common strategy throughout the company, but rather 'to strengthen the position of their own plant in the implicit competition between plants' (2000: 54). In a sector marked by high levels of unionization and production integration, EWCs 'are increasingly becoming vehicles for international labour regime competition' rather than bulwarks against social dumping (ibid.: 36). Where more effective cross-border trade union cooperation has been achieved, as in General Motors, it embodied the unions' acceptance of the management's view that a transformational corporate change was required in the face of the challenge of globalization (Fetzer, 2008, 304). Despite their relatively positive judgement of EWCs, it is telling that Arrowsmith and Marginson conclude that the Europeanization of industrial relations in the MNC, whether directly through negotiation in works councils or through international benchmarking and networking, 'seems part of a process of reconstituting collective bargaining better to fit a management-led agenda of competition and adaptability' (2006: 263).

These developments embody the growing entrenchment of so-called 'neovoluntarist' approaches to industrial relations. The nature and significance of EWCs will be determined by negotiations between management and employees. The terms of the deal agreed in any given case will reflect the negotiating strategies and relative bargaining strengths of the two sides. In contrast to the public enforcement of workplace rights in national systems, the role of EWCs will be the product of negotiations rather than a conditioning factor in them. Firms will only accede to the creation of a strong works council where they anticipate a benefit from them. They will be a contingent and particularistic product of favourable market conditions rather than a universal right (Streeck, 1997: 653). From this perspective, EWCs are an indication of the EU's incapacity to constrain MNCs and they reflect the broader retreat of state intervention before the power of market forces (Müller and Platzer, 2003: 80). European integration serves to advance a liberal reconstitution of the institutions of economic governance.

## Conclusion

Despite the 'Amsterdam exclusion', which denies it any role in relation to pay determination, the right of association and right to strike and lockout, the impact of the EU on the conduct of industrial relations is both significant and expanding. The shift to EMU generated a substantial degree of innovation in national systems of collective bargaining, exemplified in the phenomenon of social pacts. The intensification of market competition facilitated by the single market and currency projects has seen the gradual emergence of a European 'going rate for the job'. As a result, national bargaining is increasingly conducted in the shadow of Europe. Key ECJ judgments have effectively served to 'open' collective bargaining systems in some member states to competition from low-wage countries. The growth in the number of 'Euro-companies' has contributed to the erosion of the status and influence of national systems of employee representation. In short, while there is little sign of the emergence of a European system of collective bargaining, the legal challenges and market dynamics unleashed by EU policy are serving to destabilize key aspects of national industrial relations systems. Even if many of the institutional forms of European industrial relations continue to exist, their policy output seems to be considerably less favourable for labour.

The changes in the conduct of industrial relations in Europe cannot all be attributed to the EU. Wider processes of technological change and global market integration are also in operation. The growing sensitivity of collective agreements to the specific market circumstances of individual firms is a general phenomenon in the contemporary world. However, it is striking that despite its efforts to develop a form of social partnership and establish a set of employee representation rights at the European level, the overwhelming impact of EU policy is to facilitate and substantially accentuate these wider processes. Even when it does not seek to emulate Anglo-American practices, its activities serve to threaten the sustainability of more 'organized', non-liberal institutional forms of economic governance.

FURTHER READING

Marginson and Sisson (2004) provide a very comprehensive discussion of the EU's impact on industrial relations. Gold et al. (2007) analyse the more recent fate of social partnership. Natali and Pochet (2009) examine the evolution of national social pacts under EMU. Waddington (2006) and Fetzer (2008) offer contrasting case studies of the performance of EWCs.

# Conclusion: Liberal Europe and National Capitalism

The achievements of the European Union in building a common European market are undeniable. Compared to the nationally fragmented economies of the 1950s, goods, services, capital and people flow across borders far more freely. The number and range of barriers to trade have been greatly diminished. Powerful monitoring and enforcement agencies have been created at the European level to ensure that both private and public actors respect the system's rules. In many member states monetary policy has been ceded to the European Central Bank, while fiscal policy is subject to increasing European oversight and restraint. Clearly, a more open, competitive form of capitalism has been established across the Union. What is less certain, however, is whether this exercise in liberal market-building at the European level has been accompanied by a corresponding liberal reconfiguration of economic governance at the national level. As noted in chapter 1, many member states rely on non-market governance institutions to regulate the interaction of economic agents. Associational actors, complex inter-corporate networks and highly interventionist states play crucial roles in governing economies across Europe. The design and operation of key institutions such as works councils, corporate governance systems, collective bargaining regimes, etc. primarily reflect political compromises between socioeconomic actors rather than the functional demands of market exchange. In 'making Europe', is the EU enforcing the liberal remaking of such institutions at the national level and, in the process, transforming the governance of capitalism in Europe?

In the first phase of integration, stretching from 1957 into the 1980s, it is clear that the challenge presented by the EEC/EU to national institutional systems was quite modest. During these years, cross-border trade did increase substantially and basic European institutions were established and developed. However, most aspects of product, capital and labour market governance remained within the control of national policymakers. Firms cooperated or colluded and governments subsidized and conferred privileges according to national tradition and inclination. Product-market regulation continued to afford many national producers a high level of protection against imports. The financing, ownership and governance of corporations was largely unaffected by European policy. Though European law greatly extended the rights of workers who moved between member states, the broad field of labour market regulation and related welfare provision remained largely impervious to the progress of European integration.

However, with the advent of the single market and single currency projects in the 1980s and early 1990s, this picture began to change. Empowered and energized by the emergence of a political climate favouring liberal, market-oriented reforms, the EU moved to build a much more substantial European regulatory system that would facilitate a far deeper form of integration. The strategy adopted had a number of distinct elements. Firstly, it sought to circumvent many of the obstacles erected by member states to open and competitive product markets. Adopting the principle of mutual recognition allowed foreign producers simply to bypass the massed protectionist ranks of national product specifications that had formerly blocked their attempts to enter new markets. Secondly, it moved to develop much stronger policy enforcement mechanisms that would overcome resistance to the effective implementation of European policies. A strengthened competition policy was established to challenge the anti-competitive practices of both private firms and governments. Thirdly, there was a concerted effort to push European policy into areas that had previously been neglected. New directives concerning banking and financial market regulation were passed, with the aim of opening up national financial systems to foreign competition.

Initially, the single market project focused on removing non-tariff barriers to cross-border trade. However, as its implementation progressed, it began to challenge domestic institutions much more directly. Most immediately, perhaps, the drive to build a level competitive playing field for companies led the Commission to formulate a policy to restrict state aid. Long-established and deeply rooted relations of dependency between firms and states were now subject to EU oversight and control. The advent of the euro greatly intensified the impact of integration on domestic labour markets and social policies. The effort to create a truly European financial system quickly led the Commission to press for changes in the rules sustaining the closed, insider-dominated networks of corporate ownership and governance that predominated in many member states. Without such reforms, genuine market competition would be impossible and efforts to integrate national financial and corporate systems would fail. The commitment to market openness, transparency and competition inevitably led the EU to challenge ever more aspects of national political economic governance. As implementation of the single market and currency projects advanced, the Commission pressed with increasing vigour for national governments and regulatory authorities to curb their tendency to favour stability over innovation and system insiders over outsiders.

The fundamental tension between the liberal economic principles of the integration project and many national institutional arrangements has perhaps been demonstrated most clearly in recent years by a series of ECJ decisions relating to incorporation law and collective bargaining rights. In the *Centros* and *Überseering* cases, for example, the effect of its decisions has been to undermine the 'real seat' principle of incorporation and to further the cause of those who favour the development of a market for incorporation modelled on US practice. Were such a market to establish itself, it would undermine the ability of individual states to impose governance structures and obligations on firms that are unappealing to investors and companies. Supporters of German co-determination have been especially alarmed by the prospect of an 'incorporation flight' by German firms to less onerous legal jurisdictions. In the *Laval* and *Rüffert* cases, the ECJ's reasoning challenged the legal basis of voluntary collective bargaining in Sweden, Finland and, to a lesser extent, Germany. Its broader impact was manifest in the protest against foreign workers that broke out in northern England in the early part of 2009.[1] While workers 'posted' to Britain are subject to national statutory minimum-wage provisions, employers are not legally constrained to pay them at the rate agreed with local workers in collective negotiations. National systems of collective bargaining have been levered open, and a form of regime competition is emerging. The application of European law is directly threatening the sustainability of key national institutional arrangements and the balance of socioeconomic power that they embody.

Furthermore, in important areas of economic activity, the destabilizing impact of Commission and ECJ activism on national institutions is being reinforced by pressures for change generated by the day-to-day functioning of the common market and single currency. The effect of these pressures has been particularly evident in the industrial relations field, where national systems of collective bargaining and employee workplace representation are subject to growing strain. As integration deepens, for example, threats by investors and firms to move jurisdiction if national policymakers ignore their demands have gained much greater plausibility. In some states, this has prompted a liberal reform of significant aspects of labour market regulation. Similarly, as barriers to trade fall away and the costs and risks of moving the location of production diminish, employers have exploited the threat of disinvestment to drive down wages. In addition, as firms increasingly 'multinationalize' their operations, works councils at plant level find it extremely difficult to hold management to account as ultimate control migrates to international corporate headquarters. Elements of inter-plant competition have emerged. Attempts to counteract these effects have met with limited success. Moves by unions to regain bargaining power by coordinating wage negotiations across a number of countries have largely failed, at least to date. The results of efforts to recapture employee influence over management by creating a system of European Works' Councils have generally been disappointing. In most cases, the terms of reference of EWCs are markedly less favourable to employees than those found in equivalent domestic arrangements. It is generally true that established institutions continue to perform an important role. Yet it is also often the case that they come to function in significantly different ways. National 'social pacts' agreed in many countries typically rely on existing industrial relations institutions to operate. But their provisions frequently embody a substantial shift in the balance of bargaining power from labour to employers. Systems of economic governance in member states are being simultaneously threatened from above, by the strengthening of the EU's legal authority, and from below, by the expanding opportunities for business to 'regime shop'. The making of liberal Europe does appear to threaten the sustainability of many national institutions and the fundamental relations of power that they embody.

### Transformation?

The EU's liberal challenge to national institutional systems is real. Across the Union, domestic governance institutions in product, financial and labour markets are being reformed in significant ways. Yet if one is to speak of the liberal transformation of national capitalisms, these changes will have to be pressed much further. Even after decades of effort, it is telling that measures of product-market openness and competitiveness in member states reveal the persistence of significant barriers between them. Despite the Second Banking Directive and the FSAP, financial systems remain substantially national in structure and orientation. The distinctive properties of national systems of corporate ownership and governance exhibit great durability in the face of multiple EU interventions, ranging from directives enforcing greater financial transparency, through new takeover rules, to direct challenges by the Commission to the legitimacy of national decisions favouring domestic firms. Where co-determination arrangements operate, neither European laws nor market pressures have yet succeeded in undermining them. In response to the growing pressures on national employment and social policies generated by integration, governments have sought to adjust rather than transform established practices, exploiting the resources provided by their particular institutional inheritance to ease adaptation to changing conditions. Both EU policy and market developments have destabilized important aspects of many national institutions, but these changes need to go much further if a thoroughgoing liberal remaking of national capitalisms is to take place

Transformation may yet occur. Many of the more recent financial and corporate law reforms will take time to have their full impact. The capacity of ECJ judgments to have a major effect on national practice has been demonstrated repeatedly. However, there are also reasons to question the EU's capacity to press the liberal reform agenda too much further. The existence of significant political resistance to this project needs to be recognized. It is revealing that though the CAP has undergone substantial reform, a significant core group of member states continues to resist its wholesale market transformation. It is also significant that, though the USA is frequently invoked as a reference model for reform, European social policy has been markedly influenced by social and Christian democratic thinking. Most importantly of all, disagreement and equivocation about the desirability of further liberal reform is clearly evident among member states. The controversy over the Bolkestein Services Directive revealed deep differences of view between states on whether the interests of the citizen-consumer should supersede the interests of the citizen-producer.

These political obstacles at the European level are compounded by the unpredictable dynamics of Europeanization, which frequently inhibit the effective implementation of EU policy measures at national level. In many areas of policy, European initiatives will not succeed unless they attract the support of powerful domestic actors. In the case of German bank regulation, for example, it was only after the decision by Germany's powerful private banks to make a complaint to the EU that the state guarantees enjoyed by German public banks became the subject of investigation by DG Comp. Yet examples of such domestic appeals to EU actors are relatively rare. In many cases, the potential beneficiaries of reform lack the will or capacity to lobby effectively. As Franzese and Mosher (2002) have pointed out, the costs of reform are frequently more immediately apparent than the benefits. Consequently, the potential losers from change are often quicker, and better placed, to mobilize in resistance. In the competition policy field, reforms introduced in 2004 tried to address some of these problems by encouraging aggrieved parties to take private legal action against those breaching EU law. As yet, however, it is not obvious that this aspect of the reform has met with much success. Even where support for liberal-oriented reform is generally strong, there is no guarantee that particular reforms will not be blocked. In the case of the Takeover Directive, for example, positive attitudes towards securities-market reform in Germany hardened into opposition as the implications of this particular measure became clearer. The concrete and immediate risks that the new provisions generated outweighed any longer-term prospective benefits.

Perhaps the greatest obstacle to effective Europeanization stems from the frequent tendency of national governments to evade the implications of measures they have accepted in the Council of Ministers by pursuing economically nationalist implementation strategies. In many instances, the regulatory accommodation of European policy has been carefully shaped to protect important established national relationships or favoured actors. When liberalizing the networked industries, national implementation of the regulatory changes mandated by European policy has frequently been designed to further the interests of favoured domestic firms. Furthermore, even when there is no conscious act of manipulation, distinctive national administrative and judicial inheritances often 'distort' the impact of EU measures. Thus, liberal reform measures in corporate law have little resonance within the Italian judicial system. Consequently, their application to particular cases can produce outcomes that are quite at odds with what was intended by the reforms' instigators. After they have been filtered through the unique and potentially uncongenial environment of national administrative and judicial systems, the practical impact of EU policies may be quite different from their intended purpose.

These problems may be exacerbated by recent Commission initiatives to develop more effective strategies of Europeanization. The 2004 reform of EU competition policy actually increased the role of national judicial systems in its enforcement, thereby reinforcing the potential for highly divergent interpretations to develop. Similarly, the capacity of the Open Method of Coordination to achieve a significant reform of social policy is subject to grave doubt. While its defenders may emphasize its innovative quality, the evidence suggests that the processes of 'discourse formation' and 'mutual learning' on which it relies to effect change often fail in the face of substantial differences in the values and objectives of social policy across member states. While there is some evidence from the competition policy field to suggest that the EU is capable of building reformist epistemic communities encompassing national expert and bureaucratic elites, the political sensitivity of social policy raises doubts about the replicability of this process. In short, the effectiveness of many Europeanization strategies depends greatly on the existence of a congenial political, administrative or judicial context at the national level. As a result, reform is likely to be uneven across and within member states. Institutional systems may change, but a wholesale liberal reconfiguration is unlikely.

Finally, the task facing EU efforts to transform the governance of capitalism in Europe has been made even more difficult by the financial and economic crisis that began in 2008. Its shocking force has led to the introduction of many measures that run counter to common market rules. Banks have been given massive financial aid to enable them to survive. A significant number of them have been part-nationalized as an alternative to collapse. Substantial subsidies have been given to some industrial sectors to enable them to weather an unprecedented drop in demand. Most notably, perhaps, the car industry has received considerable direct and indirect support across the developed world. Governments have summarily set aside many of the competition policy gains of the previous two decades, with the Commission desperately seeking to regain control over the process. The demand by some governments that national firms favour 'home' production sites over others within the Union is particularly threatening to common market principles. The EU's monetary and fiscal regime has also come under severe strain. Overwhelmed by the combined costs of financial and industrial subsidies, falling tax revenue and rising social security payments to the unemployed, the budget deficits of Eurozone states have risen sharply. Many have burst through the 3 per cent limit set by the Stability and Growth Pact (SGP). While the Commission has moved to initiate 'excessive deficit procedures' against these states, the size of the deficits and the number of states involved has prevented it from adopting a tough stance. Indeed, the severity of the problems have gone beyond anything anticipated by the SGP; countries such as Ireland and Greece may be forced to default on their debt, throwing the very sustainability of the Eurozone's governance into doubt.

The implications of these events for the integration project are highly uncertain. If they are short-lived in duration, they may amount to little more than a temporary and relatively inconsequential suspension of the rules. Indeed, optimists could argue that many of the actions taken demonstrate the sensible flexibility of European policymakers and institutions in the face of exceptional events. In particular, the ECB has proven to be a more innovative institution than many of its critics had anticipated, intervening forcefully to sustain the European banking system once the true scale of the crisis became apparent.[2] If, as seems more likely, however, the dramas of 2008–9 are so serious that they preclude any return to the *status quo ante*, key aspects of the integration project may be called into question. Most immediately, the system of prudential financial regulation is almost certain to be revised. The compatibility of a nationally based regulatory system with an integrated financial system and a single currency has clearly been challenged. More fundamentally, the risks involved in seeking to approximate European financial markets to Anglo-American practice have become more apparent. The entire policy was predicated on the belief that creating a shareholder-friendly system of corporate ownership and governance, underpinned by a securities market-based financial system, would stimulate higher levels of investment and growth in Europe. However, it is precisely this model of financial organization and corporate governance that has been exposed by recent events. At the very least, it is likely that the proposition that further liberal reform is the only way to overcome Europe's economic problems will meet with greater opposition from some member states.

# Notes

## CHAPTER 2    THE EUROPEAN UNION AND THE EVOLUTION OF LIBERAL EUROPE

1 The Treaty of Amsterdam renumbered the Articles of the EC and EU Treaties. The Nice Treaty merged the EC Treaty and the EU Treaty into the 'Consolidated' Treaties. When directly referring to the Treaty of Rome, I will use the original numbering system. All other references to EU Treaty articles will be to the EC section of the Consolidated version and the numbering system therein.
2 ECB President, Jean-Claude Trichet, quoted in *Irish Times*, 18 July 2008.
3 Lisbon European Council, 23 and 24 March 2000, Presidency Conclusions. These can be found at www.eurofound.europa.eu/summits/us1.en.htm.
4 These initiatives will be examined in some detail in chapter 6.
5 The impact of these initiatives will be examined in some detail in chapter 5.

## CHAPTER 3    NATIONAL CAPITALISMS AND EU COMPETITION POLICY

1 Article 81, paragraph 3, Consolidated Version of the Treaty Establishing the European Community.
2 Or, more frequently, the Court of First Instance.
3 It was agreed on 21/12/1989 and came into force on 21/9/1990.
4 Specifically article 9 provided that consideration of a particular 'concentration' could be referred back to a competent state authority if:
   - a concentration threatens to affect significantly competition in a market within that Member State, which presents all the characteristics of a distinct market; or
   - a concentration affects competition in a market within that Member State, which presents all the characteristics of a distinct market and which does not constitute a substantial part of the Common Market. (Rodgers and MacCulloch, 2004: 212)
5 This particular formulation of EU policy is taken from a speech by the Commissioner responsible for Competition (2005–10), Neelie Kroes, delivered on 14 June 2005 at a conference at the University of Leiden.
6 Ibid.
7 The estimate was made in the European Commission's Competition Report (2000).
8 Case Com/37.542 Gas Natural+Endesa
9 Comp/M.3440 ENI/EDP/GDP.
10 *The Times*, 13 March 2009.
11 L'Autorità garante della concorrenza e del mercato (AGCM)
12 The Federation of German Industries was the peak representative trade body for German industry. In 2007 it joined with the equivalent German Employers' Association in a new organization, BDI/BDA.

13 This assessment is made in the European Commission's 21st Report on the Functioning of Community Product and Capital Markets, 2001.

14 These figures are provided by the Commission itself in its 2005 report on state aid measures. Report: *State Aid Scoreboard*, Spring 2005, Commission of the European Communities, p.14.

15 Ibid. p. 5.

16 Ibid. p. 37.

17 The guidelines and 'recitals' of the new merger regulation allow for greater attention to be paid to potential 'efficiency gains' from a merger. If such efficiency gains can be demonstrated, then they may be judged to 'counteract' the negative impact of a concentration on competition and consumer welfare. In effect, some mergers may be allowed that would previously have been prevented. It is still not yet clear what the impact of these provisions will be in practice (Morgan, 2006: 97).

18 Speech to the Eighth Annual Competition Conference, European University Institute, Fiesole, Florence, 17 September 2004. Europa Press Releases: Speech/04/403.

19 The basis for granting such exemptions is laid down in Article 81(3). They can apply where an agreement 'contributes to improving the production or distribution of goods or to promoting technical or economic progress, while allowing consumers a fair share of the resulting benefit' (EU Consolidated Treaties). The interests of consumers are not to be neglected but neither are they accorded an overriding importance.

## CHAPTER 4   FINANCE, CORPORATE OWNERSHIP AND GOVERNANCE IN AN INTEGRATING EUROPE

1 Universal banks can operate in every area of banking without significant restriction. In many countries, banks were confined to a narrower range of activities. In particular, the separation of commercial from investment banking was common in many countries until quite recently.

2 This is taken as a measure of the extent to which firms rely on bank borrowing rather than issuing securities to raise finance.

3 For more details concerning the composition of the supervisory board in Germany, see www.eurofound.europa.eu/emire/germany/codetermination-de.htm.

4 Share classes are different types of shares which have different voting weights.

5 This comment is contained in The Directorate General for Internal Market and Services, 'Consultation on Future Priorities for Plan on Modernising Company Law and Enhancing Corporate Governance in the European Union', published in 2006, p. 10.

6 Case numbers C-212/97, C-208/00 and C-167/01, respectively.

7 The Commissioner for the Internal Market, Charlie McCreevy, stated that the case for such a reform was 'not as obvious or as clear-cut as it may seem and Member States currently follow very different approaches to which they are strongly attached' (SPEECH/07/441; Berlin, 28 June 2007). There are clear political limits to the wholesale Europeanization of national corporate law.

8 One such development came in December 2008 with the ECJ's judgment in the *Cartesio* case (C-210/-6). This restricted the ability of a member state to prevent a company moving its registered office and real seat of business to another state allowing such transfers. Any attempt by the member state of incorporation to restrict the conversion 'by requiring the winding-up or liquidation of the company will amount to a restriction on the company's freedom of establishment contrary to Article 43, "unless it serves overriding requirements in the public interest"'(Johnson, 2009: 164–5).

9 Lisbon European Council 23 and 24 March 2000, Presidency Conclusions. These can be found at www.eurofound.europa.eu/summits/us1.en.htm.

## CHAPTER 5   FINANCE, CORPORATE OWNERSHIP AND GOVERNANCE: NATIONAL SYSTEM CHANGE

1 However, the rules for electing the Supervisory Board Chairperson favour the share-holders. In effect, this means that in the event of a standoff between shareholder and employee representatives, the former always have a decisive advantage. For more detail, see www.eurofound.europa.eu/emire/germany/codetermination/de.htm.

2 The rules also seek to guarantee that the offer price for the mandatory bid will reflect, at least partially, any rise in the value of the stock consequent to the bid.

3 This episode occurred during the final months of the centre-left coalition government of Romano Prodi. However, the advent of a new centre-right government led by Silvio Berlusconi in April 2008 did not alter the fundamental position. Thus, while a signifi-cant minority stake in Italia Telecom had been taken by the Spanish firm Telefonica, the Italian government made it clear during talks with Telefonica's CEO, Cesar Alierta, that Italia Telecom must remain an Italian company. See 'Il governo avverte Alierta Telecom deve restare italiana', *La Repubblica*, 10 September 2008.

4 'Berlusconi hints at Alitalia Deal', *Financial Times*, 24 April 2008.

5 Indeed, the Finance Minister, Domenico Siniscalco, resigned in frustration at the govern-ment's incapacity, or perhaps Berlusconi's unwillingness, to force Fazio's resignation over the issue.

6 An example of his reasoning can be found in Menichella's response to the Parliamentary Commission on Unemployment, 26 February 1953. See Cotula et al., 1997: 443–59.

7 Cesare Geronzi, President of Capitalia, quoted in the *Financial Times*, 'Comment and Analysis', 12 April 2005.

8 Ibid.

9 These statements were made to the annual assembly of the Bank of Italy, 31 May 2005: 29–30. A copy of Governor Fazio's speech can be found at www.bancaditalia.it/pubblicazioni.

10 Ibid., 30.

## CHAPTER 6   WORK AND WELFARE: NATIONAL CAPITALISM AND SOCIAL EUROPE

1 Consolidated Treaties

2 Lisbon European Council Presidency Conclusions, 23–24 March 2000, para. 37. These can be found at: www.europarl.europa.eu/summits/lis1_en.htm.

3 Measures designed to force the unemployed back into work – i.e., by shortening the period of benefit entitlements.

## CHAPTER 7   SOCIAL EUROPE AND INDUSTRIAL RELATIONS

1 Collective bargaining is defined by the ILO Convention No. 98, 1949, as 'voluntary nego-tiations between employers or employers' organisations and workers organisations with a view to the regulation of terms and conditions by collective agreements'.

2 Title X1, article 137(5), EC Treaty, Consolidated Version.

3 Though it is notable that 'social partnership' in Ireland broke down at least temporarily in the face of economic crisis in the spring of 2009. Government efforts to agree a set of severe budgetary cutbacks with trade unions were rebuffed by the latter.

4 Case C-438/05, The International Transport Workers Federation (ITF) and the Finnish Seamens' Union (FSU) v. Viking Line ABP and Oü Viking Line Eesti.

5 C-118/89.

6  The Posted Workers Directive, 96/71/EC.
7  EU07060291.
8  Case C-346/06.

## CONCLUSION:  LIBERAL EUROPE AND NATIONAL CAPITALISM

1  There is mounting pressure from trade unions for a revision of the Posted Workers Directive to eliminate these pressures: *Financial Times,* 13 February 2009.
2  The scale of support has been enormous. Though an extreme case, the €54 billion that the Irish government had to raise to fund its bank rescue plan in the autumn of 2009 was effectively underwritten by the ECB (S. Carswell, *Irish Times*, 18 September 2009). More generally, the ECB has been giving indirect support to many banks in Europe by allowing them post-domestic government debt as collateral for nearly-free central bank cash.

# References

Ackrill, R. (2000) *The Common Agricultural Policy*, Sheffield University Press, Sheffield.

Agnblad, J., E. Berglöf, P. Högfeldt and H. Svancar (2001) 'Ownership and Control in Sweden: Strong Owners, Weak Minorities, and Social Control', in Barca and Becht (eds.), *The Control of Corporate Europe*, pp. 228–58.

Allen, F. and D. Gale (2000) *Comparing Financial Systems*, MIT Press, Cambridge, MA.

Amable, B. (2003) *The Diversity of Modern Capitalism*, Oxford University Press, Oxford.

Adnett, N. and S. Hardy (2005) *The European Social Model: Modernisation or Evolution?* Edward Elgar, Cheltenham.

Armingeon, K. (2007) 'Active Labour Market Policy, International Organizations and Domestic Politics', *Journal of European Public Policy*, 14/6: 905–32.

Armstrong, K., I. Begg and J. Zeitlin (2008) 'JCMS Symposium: EU Governance After Lisbon', *Journal of Common Market Studies*, 46/2: 413–50.

Armstrong, K and S. Bulmer (1998) *The Governance of the Single Market*, Manchester University Press, Manchester.

Arrowsmith, J. and P. Marginson (2006) 'The European Cross-border Dimension to Collective Bargaining in Multinational Companies', *European Journal of Industrial Relations*, 13/2: 245–66.

Artis, M. (2007) 'The ECB's Monetary Policy', in Artis, and Nixson (eds.), *The Economics of the European Union*, pp. 263–79.

Artis, M. and F. Nixson (eds.) (2007) *The Economics of the European Union*, Oxford University Press, Oxford.

Baldi, G. (2006) 'Europeanising Antitrust: British Competition Policy Reform and Member State Convergence', *British Journal of Politics and International Relations*, 8: 503–18.

Banca d'Italia (2005) *Relazione Annuale sul 2004*, Rome.

Barca, F. (ed.) (1997a) *Storia del Capitalismo Italiano: Dal Dopoguerra a Oggi Donzelli*, Rome.

Barca, F. (1997b) 'Compromesso Senza Riforme nel Capitalismo Italiano', in Barca, *Storia del Capitalismo Italiano: Dal Dopoguerra a Oggi*, pp. 4–117.

Barca, F. and Becht, M. (eds.) (2001) *The Control of Corporate Europe*, Oxford University Press, Oxford.

Barros, P. P., E. Berglöf, P. Fulghieri, J. Gual, C. Mayer and X. Vives (2005) *Integration of European Banking: The Way Forward*, Monitoring European Deregulation 3, Centre for Economic Policy Research, Fundación BBVA, Madrid.

Bartolini, S. (2005) *Restructuring Europe: Centre Formation, System Building, and Political Structuring Between the Nation State and the European Union*, Oxford University Press, Oxford.

Barysch, K., S. Tilford and P. Whyte (2008) *The Lisbon Scorecard VIII: Is Europe Ready for an Economic Storm?* Centre for European Reform, London.

Bauby, P. and F. Varone (2007) 'Europeanization of the French Electricity Policy: Four Paradoxes', *Journal of European Public Policy*, 14/7: 1048–60.

Becht, M. (2003) 'European Disclosure for the New Millennium', in Hopt and Wymeersch (eds.), *Capital Markets and Company Law*, pp. 87–92.

Becht, M., A. Chapelle and L. Renneboog (2001) 'Shareholding Cascades: The Separation of Ownership and Control in Belgium', in Barca and Becht (eds.), *The Control of Corporate Europe*, pp. 71–105.

Becht, M. and E. Böhmer (2001) 'Ownership and Voting Power in Germany', in Barca and Becht (eds.), *The Control of Corporate Europe*, pp. 128–53.

Becht, M., C. Mayer and H. F. Wagner (2007) 'Where Do Firms Incorporate? Deregulation and the Cost of Entry', European Corporate Governance Network, Working Paper No. 70.

Belli, F., F. Mazzini and R. Tedeschi (1998) *Il Testo Unico della Finanza*, Il Sole 24Ore, Milan.

Bercusson, B. (2007) 'The Trade Union Movement and the European Union: Judgement Day', *European Law Journal*, 15/3: 279–308.

Beyer, J. and M. Höpner (2003) 'The Disintegration of Organised Capitalism: German Corporate Governance in the 1990s', *West European Politics*, 26/4: 179–98.

Bianchi, M. and P. Casavola (1996) 'Piercing the Corporate Veil', Nota di Lavoro 6.96, Milan, Fondazione Eni Enrico Mattei.

Bianchi, M and L. Enriques (2001) 'Corporate Governance in Italy After the 1998 Reform: What Role For Institutional Investors?', *Quanderni Di Finanza*, Consob, 43.

Bianchi, M., M. Bianco and L. Enriques (2001) 'Pyramidal Groups and the Separation Between Ownership and Control in Italy', in Barca and Becht (eds.), *The Control of Corporate Europe*, pp. 154–87.

Bianco, M., C. Gola and L. F. Signorini (1996) 'Dealing with Separation Between Ownership and Control: State, Family, Coalitions and Pyramidal Groups in Italian Corporate Governance', Nota di Lavoro 5.96, Milan, Fondazione Eni Enrico Mattei.

Bladen–Hovell, R. (2007) 'The Creation of EMU', in Artis and Nixson (eds.), *The Economics of the European Union*, pp. 245–62.

Block, T. and J. Grahl (2009) 'The Official Case for Financial Integration', in Grahl (ed.), *Global Finance and Social Europe*, pp. 137–49.

Borsch, A. (2004) 'Globalisation, Shareholder Value, Restructuring: The (Non)-Transformation of Siemens', *New Political Economy*, 9/3: 367–84.

Börzel, T. and T. Risse (2000) 'When Europe Hits Home: Europeanization and Domestic Change', EUI Working Papers, RSC No. 2000/56.

Budzinski, O. (2008) 'Monoculture Versus Diversity in Competition Economics', *Cambridge Journal of Economics*, 32: 295–324

Budzinski, O. and A. Christiansen (2005) 'Competence Allocation in the EU Competition Policy System as an Interest-Driven Process', *Journal of Public Policy*, 25/3: 313–37.

Bulmer, S. (2007) 'Theorizing Europeanization', in Graziano and Vink (eds.), *Europeanization: New Research Agendas*, pp. 46–58.

Busch, A. (2004) 'National Filters: Europeanisation, Institutions, and Discourse in the Case of Banking Regulation', *West European Politics*, 27/2: 310–33.

Büthe, T. (2007) 'The Politics of Competition and Institutional Change in the European Union: The First Fifty Years', in Meunier and McNamara (eds.), *Making History: European History and Institutional Change at Fifty*, pp. 195–4.

Butt Philips, A. (1986) 'Europe's Industrial Policies: An Overview', in Hall (ed.), *European Industrial Policy*.

Callaghan, H. and M. Höpner (2005) 'European Integration and the Clash of Capitalisms: Political Cleavages over Takeover Liberalization', *Comparative European Politics*, 3: 37–332.

Casey, B. (2004) 'The OECD Jobs Strategy and the European Employment Strategy: Two Views of the Labour Market and the Welfare State', *European Journal of Industrial Relations*, 10/3: 329–52.

Catelani, E. (2005) *Il Futuro delle Fondazioni Bancarie:Tra Holding di Partecipazioni Creditizie ed Elargizioni al Terzo Settore*, Franco Angeli, Milan.

Cerny, P. G. (1997) 'International Finance and the Erosion of Capitalist Diveristy', in Crouch and Streeck (eds.), *The Political Economy of Modern Capitalism*, pp. 173–81.

Chalmers, D. and M. Lodge (2003) 'The Open Method of Co-ordination and the European Welfare State', ESRC Centre for Analysis of Risk and Regulation, Discussion Paper No. 11.

Chang, M. (2009) *Monetary Integration in the European Union*, Palgrave Macmillan, Basingstoke.

Cini, M. and L. McGowan (1998) *Competition Policy in the European Union*, Palgrave Macmillan, Basingstoke.

Cini, M. and L. McGowan (2009) *Competition Policy in the European Union*, 2nd edn., Palgrave Macmillan, Basingstoke.

Ciocca, P. (2005) *The Italian Financial System Remodelled*, Palgrave Macmillan, Basingstoke.

Cioffi, J. (2002) 'Restructuring "Germany Inc.": The Politics of Company and Takeover Law Reform in Germany and the European Union', Working Paper PEIF-1, University of California.

Clarich, M. and A. Pisaneschi (2001) *Le Fondazioni Bancarie: Dalla Holding Creditizia all'ente Non-profit*, Il Mulino, Bologna.

Clarke, R. (2006) 'Dominant Firms and Monopoly in the UK and EU', in Clarke and Morgan (eds.), *New Developments in UK and EU Competition Policy*, pp. 22–50.

Clarke, R. and E. J. Morgan (2006a) 'Horizontal Agreements and Restrictive Practices in the UK and EU', in Clarke and Morgan (eds.), *New Developments in UK and EU Competition Policy*, pp. 110–41.

Clarke, R. and E. J. Morgan (eds.) (2006b) *New Developments in UK and EU Competition Policy*, Edward Elgar, Cheltenham.

Coates, D. (2005) 'Paradigms of Explanation', in D. Coates (ed.), *Varieties of Capitalism, Varieties of Approaches*, Palgrave Macmillan, Basingstoke, pp. 1–25.

Cobham, D., S. Cosci and F. Mattsini (1999) 'The Italian Financial System: Neither Bank Based Nor Market Based', *The Manchester School*, 67/3: 325–45.

Coleman, W. D. and G. Underhill (1998) 'Globalization, Regionalism and the Regulation of Securities Markets', in G. Underhill and W. D. Coleman (eds.), *Regionalism and Global Economic Integration: Europe, Asia and the Americas*, Routledge, London, pp. 221–48

Colman, D. (2007) 'The Common Agricultural Policy', in Artis and Nixson (eds.), *The Economics of the European Union*, pp. 77–103.

Conti, G. and G. Ferri (1997) 'Banche Locali e Sviluppo Economico Decentrato', in Barca (ed.), *Storia del Capitalismo Italiano: Dal Dopoguerra a Oggi*, pp. 429–66.

Cotula, F., C. Gelsomino and E. A. Gigliobianco (1997) *Donato Menichella: Stabilita e Sviluppo dell'Economia Italiana 1946–1960*, Laterza, Bari.

Cubbin, J. (2006) 'Competition and Regulated Industries', in Clarke and Morgan (eds.), *New Developments in UK and EU Competition Policy*, pp. 169–201.

Culpepper, P. D. (2005) 'Institutional Change in Contemporary Capitalism: Coordinated Financial Systems since 1990', *World Politics*, 57/2: 173–99.

Crouch, C. and W. Streeck (1997) *Political Economy of Modern Capitalism*, Sage, London.

Daly, M. (2006) 'EU Social Policy after Lisbon', *Journal of Common Market Studies*, 44/3: 461–81.

Deakin, S. (2006) 'Legal Diversity and Regulatory Competition: Which Model for Europe?', *European Law Journal*, 12/4: 440–54.

De Boer, R., H. Benedictus and M. van der Meer (2005) 'Broadening Without Intensification: The Added Value of the European Social and Sectoral Dialogue', *Journal of European Industrial Relations*, 11/1: 51–70.

De Búrca, G. (ed.) (2005) *EU Law and the Welfare State: In Search of Solidarity*, Oxford University Press, Oxford.

Dedman, M. (2010) *The Origins and Development of the European Union, 1945–2008: A History of European Integration*, 2nd edn., Routledge, London.

Deeg, R. (1999) *Finance Capitalism Unveiled: Banks and the German Political Economy*, University of Michigan Press, Ann Arbor.

Deeg, R. (2001) 'Institutional Change and the Uses and Limits of Path Dependency: The Case of German Finance', MPIfG Discussion Paper, 01/6.

Deeg, R. (2005a) 'The Comeback of *Modell Deutschland*? The New German Political Economy in the EU', *German Politics*, 14/3: 332–53.

Deeg, R. (2005b) 'Remaking Italian Capitalism? The Politics of Corporate Governance Reform', *West European Politics*, 28/3: 521–48.

Decressin, J. and B. Kudela (2007) 'Comparing Europe and the United States', in Decressin et al. (eds.), *Integrating Europe's Financial Markets*, pp. 64–85.

Decressin, J., H. Faruqee and W. Fonteyne (eds.) (2007) *Integrating Europe's Financial Markets*, International Monetary Fund, Washington.

De Beus, J. (2004) 'The Netherlands: Monetary Integration and the *Polder* model', in Martin and Ross (eds.), *Euros and Europeans*, pp. 174–200.

De Jong, H. (1997) 'The Governance Structure and Performance of Large European Corporations', *Journal of Management and Governance*, 1: 5–27.

De Jong, R. Kabir, T. Marra, and A. Röell (2001) 'Ownership and Control in the Netherlands', in Barca and Becht (eds.), *The Control of Corporate Europe*, pp. 188–206.

De la Porte, C. and P. Pochet (2004) 'The European Employment Strategy: Existing Research and Remaining Questions', *Journal of European Social Policy*, 14/1: 71–8.

Della Salla, V. (2004) 'The Italian Model of Capitalism: On the Road Between Globalization and Europeanization?', *Journal of European Public Policy*, 11/6: 1020–40

Dermine, J. (2005) 'European Banking Integration: Don't Put the Cart before the Horse', Insead, *papers.ssrn.com/sol3/papers.cfm?abstract_id=896823.*

Dinan, D. (2004) *Europe Recast: A History of the European Union*, Palgrave Macmillan, Basingstoke.

Dølvik, J. E. (2004) 'Industrial Relations in EMU: Are Renationalization and Europeanization Two Sides of the Same Coin?', in Martin and Ross (eds.), *Euros and Europeans*, pp. 278–208.

Dyson, K. (2000) *The Politics of the Euro-zone*, Oxford University Press, Oxford.

Dyson, K. (2007) 'Economic Policy', in Graziano and Vink (eds.), *Europeanization: New Research Agendas*, pp. 281–94.

Dyson, K. and K. Featherstone (1996) 'Italy and EMU as a "Vincolo Esterno": Empowering the Technocrats, Transforming the State', *South European Politics and Society*, 1/2: 272–99.

Dyson, K. and K. Featherstone (1998) *The Road to Maastricht: Negotiating Economic and Monetary Union*, Oxford University Press, Oxford.

Ebbinghaus, B. (1999) 'Does a European Social Model Exist and Can it Survive?', in G. Huemer, M. Mesch and F. Traxler (eds.), *The Role of Employer Associations and Labour Unions in the EMU*, Ashgate, Aldershot, pp. 1–26.

Ehlermann, C.D. (2000) 'The Modernization of EC Anti-Trust Policy: A Legal and Cultural Revolution', *Common Market Law Review*, 37: 537–90.

Enriques, L. (2001) 'Il Nuovo Diritto Societario Nelle Mani dei Giudici: Una Ricognizione Empirica', *Stato e Mercato*, 61/1: 79–133.

Enriques, L. 2005, 'EC Company Law Directives and Regulations: How Trivial Are They?' ECGI, Law Working Paper No. 39/2005.

EIROnline (1999) 'Posted Workers and the Implementation of the Directive', www. eurofound,europa.eu/eiro/1999/study/tn9909201s.htm.

EIROnline (2008) 'Unions fear ECJ ruling in Laval case could lead to social dumping', www.eurofound,europa.eu/eiro/2008/01/articles/eu08010191i.htm.

European Commission (1985) *Completing the Single Market*, Brussels.

European Commission (1993) *Growth, Competitiveness and Employment*, Brussels.

European Commission (1999) *Financial Services: Implementing the Framework for Financial Markets: Action Plan*, Brussels.

European Commission (2000) *Report on Competition Policy*, Brussels.

European Commission (2001) *21st Report on Functioning of Community Product and Capital Markets*, Brussels.

European Commission (2003) *Modernising Company Law and Enhancing Corporate Governance in the EU: Action Plan*, Brussels

European Commission (2004) *Industrial Relations in Europe*, Luxembourg.

European Commission (2005a) *Single Market in Financial Services, Progress Report*, 2004–2005. Brussels.

European Commission (2005b) *State Aid Scoreboard*, June 2005 Update, Brussels.

European Commission (2006a) *Consultation on Future Priorities for the Action Plan on Modernising Company law and Enhancing Corporate Governance in the European Union*, Brussels.

European Commission (2006b) *EU Integration Seen Through Statistics*, Luxembourg.

European Commission (2006c) *Industrial Relations in Europe*, Luxembourg.

European Commission (2008) *Industrial Relations in Europe*, Luxembourg.

Evans, T. (2009a) 'Money and Finance Today', in Grahl (ed.), *Global Finance and Social Europe*, pp. 1–28.

Evans, T. (2009b) 'International Finance', in Grahl (ed.) *Global Finance and Social Europe*, pp. 29–52.

Eyre, S. and M. Lodge (2000) 'National Tunes and a European melody? Competition Law Reform in the UK and Germany', *Journal of European Public Policy*, 7/1: 63–79.

Falkner, G. (2001) 'Policy Networks in a Multi-Level System: Convergence Towards Moderate Diversity?', *West European Politics*, 23/4: 94–120.

Falkner, G. (2003) 'The Interprofessional Social Dialogue at European Level: Past and Future', in Keller and Platzer (eds), *Industrial Relations and European Integration*, pp. 11–29.

Faruqee, H. (2007) 'Equity Market Integration', in Decressin et al. (eds.), *Integrating Europe's Financial Markets*, pp. 86–115.

Fennell, R. (1997) *The Common Agricultural Policy: Continuity and Change*, Clarendon Press, Oxford.

Ferrara , M. (2005) *The Boundaries of Welfare: European Integration and the New Spatial Politics of Social Protection*, Oxford University Press, Oxford.

Ferrarini, G. (2003) 'Shareholder Value and the Modernization of European Company Law', in Hopt and Wymeersch, *Capital Markets and Company Law*, pp. 223–60.

Ferrarini, G. (2005) 'Corporate Governance Changes in the 20th Century: A View from Italy', ECGI, Working Paper No. 29/2005.

Fetzer, T. (2008) 'European Works Councils as Risk Communities: The Case of General Motors', *European Journal of Industrial Relations*, 14/3: 289–308.

Fleckenstein, T. (2006) 'Europeanisation of German Labour Market Policy? The European Employment Strategy Scrutinised', *German Politics*, 15/3: 284–301

Fonteyne, W. (2007) 'Towards a Single Financial Market', in Decressin et al. (eds.), *Integrating Europe's Financial Markets*, pp. 1–14.

Frangakis, M. (2009a) 'Europe's Financial Systems Under Pressure', in Grahl (ed.), *Global Finance and Social Europe*, pp. 53–90.

Frangakis, M. (2009b) 'EU Financial Market Integration Policy', in Grahl (ed.), *Global Finance and Social Europe*, pp. 91–114.

Franks, J.. C. Mayer, P. Volpin and H. F. Wagner (2008) 'Evolution of Family Capitalism: A Comparative Study of France, Germany, Italy and Britain', www.bancaitalian.it/studiricerche/convegni/atti/corpigov_it/session1/mayer.pdf.

Franzese, R. J. and J. M. Mosher (2002) 'Comparative Institutional and Policy Advantage: The Scope for Divergence within European Economic Integration', *European Union Politics,* 3/2: 177–203.

Frieden, J. and R. Rogowski (1996) 'The Impact of the International Economy on National Policies: An Analytical Overview', in Keohane and Milner (eds.), *Internationalization and Domestic Politics*, pp. 25–47.

Garrett, G. and P. Lange (1996) 'Internationalization, Institutions and Political Change', in Keohane and Milner (eds.), *Internationalization and Domestic Politics*, pp. 48–75.

Gerschenkron, A. (1966) *Economic Backwardness in Historical Perspective*, Cambridge University Press, Cambridge.

Giacomelli, S. and S. Trento (2005) 'Proprietà, Controllo è Trasferimenti nelle Imprese Italiane. Cosa è Cambiato nel Decennio 1993–2003?', Banca D'Italia, Temi di Discussione 550, www.bancaitalian.it/studiricerche

Gillingham, J. (2003) *European Integration 1950–2003: Superstate or New Market Economy*, Cambridge University Press, Cambridge.

Giraudi, G. (2003) 'L'Europeizzazione della Politica della Concorrenza e dell'autorità Garante della Concorrenza e del Mercato', in S. Fabbrini (ed.), *L'Europeizzazione dell'Italia*, Laterza, Bari, pp. 139–63.

Gjersem, Carl (2004) 'Policies Bearing on Product Market Competition and Growth in Europe', OECD, Working Paper No. 378.

Goddard, J., P. Molyneux, J. O. S. Wilson and M. Tavakoli (2007) 'European Banking: An Overview', *Journal of Banking and Finance*, 31: 1911–35.

Goetschy, J. (2003) 'The European Employment Strategy, Multi-level Governance, and Policy Coordination: Past, Present, Future', in Zeitlin and Truebek (eds.), *Governing Work and Welfare in a New Economy*, pp. 59–87.

Goergen, M. and L. Renneboog (2001) 'Strong Managers and Passive Institutional Investors in the United Kingdom', in F. Barca and M. Becht (eds.), *The Control of Corporate Europe*, pp. 259–284.

Gold, M., P. Cressey and E. Léonard (2007) 'Whatever Happened to Social Partnership? From Partnership to Managerialism in the EU Employment Agenda', *European Journal of Industrial Relations*, 13/1: 7–25.

Gordon, J. N. (2002) ' An International Relations Perspective on the Convergence of Corporate Governance: German Shareholder Capitalism and the European Union, 1990–2000', Johann Wolfgang Goethe-University, Frankfurt am Main, Working Paper No. 108, *papers.ssrn.com/sol3/papers.cfm?abstract_id=374620*.

Gourevitch, P. (2003a) 'Corporate Governance: Global Markets, National Politics', in M. Kahler and D. Lake (eds.), *Governance in a Global Economy*, Princeton, Princeton University Press, pp. 305–31

Gourevitch, P. (2003b) 'The Politics of Corporate Governance Regulation', *Yale Law Journal*, 112/7: 1829–80

Grahl, J. (ed.) (2009a) *Global Finance and Social Europe*, Edward Elgar, Cheltenham.

Grahl, J. (2009b) 'Lisbon, finance and the European social model', in Grahl (ed.), *Global Finance and Social Europe*, pp. 115–136.

Grahl, J. (2009c) 'Finance and the Household', in Grahl (ed.), *Global Finance and Social Europe*, pp. 207–18.

Grahl, J. (2009d) 'The Impact of Financial Change on European Employment Relations', in Grahl (ed.), *Global Finance and Social Europe*, pp. 219–33.

Grahl, J. and P. Teague (2003) 'The Eurozone and Financial Integration: The Employment Relations Issues', *Industrial Relations Journal*, 34/5: 396–410.

Grahl, J. and P. Teague (2005) 'Problems of Financial Integration in Europe', *Journal of European Public Policy*, 12/6: 1005–21.

Grant, J. and T. Kirchmaier (2004) 'Who Governs? Corporate Ownership and Control Structures in Europe', SSRN Working Papers, ssrn.com/abstract=555877.

Grant, W. (1997) *The Common Agricultural Policy*, Palgrave, Basingstoke.

Graziano, P and M. P. Vink (eds.) (2007) *Europeanization: New Research Agendas*, Palgrave Macmillan, Basingstoke.

Green Cowles, M. and D. Dinan (eds.) (2004) *Developments in the European Union*, Palgrave Macmillan, Basingstoke.

Green Cowles, M., J. Caporaso and T. Risse (2001) *Transforming Europe: Europeanization and Domestic Change*, Cornell University Press, Ithaca.

Green, R. (2007) 'EU Regulation and Competition Policy Among the Energy Utilities', Discussion Paper, Birmingham University, ftp://ftp.bham.ac.uk/pub/repec/pdf/08-01.pdf.

Grossman, E. (2006) 'Europeanization as an Interactive Process: German Public Banks Meet EU State Aid Policy', *Journal of Common Market Studies*, 44/2: 325–48.

Gugler, K., S. Kalss, A. Stomper and J. Zechner (2001) 'The Separation of Ownership and Control in Austria', in Barca and Becht (eds.), *The Control of Corporate Europe*, pp. 46–71.

Haas, F. (2007) 'Current State of Play', in Decressin et al. (eds.), *Integrating Europe's Financial Markets*, pp. 41–63.

Hall, G. (ed.), *European Industrial Policy*, Croom Helm, Kent.

Hall, P. (2007) 'The Evolution of Varieties of Capitalism in Europe', in Hancké et al. (eds.), *Beyond Varieties of Capitalism*, pp. 39–85.

Hall, P. and D. W. Gingerich (2004) 'Varieties of Capitalism and Institutional Complementarities in the Macroeconomy: An Empirical Analysis', MPIfG Discussion Paper No. 04/5, Cologne.

Hall, P. and D. Soskice (2001a) 'An Introduction to Varieties of Capitalism', in Hall and Soskice (eds.), *Varieties of Capitalism: The Institutional Foundations of Comparative Advantage*, pp. 1–70.

Hall, P. and D. Soskice (eds.) (2001b) *Varieties of Capitalism: The Institutional Foundations of Comparative Advantage*, Oxford University Press, Oxford.

Halbhuber, H. (2001) 'National Doctrinal Structures and European Company Law', *Common Market Law Review*, 38: 1385–1420.

Hancher, L. (1996) 'The Regulatory role of the European Union', in Kassim and Menon (eds.), *The European Union and National Industrial Policy*, pp. 52–69.

Hancké, B. (2000) 'European Works Councils and Industrial Restructuring in the European Motor Industry', *European Journal of Industrial Relations*, 6/1: 35–59.

Hancké, B., Rhodes, M. and M. Thatcher (eds.) (2007) *Beyond Varieties of Capitalism*, Oxford University Press, Oxford.

Hansmann, H. and Kraakman, R. (2002) 'Towards a Single Model of Corporate Law?', in McCahery et al. (eds.), *Corporate Governance Regimes: Convergence and Diversity*, pp. 56–82.

Hantrais, L. (2007) *Social Policy in the European Union*, 3rd edn., Palgrave Macmillan, Basingstoke.

Hardie, I. and D. Howarth (2009) '*Die Krise* but not *La Crise*? The Financial Crisis and the Transformation of German and French Banking Systems', *Journal of Common Market Studies*, 47/5: 1017–39.

Hassel (2002) 'The Erosion Continues: A Reply', *British Journal of Industrial Relations*, 40/2: 309–17.

Hassel, A. (2003) 'The Politics of Social Pacts', *British Journal of Industrial Relations*, 41/4: 707–26.

Hassel, A. (2009) 'Policies and Politics in Social Pacts in Europe', *European Journal of Industrial Relations*, 15/1: 7–26.

Hemerijck, A. and M. Ferrera (2004) 'Welfare Reform in the Shadow of EMU', in Martin and Ross (eds.), *Euros and Europeans*, pp. 248–77.

Hirst, P. and G. Thompson (2000) 'Globalisation in One Country? The Peculiarities of Britain', *Economy and Society*, 29/3: 335–56.

Hix, S. (2005) *The Political System of the European Union*, 2nd edn., Palgrave Macmillan, Basingstoke.

HM Treasury (2004) *The EU Financial Services Action Plan: Delivering the FSAP in the UK*, The Treasury, London.

Hodson, D. and I. Maher (2001) 'The Open Method as a New Mode of Governance: The Case of Soft Economic Policy Co-ordination', *Journal of Common Market Studies*, 39/4: 719–46.

Hodson, D. and I. Maher (2004) 'Soft Law and Sanctions: Economic Policy Co-ordination and Reform of the Stability and Growth Pact', *Journal of European Public Policy*, 11/5: 798–813.

Hollingsworth, J. Rodgers and W. Streeck (1994) 'Countries and Sectors: Concluding Remarks on Performance, Convergence and Competitiveness' in J. Rodgers Hollingsworth, P. C. Schmitter and W. Streeck (eds.), *Governing Capitalist Economies: Performance and Control of Economic Sectors*, Oxford University Press, pp. 270–300.

Hollingsworth, J. Rogers and R. Boyer (1997) 'Coordination of Economic Actors and Social Systems of Production', in J. Rogers Hollingsworth and R. Boyer (eds.), *Contemporary Capitalism: The Embeddedness of Institutions*, Cambridge University Press, Cambridge, pp. 1–48.

Hooghe, L. and G. Marks (1999) 'The Making of a Polity: The Struggle over European Integration', in H. Kitschelt, P. Lange, G. Marks and J. D. Stephens (eds.), *Continuity and Change in Contemporary Capitalism*, Cambridge University Press, Cambridge, pp. 70–97.

Höpner, M. (2003) 'European Corporate Governance Reform and the German Party Paradox', MPIfG Discussion Paper No. 03/1, Cologne.

Höpner, M. (2007) 'Coordination and Organization: The Two Dimensions of Non-liberal Capitalism', MPIfG Discussion Paper No. 07/12, Cologne.

Höpner, M. and A. Schäfer (2007) 'A New Phase of European Integration: Organized Capitalisms in Post-Ricardian Europe', MPIfG Discussion Paper No. 07/4, Cologne.

Hopt, K. and E. Wymeersch (2003) *Capital Markets and Company Law*, Oxford University Press, Oxford.

Inzerillo, U. and Messori, M (2000) 'Le Privatizzazioni Bancarie in Italia', in S. Nardis (ed.), *Le Privatizzazioni Italiane*, Bologna, il Mulino.

Jacobsson, K. (2004) 'Soft Regulation and the Subtle Transformation of States: The Case of EU Employment Policy', *Journal of European Social Policy*, 14/4: 355–70.

Jackson. G and R. Deeg (2006) 'How Many Varieties of Capitalism? The Comparative Institutional Analysis of Capitalist Diversity', MPIfG Discussion Paper No. 06/2, Cologne.

Jappelli, T. and M. Pagano (2008) 'Financial Market Integration Under EMU', Economic Papers 312, European Commission, Economic and Social Affairs, Brussels.

Johnson, A (2005) *European Welfare States and Supranational Governance of Social Policy*, Palgrave Macmillan, Basingstoke.

Johnson, A. (2007) 'EU Social Policy, or, How Far Up Do You Like Your Safety Net?', in Meunier and McNamara (eds.), *Making History: European History and Institutional Change at Fifty*, pp. 247–64.

Johnson, A. (2009) *EC Regulation of Corporate Governance*, Cambridge University Press, Cambridge.

Johnson, S., R. La Porta, F. Lopez-de-Silanes and A. Shleifer (2003) 'Tunnelling', in Hopt and Wymeersch (eds.), *Capital Markets and Corporate Law*, pp. 611–18.

Jordana, J., D. Levi-Faur and I. Puig (2006) 'The Limits of Europeanization: Regulatory Reforms in the Spanish and Portuguese Telecommunications and Electricity Sectors', *Governance*, 19/3: 437–64.

Kassim, H. and A. Menon (eds.) (1996) *The European Union and National Industrial Policy*, Routledge, London.

Keller, B. (2003) 'Social Dialogues at Sectoral Level: The Neglected Ingredient of European Industrial Relations', in Keller and Platzer (eds.), *Industrial Relations and European Integration*, pp. 30–57.

Keller, B. and H. Platzer (eds.) (2003) *Industrial Relations and European Integration*, Ashgate, Aldershot.

Keohane, R. and H. Milner (eds.) (1996) *Internationalization and Domestic Politics*, Cambridge, Cambridge University Press

Kirchmaier, T. and J. Grant (2008) 'Financial Tunnelling and the Mandatory Bid Rule', FMG Discussion Papers No. 536. Available at SSRN, ssrn.com/abstract=613945 or DOI.

Knill, C. and D. Lehmkuhl (2002) 'The National Impact of European Union Regulatory Policy: Three Europeanization Mechanisms', *European Journal of Political Research*, 41: 255–80.

Kruse, T. (2005) 'Ownership, Control and Shareholder Value in Italy: Olivetti's Hostile Takeover of Telecom Italia', ECGI Working Paper No. 83/2005.

Larsen, T. P. and P. Taylor-Gooby (2004) 'New Risks at the EU level; A Spillover from Open Market Policies?', in P. Taylor-Gooby (ed.), *New Risks/New Welfare: The Transformation of the European Welfare State*, Oxford University Press, Oxford, pp. 181–208.

Larsson, A. (1998) 'The European Employment Strategy and the EMU: You Must Invest to Save', *Economic and Industrial Democracy*, 19: 391–415.

Leblond, P. (2006) 'The Stability and Growth Pact is Dead: Long Live the Stability and Growth Pact', *Journal of Common Market Studies*, 44/5: 969–90.

Leibfried, S. (2005) 'Social Policy', in Wallace et al. (eds.), *Policy-Making in the European Union*, pp. 243–78.

Lodovici, M. S (2000) 'The Dynamics of Labour Market Reform in Europe', in G. Esping-Andersen and M. Regini (eds.), *Why Deregulate Labour Markets?*, Oxford University Press, Oxford, pp. 30–65.

Lütz, S. (2005) 'The Financial Sector in Transition: A Motor for Economic Reform?', *German Politics*, 14/2: 140–56.

Maher, M. and T. Andersson (2002) 'Corporate Governance: Effect on Firm Performance and Economic Growth', in McCahery et al. (eds.), *Corporate Governance Regimes: Convergence and Divergence*, pp. 386–418.

Marrelli, M. and F. Stroffolini (1998) 'Privatization in Italy: A Tale of "Capture"', in D. Parker (ed.), *Privatization in the European Union: Theory and Policy Prospects*, Routledge, London, pp. 248–61.

Marginson, P. (2000) 'The Eurocompany and Euro Industrial Relations', *European Journal of Industrial Relations*, 6/1: 9–34.

Marginson, P. and K. Sisson (2004) *European Integration and Industrial Relations: Multi-level Governance in the Making*, Palgrave Macmillan, Basingstoke.

Martin, S. (2007) 'Competition Policy', in Artis and Nixson (eds.), *The Economics of the European Union*, pp. 105–27.

Martin, A. and G. Ross (2004a) *Euros and Europeans: Monetary Integration and the European Model of Society*, Cambridge University Press, New York.

Martin, A. and G. Ross (2004b) 'Introduction: EMU and the European Social Model', in Martin and Ross (eds.), *Euros and Europeans*, pp. 1–19.

McCahery, J. A., P. Moreland, T. Raajimakers and L. Renneboog (eds.) (2002) *Corporate Governance Regimes: Convergence and Diversity*, Oxford University Press, Oxford.

McCann, D. (2000) 'The "Anglo-American" Model, Privatization and the Transformation of Private Capitalism in Italy', *Modern Italy*, 5/1: 47–61.

McCann, D. (2007) 'Globalization, European Integration and Regulatory Reform in Italy: Liberalism, Protectionism or Reconstruction?' *Journal of Modern Italian Studies*, 12/1: 101–17.

Menz, G. (2003) 'Re-regulating the Single Market: National Varieties of Capitalism and Their Responses to Europeanization', *Journal of European Public Policy*, 10/4: 532–55.

McGowan, Lee (2005) 'Europeanization Unleashed and Rebounding: Assessing the Modernization of EU Cartel Policy', *Journal of European Public Policy*, 12/6: 986–1004.

McNamara, K. (1998) *The Currency of Ideas: Monetary Politics in the European Union*, Cornell University Press, Ithaca.

McNamara, K. (2005) 'Economic and Monetary Union', in Wallace et al. (eds.), *Policy-Making in the European Union*, pp. 141–60.

Meunier, S. and K. R. McNamara (eds.) (2007) *Making History: European History and Institutional Change at Fifty*, Oxford University Press, Oxford.

Milward, A. (2000) *The European Rescue of the Nation-State*, Routledge, London.

Moerland, P. (2002) 'Complete Separation of Ownership and Control: The Structure-Regime and Other Defensive Mechanisms in the Netherlands', in McCahery et al. (eds.), *Corporate Governance Regimes: Convergence and Divergence*, pp. 287–96.

Molyneux P. (1996) 'Banking and Financial Services', in Kassim and Menon (eds.), *The European Union and National Industrial Policy*, pp. 247–66.

Moravscik, A. (1998) *The Choice for Europe: Social Purpose and State Power from Messina to Maastricht*, UCL, London.

Morgan, E. J. (2006) 'Merger Policy in the EU', in Clarke and Morgan (eds.), *New Developments in UK and EU Competition Policy*, pp. 78–109.

Morris, R., H. Ongena and B. Winkler (2007) 'Fiscal Policy', in Artis and Nixson (eds.), *The Economics of the European Union*, pp. 280–321.

Müller, T. and H. W. Platzer (2003) 'European Works Councils: A New Mode of EU Regulation and the Emergence of a European Multi-level Structure of

Workplace Industrial Relations', in Keller and Platzer (eds.,), *Industrial Relations and European Integration*, pp. 58–84.

Natali, D. and P. Pochet (2009) 'The Evolution of Social Pacts in the EMU Era: What Type of Institutionalization?', *European Journal of Industrial Relations*, 15/2: 147–66.

Nicolaïdis, K. and S. K. Schmidt (2007) 'Mutual Recognition "On Trial": The Long Road to Services Liberalization', *Journal of European Public Policy*, 14/4: 717–34.

Nicoletti, G., S. Scarpetta and O. Boylaud (2000) 'Summary Indicators of Product Market Regulation with an Extension to Employment Protection Legislation', OECD Working Paper No. 226, Paris.

Noaksson, N. and K. Jacobsson (2003) 'The Production of Ideas and Expert Knowledge in OECD: The OECD Jobs Strategy in Contrast with the EU Employment Strategy', Stockholm Centre for Organisation Research, Stockholm University, Stockholm.

OECD (1994) *Jobs Study: Facts, Analysis, Strategies*. OECD, Paris.

Pagoulatos, G. (2005) 'The Politics of Privatization: Redrawing the Public–Private Boundary', *West European Politics*, 28/2: 358–80.

Pellé, P. (2008) 'Companies Crossing Borders Within Europe', *Utrecht Law Review*, 4/1: 6–12.

Pierson, P. (ed.) (2001) *The New Politics of the Welfare State*, Oxford University Press, Oxford.

Pisani-Ferry, J. (2006) 'Only One Bed for Two Dreams: A Critical Retrospective on the Debate over the Economic Governance of the Euro Area', *Journal of Common Market Studies*, 44/4: 823–44.

Pollack, M. (1998) 'Beyond Left and Right? Neoliberalism and Regulated Capitalism in The Treaty of Amsterdam', University of Wisconsin-Madison, Working Paper Series in European Studies 2, No. 1.

Pontusson, J. (2005) *Inequality and Prosperity: Social Europe vs Liberal America*, Cornell University Press, Ithaca.

Purdy, D. (2007) 'Social Policy', in Artis and Nixson (eds.), *The Economics of the European Union*, pp. 200–22.

Radaelli, C. M. (2003) 'The Europeanization of Public Policy', in K. Featherstone and C. M. Radaelli (eds.), *The Politics of Europeanization*, Oxford University Press, Oxford.

Radaelli, C. and R. Pasquier (2007) 'Conceptual Issues', in Graziano, and Vink (eds.), *Europeanization: New Research Agendas*, pp. 35–45.

Raess, D. and B. Burgoon (2006) 'The Dogs that Sometimes Bark: Globalization and Works Council Bargaining in Germany', *European Journal of Industrial Relations*, 12/3: 287–309.

Raveaud, G. (2007) 'The European Employment Strategy: Towards More and Better Jobs?', *Journal of Common Market Studies*, 45/2: 411–34.

Regalia, I. (1995) 'The costs and benefits of informality', in J. Rogers and W. Streeck (eds.), *Works Councils: Consultation, Representation and Cooperation in Industrial Relations*, Chicago, Chicago University Press, pp. 217–42.

Reich, N. (2008) 'Free Movement v. Social Rights in an Enlarged Union: The *Laval* and *Viking* Cases Before the ECJ', *German Law Journal*, 9/2: 125–61.

Rhodes, M. (2003) 'National "Pacts" and EU Governance in Social Policy and the Labour Market', in Zeitlin and Truebek (eds.), *Governing Work and Welfare in a New Economy*, pp. 129–57.

Rhodes, M. (2005) 'Employment Policy', in Wallace et al. (eds.), *Policy-Making in the European Union*, pp. 279–304.

Rieger, E. (2005) 'Agricultural Policy', in Wallace et al. (eds.), *Policy-Making in the European Union*, pp. 161–90.

Riley, A. (2003) 'EC Antitrust Modernisation: The Commission Does Very Nicely – Thank You! Part 1: Regulation 1 and the Notification Burden', *European Competition Law Review*, 11: 604–15.

Rodger, B. J. and A. MacCulloch (2004) *Competition Law and Policy in the EC and UK*, 3rd edn., Cavendish, London. (4th edn., 2009.)

Roe, M. (2003) *Political Determinants of Corporate Governance*, Oxford University Press, Oxford.

Sandholtz, W. and J. Zysman (1989) 'Recasting the European Bargain', *World Politics*, 42/1: 95–128.

Sandholtz, W. and A. Sweet Stone (eds.) (1998) *European Integration and Supranational Governance*, Oxford University Press, Oxford.

Sapir, A. (2006) 'Globalization and the Reform of European Social Models', *Journal of Common Market Studies*, 44/2: 369–90.

Sbragia, A. (2004) 'Shaping a Polity in an Economic and Monetary Union: The EU in Comparative Perspective', in Martin and Ross (eds.), *Euros and Europeans*, pp. 51–75.

Scharpf, F. (1999) *Governing in the New Europe: Effective and Democratic?* Oxford University Press, Oxford.

Scharpf, F. (2002) 'The European Social Model: Coping with the Challenges of Diversity', *Journal of Common Market Studies*, 40/4: 645–70.

Schmidt, S. K. (2005) 'Reform in the Shadow of Community Law: Highly Regulated Economic Sectors', *German Politics*, 14/2: 157–73.

Schmidt, S. K. (2007) 'Mutual Recognition as a New Mode of Governance', *Journal of European Public Policy*, 14/5: 667–81.

Schmidt, V (2002a) 'Europeanization and the Mechanics of Economic Policy Adjustment', *Journal of European Public Policy*, 9/6: 894–912.

Schmidt, V. (2002b) *The Futures of European Capitalism*, Oxford University Press, Oxford.

Schulten, T. (2003) 'Europeanisation of Collective Bargaining: Trade Union Initiatives for the Transnational Coordination of Collective Bargaining', in Keller and Platzer (eds.), *Industrial Relations and European Integration*, pp. 112–36.

Siglenti, S. (1996) *Una Privatizzazione Molto Privata: Stato, Mercato e Gruppi Industriali: Il Caso Comit*, Mondadori, Milan.

Smith, M. P. (2001) 'Europe and the German Model: Growing Tension or Symbiosis?' *German Politics*, 10/3: 119–40.

Stapleton, G. P. (1996) *Institutional Investors and Corporate Governance*, Clarendon Press, Oxford.

Story, J. and I. Walter (1997) *Political Economy of Financial Integration in Europe: The Battle of the Systems*, Manchester University Press, Manchester.

Streeck, W. (1997) 'Industrial Citizenship Under Regime Competition: The Case of the European Works Councils', *Journal of European Public Policy*, 4/4: 643–64.

Streeck, W. (1998) 'The Internationalization of Industrial Relations in Europe: Problems and Prospects', MPIfG Discussion Paper 98/2, Cologne.

Streeck, W. (2001) 'Introduction: Explorations into the Origins of Nonliberal Capitalism in Germany and Japan', in W. Streeck and K. Yamamura (eds.), *The Origins of Nonliberal Capitalism*, Cornell University Press, Ithaca, pp. 1–38.

Suzuki, K. (2000) 'Reform of British Competition Policy: Is European Integration the Only Major Factor?', Working Paper No. 94, Stockholm School of Economics, Stockholm.

Tamburini, F. (1992) *Un Siciliano a Milano*, Longanesi, Milan.

Taylor-Gooby, P. (2004) 'Introduction: Open Markets versus Welfare Citizenship: Conflicting Approaches to Policy Convergence in Europe', in P. Taylor-Gooby (ed.), *Making a European Welfare State? Convergences and Conflicts over European Social Policy*, Blackwell, Oxford, pp. 1–16.

Thatcher, M. (2001) 'The Commission and National Governments as Partners: EC Regulatory Expansion in Telecommunications 1979–2000', *Journal of European Public Policy*, 8/4: 558–84.

Thatcher, M. (2004) 'Varieties of Capitalism in an Internationalized World: Domestic Institutional Change in European Telecommunications', *Comparative Political Studies*, 37/7: 751–80.

Thatcher, M. (2007a) 'Europe and the Reform of National Regulatory Institutions: A Comparison of Britain, France and Germany', in Hancké et al. (eds.), *Beyond Varieties of Capitalism*, pp. 147–173.

Thatcher, M. (2007b) 'Regulatory Agencies, the State and Markets: A Franco-British Comparison', EUI Working Papers, Robert Schuman Centre for Advanced Studies, RSCS, 2007/1, Florence.

Thatcher, M. (2007c) *Internationalization and Economic Institutions: Comparing National Experiences*, Oxford University Press, Oxford.

Thelen, K. and I. Kume (1999) 'The Effects of Globalization on Labor Revisited: Lessons from Germany and Japan', *Politics and Society*, 27/4: 477–505.

Timmermans, C. (2003) 'Harmonization in the Future of Company Law in Europe', in Hopt and Wymeersch (eds.), *Capital Markets and Company Law*, pp. 623–38.

Toporowski, J. (2009) 'International Finance and Instability in the EU', in Grahl (ed.), *Global Finance and Social Europe*, pp. 150–66.

Traxler, F. (2003) 'Bargaining, State Regulation and the Trajectories of Industrial Relations', *European Journal of Industrial Relations*, 9/2: 141–61.

Traxler, F. and B. Woitech (2000) 'Transnational Investment and National Labour Market Regimes: A Case of "Regime Shopping"?', *European Journal of Industrial Relations*, 6/2: 141–59.

Traxler, F., B. Brandl, V. Glassner and A. Ludvig (2008) 'Can Cross-Border Bargaining Coordination Work? Analytical Reflections and Evidence from the Metals Industry in Germany and Austria', *European Journal of Industrial Relations*, 14/2: 217–37.

Trubek, D. M. and J. S. Mosher (2003) 'New Governance, Employment Policy, and the European Social Model', in Zeitlin and Truebek (eds), *Governing Work and Welfare in a New Economy*, pp. 33–57.

Tsoukalis, L. (1993) *The New European Economy: The Politics and Economics of Integration*, Oxford University Press, Oxford.

Tsoukalis, L. (2003) *What Kind Of Europe?*, Oxford University Press, Oxford.

Van Apeldoorn, B. (2002) *Transnational Capitalism and the Struggle over European Integration*, Routledge, London.

Van Waarden, F. and M. Drahos (2002) 'Courts and (Epistemic) Communities in the Convergence of Competition Policy', *Journal of European Public Policy*, 9/6: 913–34.

Verdun, A. (2004) 'The Euro and the European Central Bank', in Green Cowles and Dinan (eds.), *Developments in the European Union*, pp. 85–99.

Verdun, A. (2007) 'EMU: A Journey With Many Crossroads', in Meunier and McNamara (eds.), *Making History: European History and Institutional Change at Fifty*, pp. 195–209.

Verdier, D. (2001) 'Corporate Mobility and the Origins of Stock Markets', *International Organization*, 55: 327–56.

Visser, J. (1996) 'Transitions and Traditions in Industrial Relations', in J. Van Ruysseueldt and J. Visser (eds.), *Industrial Relations in Europe: Transitions and Traditions*, Sage, London, pp. 1–17.

Visser, J (2001) 'From "Kenynesianism" to the "Third Way": Labour Relations and Social Policy in Postwar Western Europe', *Economic and Industrial Democracy*, 21: 421–57.

Visser, J. (2005) 'Beneath the Surface of Stability: New and Old Modes of Governance in European Industrial Relations', *European Journal of Industrial Relations*, 11/3: 257–306.

Vogel, S (2002) 'The Crisis of German and Japanese Capitalism: Stalled on the Road to the Liberal Market Model', *Comparative Political Studies,* 34/10: 1103–33.

Vos, K. (2006) 'Europeanization and Convergence in Industrial Relations', *European Journal of Industrial Relations*, 12/3: 311–27.

Vossestein, G. J. (2008) 'Transfer of the Registered Office. The European Commission's Decision not to Submit a Proposal for a Directive', *Utrecht Law Review*, 4/1: 53–65.

Waddington, J. (2006) 'Contesting the Development of European Works Councils in the Chemicals Sector', *European Journal of Industrial Relations*, 12/3: 329–52.

Walkner, C. and J. P. Raes (2005) 'Integration and Consolidation in EU Banking: An Unfinished Business', Economic Papers, European Commission, Brussels.

Wallace, A. (2004) 'Completing the Single Market: The Lisbon Strategy', in Green Cowles and Dinan (eds.), *Developments in the European Union*, pp. 100–18.

Wallace, H., W. Wallace and M. A. Pollack (eds.) (2005) *Policy-Making in the European Union*, 5th edn., Oxford University Press, Oxford.

Watt, A. (2004) 'Reform of the European Employment Strategy after Five Years: A Change of Course or Merely of Presentation?', *European Journal of Industrial Relations*, 10/2: 117–37.

Whitley, R. (1999) *Divergent Capitalisms: The Social Structuring and Change of Business Systems*, Oxford University Press, Oxford.

Whittal, M. (2000) 'The BMW European Works Council: A Cause for European Industrial Relations', *European Journal of Industrial Relations*, 6/1: 61–83.

Wigger, A. and A. Nölke (2007) 'Enhanced Roles of Private Actors in the EU Business Regulation and the Erosion of Rhenish Capitalism: The Case of Antitrust Enforcement', *Journal of Common Market Studies*, 45/2: 487–514.

Wilks, S. (2005a) 'Competition Policy', in Wallace et al. (eds.), *Policy-Making in the European Union*, pp. 113–40.

Wilks, S. (2005b) 'Agency Escape: Decentralization or Dominance of the European Commission in the Modernization of Competition Policy?', *Governance*, 18/3: 431–52.

Wilks, S. and I. Bartle (2002) 'The Unanticipated Consequences of Creating Independent Competition Agencies', *West European Politics*, 25/1: 148–72.

Wishlade, F. (2006) 'EU State Aid Control', in Clarke and Morgan (eds.), *New Developments in UK and EU Competition Policy*, pp. 232–61.

Wood, S. (2001) 'Labour Market Regimes Under Threat? Sources of Continuity in Germany, Britain and Sweden', in Pierson (ed.) *The New Politics of the Welfare State*, pp. 368–409.

Wouters, J. (2000) 'European Company Law: *Quo Vadis*?', *Common Market Law Review*, 37, pp. 257–307.

Wymeersch, E. (2003) 'Do We Need a Law on Groups of Companies?', in Hopt and Wymeersch (eds.), *Capital Markets and Company Law*, pp. 573–600.

Young, A. R. (2005) 'The Single Market', in Wallace et al. (eds.), *Policy-Making in the European Union*, pp 93–112.

Zahariadis, N. (2004) 'European Markets and National Regulation: Conflict and Cooperation in British Competition Policy', *Journal of Public Policy*, 24/1: 49–73.

Zahariadis, N. (2005) 'Adaptation Without Pressure? European Legislation and British Merger Policy', *Policy Studies Journal*, 33/4: 657–74.

Zahn, R (2008) 'The *Viking* and *Laval* Cases in the Context of European Enlargement', *Web Journal of Current Legal Issues*, http://webjcli.ncl.ac.uk/2008/issue3/zahn3.html.

Zeitlin, J. (2005) 'Social Europe and Experimentalist Governance: Towards a New Constitutional Compromise', in G. De Búrca (ed.), *EU Law and the Welfare State: In Search of Solidarity*, pp. 213–42.

Zeitlin, J. and D. M. Trubek (eds.) (2003) *Governing Work and Welfare in a New Economy: European and American Experiments*, Oxford University Press, Oxford.

Ziegler, J. N. (2001) 'Corporate Governance in Germany: Towards a New Transnational Politics?', in S. Weber (ed.), *Globalization and the European Political Economy*, Columbia University Press, New York, pp. 197–228.

Zysman, J. (1983) *Governments, Markets and Finance*, Cornell University Press, Ithaca.

Zysman, J. (1994) 'How Institutions Create Historically Rooted Trajectories of Growth', *Industrial and Corporate Change*, 3/1: 243–83.

# Index